MENOPAUSE

CONTEMPORARY ENDOCRINOLOGY

P. Michael Conn, SERIES EDITOR

MENOPAUSE

Endocrinology and Management

Edited by

DAVID B. SEIFER, MD

*UMDNJ–Robert Wood Johnson Medical School,
New Brunswick, NJ*

and

ELIZABETH A. KENNARD, MD

The Ohio State University, Columbus, OH

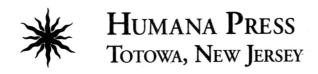

HUMANA PRESS
TOTOWA, NEW JERSEY

© 1999 Humana Press Inc.
999 Riverview Drive, Suite 208
Totowa, New Jersey 07512

For additional copies, pricing for bulk purchases, and/or information about other Humana titles, contact Humana at the above address or at any of the following numbers: Tel: 973-256-1699; Fax: 973-256-8341; E-mail: humana@humanapr.com or visit our website at http://humanapress.com

This publication is printed on acid-free paper. ∞
ANSI Z39.48-1984 (American National Standards Institute)
Permanence of Paper for Printed Library Materials.

Cover design by Patricia F. Cleary

Printed in the United States of America. 10 9 8 7 6 5 4 3 2 1
Menopause: endocrinology and management /edited by David B. Seifer and Elizabeth A. Kennard.
       p.cm.—(Contemporary endocrinology; 18)
       Includes bibliographical references and index.
       ISBM 0-89603-677-4 (alk. paper)
       1. Menopause. 2. Menopause—Hormone therapy. 3. Estrogen—Therapeutc use.
       I. Seifer, David B., 1955– . II. Kennard, Elizabeth A. III. Series: Contemporary endocrinology (Totowa, NJ); 18.
       RG186.M4817 1999
       618.1'75—dc21
                                           99-32278
                                         CIP

PREFACE

Although the life expectancy of women continues to increase, medical science has not been able to alter the average age of the onset of menopause. Thus, for the foreseeable future, a greater fraction of life will occur following the onset of menopause. Although these can be fulfilling and wonderful years, they often present many physiological challenges. Women must cope with a decline in the endocrinological processes responsible for the maintenance of normal function in several organ systems.

The management of menopause requires a basic understanding of the underlying endocrinology. The contributors to *Menopause: Endocrinology and Management* have focused on describing their contemporary understanding of this important scientific area. Estrogen-sensitive tissues are found throughout the body and issues of cardiovascular, bone, brain, and genitourinary changes are reviewed in detail. The risks, benefits, and alternatives of conventional hormone replacement are examined. Selective estrogen receptor modulators (SERMs), androgen replacement, calcium supplementation, and the role of diet are reviewed. Keeping in mind the need to address the needs of the entire patient, Chapter 16 is directed toward the general clinical care of menopausal women.

Future inroads into acquiring more effective interventions for the effects of estrogen deprivation will require several strategies, coupled with further clinical and basic science research. Earlier detection of diminished end-organ response through the development of increasingly sensitive technologies may allow for earlier intervention. Therapies that are better directed at specific sites of benefit without deleterious effects on other nontargeted tissues will be refined. Alternative methods and types of hormone replacement will continue to be developed. As we become more knowledgeable and sophisticated in our ability to manage menopause, our patients' compliance, we hope, will improve. We have learned a great deal about the problems of menopause. In the future, we shall increase our ability to understand and effectively approach many of the challenges posed by this important era of women's lives.

David B. Seifer, MD
Elizabeth A. Kennard, MD

CONTENTS

CONTRIBUTORS

MELISSA E. ABRAHAM, MD, *Department of Epidemiology, Harvard School of Public Health, Boston, MA*

SARAH L. BERGA, MD, *Departments of Obstetrics, Gynecology and Reproductive Sciences and Psychiatry, The University of Pittsburgh School of Medicine, Pittsburgh, PA*

RENEE M. CAPUTO, MD, *Department of Obstetrics and Gynecology, The Ohio State University, Columbus, OH*

DANIEL W. CRAMER, MD, SCD, *Department of Obstetrics and Gynecology, Harvard Medical School, Boston, MA*

CYNTHIA EVANS, MD, *Department of Obstetrics and Gynecology, The Ohio State University, Columbus, OH*

ELIZABETH S. GINSBURG, MD, *Department of Obstetrics, Gynecology and Reproductive Biology, Harvard Medical School, Boston, MA*

ROGER P. GOLDBERG, MD, *Department of Obstetrics, Gynecology and Reproductive Biology, Harvard Medical School, Boston, MA*

BERNARD L. HARLOW, PHD, *Obstetrics and Gynecology Epidemiology Center, Brigham and Women's Hospital, Harvard Medical School, Boston, MA*

BRENDA S. HOUMARD, MD, *Department of Obstetrics and Gynecology, The Ohio State University, Columbus, OH*

REBECCA D. JACKSON, MD, *Division of Endocrinology, Diabetes and Metabolism, The Ohio State University, Columbus, OH*

BRINDA N. KALRO, MD, *Department of Reproductive Endocrinology, The University of Pittsburgh School of Medicine, Pittsburgh, PA*

ELIZABETH A. KENNARD, MD, *Department of Obstetrics and Gynecology, The Ohio State University, Columbus, OH*

MARK P. LEONDIRES, MD, *Endocrinology and Reproduction Research Branch, National Institute of Child Health and Human Development, National Institutes of Health, Rockville, MD*

GEETHA MATTHEWS, MD, *Department of Reproductive Endocrinology, Fertility and Menopause, University of Massachusetts Memorial Health Care System, Worcester, MA*

ANNE W. MOULTON, MD, *Department of Medicine, Brown University School of Medicine, Providence, RI*

ALAN S. PENZIAS, MD, *Department of Obstetrics, Gynecology and Reproductive Biology, Harvard Medical School, Boston, MA*

VERONICA A. RAVNIKAR, MD, *Department of Reproductive Endocrinology, Fertility and Menopause, University of Massachusetts Memorial Health Care System, Worcester, MA*

NANETTE SANTORO, MD, *Department of Obstetrics and Gynecology, Albert Einstein College of Medicine, Bronx, NY*

JAMES H. SEGARS, MD, *Office of the Scientific Director, Institute of Child Health and Human Development, National Institutes of Health, Rockville, MD*

DAVID B. SEIFER, MD, *Department of Obstetrics, Gynecology and Reproductive Sciences and Division of Reproductive Endocrinology and Infertility, UMDNJ–Robert Wood Johnson Medical School, New Brunswick, NJ*

IAN H. THORNEYCROFT, MD, PHD, *Department of Obstetrics and Gynecology, University of South Alabama College of Medicine, Mobile, AL*

LAURA J. TIVIS, PHD, *Center for Alcohol and Drug Related Studies, University of Oklahoma Health Science Center, Oklahoma City, OK*

DREW V. TORTORIELLO, MD, *Department of Obstetrics and Gynecology, UMDNJ, The New Jersey Medical School, South Orange, NJ*

BRIAN W. WALSH, MD, *Department of Gynecology and Reproductive Biology, Harvard Medical School, Boston, MA*

1

Predicting the Onset of Menopause

Brenda S. Houmard, MD, PhD
and David B. Seifer, MD

INTRODUCTION

The menopausal transition represents a continuum of change from regular menstrual cyclicity and fertility in the premenopausal woman to amenorrhea and loss of fecundability in the postmenopausal female. Understanding and predicting the onset of this transition has become increasingly important as the 21st century approaches. Demographic studies estimate that, in 1990, there were 467 million postmenopausal women in the world. Population projections based on these demographic studies predict that, by the year 2030, the number of postmenopausal women will increase to 1.2 billion *(1)*. At this time, approx 47 million women will be entering menopause each year *(1)*. Furthermore, it is estimated that women in developed countries will spend about 30 yr of their life in the postmenopausal state *(2)*.

The median age of menopause in the Massachusetts Women's Health Study of 2570 women was 51.3 yr *(3)*; however, individual variation in the onset of menopause is significant. Predicting the onset of menopause in individual women has important health implications. It allows us to predict age-related infertility and responsiveness to fertility therapy, to appropriately time initiation of hormone replacement therapy (HRT), and to assess risks of chronic diseases.

Predicting the onset of menopause and the period of impaired fertility that proceeds it has become increasingly important as women delay childbearing to their late 30s and 40s. With aging of the Baby Boom generation, it is estimated that the number of women aged 35–45 will increase from 13 million in 1980 to 18.5 million in 2010 *(4)*. Further-

From: *Contemporary Endocrinology: Menopause: Endocrinology and Management*
Edited by: D. B. Seifer and E. A. Kennard © Humana Press Inc., Totowa, NJ

more, these women are delaying childbearing, as reflected by a 33% increase from 1982 to 1988 in the number of women aged 25–34 yr who have never had a child *(5)*.

It has long been known that fertility declines with age, particularly over the age of 30–35 *(6)*. As more women who have delayed childbearing to their late 30s and 40s desire pregnancy, the demand for infertility treatment will increase. Recent data from the Society for Assisted Reproductive Technology (SART) suggest that approximately one-sixth of the assisted reproductive technology (ART) cycles were performed on women aged > 40 yr *(7)*. As expected, delivery rate per oocyte retrieval were considerably lower in women > 40 yr (about 8–12%) as compared to women < 40 yr (20–33%). Given the monetary, physical and emotional expenses of these advanced therapies, it would be helpful in individual women to identify predictors of menopause and the reduced fertility that proceeds it.

The increase in the incidence of certain chronic diseases after menopause has becoming increasingly apparent. As emphasized by a recent review *(8)*, the menopausal state is an important risk factor for cardiovascular disease and its associated risk factors such as obesity and hypertension, and for osteoporosis and joint disease, urogenital dysfunction, Alzheimer's disease, and depression. These associations are also explored in depth in other chapters of this textbook. It is important to note that, in addition to morbidity from the often life-threatening and debilitating diseases listed earlier, the perimenopausal woman sometimes experiences significant discomfort and distress from the psychosocial and "hot flush" symptomatology of the climacteric.

Given the diverse impact that the menopausal transition may have on some women's overall health and well being, it seems logical that an improved ability to predict the onset of menopause may be helpful in timing surveillance, prevention and treatments for these chronic diseases and conditions. In particular, timing the initiation of hormone replacement therapy may be improved by more accurate prediction of the onset of menopause.

This chapter seeks to identify and evaluate various epidemiologic, endocrinologic, and anatomic parameters as predictors of the onset of menopause. It is important, however, to first begin by reviewing the definitions of common terms used to discuss the menopausal transition.

DEFINITIONS

Menopause is defined as cessation of menstruation because of depletion of follicular stores. It is retrospectively determined after 12 mo of amenorrhea during the midlife period. The *perimenopause* (often called the *climacteric*) is the period of transition that precedes and follows this final menses. The perimenopause, marked by menstrual irregularity, was reported in one Caucasian population to be about 4 yr in length *(3)*.

It is known that, as a woman's chronological age increases, her hormonal response to ovulation induction *(9–11)*, the number of oocytes retrieved *(12–14)*, fertilization and pregnancy rates *(9,12,13,15–18)* decrease. This often occurs despite regular menstrual cycles. Recently, the concept of *ovarian reserve (19)*, as reflected by d 3 serum follicle-stimulating hormone (FSH) level *(9,20)*, has been introduced as a more accurate predictor of decreased fecundity than chronological age. The success of ovulation induction *(21)* and in vitro fertilization *(9,22)* decline with diminishing ovarian reserve, as assessed indirectly by elevated d 3 FSH levels. Thus, the transition from optimal fertility in the premenopausal period to menopause begins as a period of diminished ovarian reserve

Table 1
Epidemiologic Predictors of Menopause

Sufficient Literature Suggesting Association *(References)*
• Cigarette Smoking *(24–33)*
• Multiparity *(25,31–33,49–52)*
• Age of Maternal Menopause *(32,55–57)*
Sufficient Literature Refuting Association
• Age of Menarche *(31,33,50,52)*
• Oral Contraceptive Use *(24,25)*
Possible Association—Insufficient/Conflicting Literature Available
• Lifelong Menstrual Cycle Characteristics *(31,51,52)*
• Relative Body Weight *(24,25,29,32,33,51,62–64)*
• Alcohol/Meat Consumption *(32)*
• Race *(25,63)*
• Toxic Exposures (Radiation, Chemotherapy, DES) *(66,67,74)*

with regular menstrual cyclicity. This is then followed by the menstrual irregularity of the climateric and, finally, by the amenorrhea of menopause.

In evaluating various parameters as predictors of menopause, it is important to keep these particular definitions in mind. This is because some of the investigations, particularly regarding endocrinologic and anatomic parameters, often select prediction of ovarian reserve rather than age at menopause as the endpoint of their studies. It seems logical that predicting the onset of diminished ovarian reserve may also be predictive of the onset of menopause; however, the exact relationship between the period of diminished ovarian reserve and the onset of menopause remains unstudied at this time.

The preceding definitions refer to *natural menopause. Surgical menopause* is defined by the World Health Organization *(23)* as cessation of menses because of removal of both ovaries, with or without removal of the uterus. Obviously, this state is quite different from natural menopause. However, surgical menopause resulting from ablation of ovarian function is similar to medically induced amenorrhea from treatment with GnRH agonists, in that both rapidly initiate a hypoestrogenic hormonal milieu. Both of these states pose problems similar to those encountered by women undergoing natural menopause: "hot flush" symptomatology and risks of chronic diseases, such as osteoporosis and cardiovascular disease. Because predicting the onset of these iatrogenic types of menopause is not an issue, the remaining parts of this chapter focus on determining useful parameters for predicting the onset of natural menopause.

EPIDEMIOLOGIC PREDICTORS

Many epidemiologic factors have been studied for their association with the age at menopause. These include smoking, reproductive parameters, genetic factors, nutritional factors, socioeconomic factors, and toxic exposures (Table 1).

The limitations of many epidemiologic studies also apply to these investigations. Many are retrospective studies, although some recent prospective studies have been reported *(24,25)*. The problems of selection bias and confounding variables must be addressed in most studies. Despite these limitations, these epidemiologic studies do provide useful insight into the prediction of the onset of menopause.

Smoking

One of the most well studied and consistent associations with earlier age at menopause is cigarette smoking *(3,24–33)*. These studies have reproducibly shown that menopause occurs 1–2 yr earlier in women who smoke as compared to nonsmokers.

Epidemiologic studies also show an association between smoking and reduced fertility *(34,35)*, independent of age and socioeconomic class. Studies of outcomes of IVF in smokers versus nonsmokers, however, have been conflicting. Some studies report reduced fertilization and pregnancy rates *(36,37)*, whereas others show no effect *(38–40)*. Interestingly, two recent studies have shown that cigarette smoking may decrease ovarian reserve, as evidenced by increased basal FSH levels *(41)* or an abnormal clomiphene citrate challenge test *(42)*. This effect of smoking on ovarian reserve would be consistent with its effect upon the timing of menopause.

Various mechanisms have been proposed to explain the effect of smoking on ovarian functional longevity. Lower circulating estradiol levels in smokers *(40,43)* may be because of altered production *(44)* or metabolism *(45)* of this estrogen. In addition, smoking alters estrogen binding to its receptor *(46)*. Constituents of the tobacco may also exert a direct toxic effect on oocytes *(47,48)*. Thus, smoking may effect ovarian reserve and, ultimately, age at menopause via multiple mechanisms.

Reproductive Factors

The literature addressing the effects of various reproductive parameters upon age of menopause are less consistent. Proposed predictors of menopausal age have included parity, age of menarche, age of maternal menopause, cycle characteristics, and use of oral contraceptives.

Menopause has been shown in most studies to occur later in multiparous women as compared to nulliparas *(25,31–33,49–51)*. This effect may even increase with increasing parity *(32)*. The physiological basis for this association is not well defined.

Study of population trends show that an earlier age at menarche may be associated with a later age of menopause *(52,53)* in the population as a whole. Thus, it has been postulated *(53)* that age of menarche and age of menopause might also be inversely related in individual women. Recent studies of large numbers of women, however, have failed to show an association between age of menarche and age of menopause *(31,33,51,54)*.

Age of maternal menopause appears to significantly correlate with the menopausal age of daughters *(32,55–57)*. In fact, a woman whose mother underwent menopause before 46 yr of age is 5–6 times more likely to experience menopause at an earlier age *(55,57)*. Similarly, age at menopause correlates among siblings *(55)*. A genetic basis for menopausal age is supported by several recent case reports showing deletional abnormalities in the long arm of the X chromosome in families of women with premature ovarian failure *(58,59)*. Further studies are necessary to determine whether genes in this area of the X chromosome also influence the timing of menopause when it occurs in the normal range.

Various menstrual cycle characteristics have been reported to be associated with earlier age of menopause, including short menstrual cycle length at ages 20–35 *(51)* and menstrual irregularity before age 25 *(50)*. In these studies, it is difficult to exclude confounding factors such as smoking, nutritional factors and parity. A more recent multivariate analysis failed to show an association between lifelong menstrual patterns and age at menopause *(31)*. Thus, the ability of lifelong menstrual patterns to predict age of menopause remains unclear. It is known, however, that as a woman approaches the time of diminished ovarian reserve and the perimenopause, menstrual cycles become irregular *(25,60)* and shorter in length *(41)*. Therefore, changes in menstrual characteristics toward the end of a woman's reproductive life may signal impending menopause.

The effect of oral contraceptive use on age at menopause is controversial. The use of oral contraceptives has been reported to postpone the age of menopause *(33)*. However, other studies have failed to find any association *(49)* or have noted that this association is confounded by many other variables *(50)*. These include factors known to influence onset of menopause: age, smoking, and parity. Recent data from two prospective studies *(24,25)* have failed to show any independent effect of oral contraceptive use on age at menopause. Thus, it appears that use of oral contraceptives does not significantly alter menopausal age.

Nutritional Factors

The interactions between nutritional status and reproductive functioning, particularly with respect to anovulation, amenorrhea, and the onset of puberty, are well known. Various nutritional parameters have also been studied for their association with the onset of menopause. Certainly, severe malnutrition can lead to earlier onset of a woman's last menstrual period *(61)*. However, it is difficult in these epidemiologic studies to distinguish nutritional amenorrhea secondary to hypothalamic dysfunction from early menopause with oocyte depletion.

Various investigators have shown increased relative weight to be associated with either earlier *(62)* or later *(63,64)* onset of menopause. It is important to note that smoking history was not considered in these studies. Numerous investigations have failed to show an independent relationship between weight or body mass index and menopausal age when smoking is considered as a confounding variable *(24,25,29,32,33,50)*.

Recently, several other nutritional associations with menopausal age have been described. Increased consumption of either alcohol or meat was found in women with later onset of menopause, independent of other determinants of menopausal age *(32)*. Women who prospectively reported following a weight reduction diet underwent menopause one year earlier than the average *(25)*. Further studies are necessary to clarify the role of these nutritional factors in determining menopausal age.

Socioeconomic Factors

Substantial effort has been put forth to study the socioeconomic factors that appear to correlate with age of menopause. Menopause has been reported to occur later in married women of higher socioeconomic class and educational background *(30,32,33,49, 50,54,65)*. Clearly, marital status, educational background and socioeconomic class are interrelated. These factors are also related to nutritional and reproductive factors, as well as to tobacco use. Recent studies *(24,25,31)* have challenged the notion that these socioeconomic parameters are independently useful for predicting the onset of menopause.

The issue of racial differences in menopausal age remains unclear. Studies on determinants of menopausal age have predominantly involved Caucasian women. The study of menopause in African-American women has been hampered by the high rate of premenopausal hysterectomy in this population. Limited studies suggest that natural age at menopause is somewhat earlier in African-American women *(25,63)*. Further evaluation is necessary to substantiate this finding and to determine the extent to which menopausal age is influenced in African-American women by variables such as smoking, parity, and nutrition.

Toxic Exposures

In addition to cigarette smoke, exposure to other toxic substances can predispose a woman to premature ovarian failure or early menopause. Premature ovarian failure and its etiologies are reviewed in detail elsewhere in this text. However, perhaps similar toxic exposures can alter the timing of natural menopause.

Radiation exposure is known to have variable effects on female reproductive functioning depending on the age at exposure and the ovarian dose received. These effects range from no deleterious effect to transient amenorrhea to premature ovarian failure and infertility *(66,67)*. A similar range of effects has been described for chemotherapy exposures, depending on the type of agent, dose of the drug and age of the patient *(67)*. The influence of these exposures on the age at natural menopause in women who initially experience little effect or only transient amenorrhea has not been well studied. It seems plausible that these women would be at risk for earlier menopause because of partial depletion of the oocyte pool, but this remains to be proven.

Prenatal exposure to diethylstilbestrol (DES) has been associated with various adverse effects on reproductive functioning in women: structural anomalies of the reproductive tract, infertility, and poor pregnancy outcome *(68–71)*. Animal studies have shown that prenatal exposure to DES can also lead to follicular depletion in the ovary *(72,73)*. A recent study *(74)* investigated the effects of prenatal DES exposure on the incidence of premature ovarian failure and menopausal symptoms. No significant differences in these parameters were found between exposed and unexposed women. However, these women were only about age 40 at the time of the study. It remains to be seen whether DES-exposed women have diminished ovarian reserve or experience natural menopause at an earlier age.

ENDOCRINOLOGIC PREDICTORS OF DIMINISHED OVARIAN RESERVE—THE EARLIEST SIGN OF THE ONSET OF PERIMENOPAUSE

Complex endocrinologic changes occur with the transition into menopause. For many years, hormonal parameters such as elevated follicle-stimulating hormone (FSH) levels and low estradiol levels, have been used to confirm the postmenopausal state. Recently, various endocrine tests have been studied for their predictive value with respect to the process of reproductive aging in normally cycling women. These tests have included measurement of basal or stimulated levels of gonadotropins, estradiol, and inhibin. Whereas these tests have been employed mainly to predict ovarian reserve and success during ART treatments, they may eventually be more widely applicable to the prediction of the onset of menopause. Certainly, these endocrine predictors have the potential to provide a more objective means to detect the onset of menopause than epidemiologic factors.

A brief review of the endocrinologic changes associated with the perimenopausal transition will help to set the stage for analyzing various endocrine tests as predictors of reproductive aging. The reader is also referred to the subsequent chapter of this text that thoroughly reviews the endocrinology of the climacteric.

The endocrinologic changes of menopause result from interplay between declining ovarian function and reciprocal changes in circulating gonadotropins. Both steroids and protein hormones from the ovary control pituitary production and secretion of LH and FSH. The principal ovarian steroid hormones are estradiol (predominant in the follicular phase) and progesterone (predominant in the luteal phase). These steroids regulate gonadotropin production and release via feedback loops of the hypothalamic–pituitary–ovarian axis. In addition, several peptide hormones (inhibin, activin, and follistatin) produced by granulosa cells influence FSH synthesis and secretion *(75)*.

The role of inhibin in the regulation of FSH secretion has received considerable attention given the dynamic changes in serum concentrations that occur over the menstrual cycle. There are two types of inhibin, each consisting of the same α-subunit combined with a either βA- or βB-subunit to form inhibin-A and inhibin-B, respectively. These dimeric inhibins show different patterns of secretion during the menstrual cycle. Levels of inhibin-A are low during the follicular phase, rise with ovulation, and peak during the luteal phase *(76)*. In contrast, inhibin-B levels are highest during the midfollicular phase, decline at midcycle, and display a transient rise shortly after the LH surge *(77)*.

One of the most consistent endocrinologic changes associated with onset of the perimenopause is the monotropic rise in FSH *(78–82)*. It has been hypothesized that this change in FSH may result from diminished function of the granulosa cell compartment of the ovary, manifested by decreased production of estradiol, inhibin, and/or insulin-like growth factors (IGFs).

Early studies showed that elevations in FSH are often accompanied by decreases in circulating levels of estradiol *(79,83,84)* and inhibin *(83–86)*. Other studies of the perimenopausal transition have shown no significant change in estradiol levels *(80,81)* or elevated estrogen levels *(87–89)*. These apparent conflicts in the literature may reflect differences in the timing of the sample collections over the perimenopausal transition. Perhaps, initially, the increase in FSH compensates for decreasing ovarian function and results in increased estradiol levels. Then, as the ovary continues to age in the latter part of the perimenopausal transition, a decline in estradiol occurs. Declining inhibin rather than estradiol production by the granulosa cells during the early phase of the perimenopause may be important in initiating the monotropic rise in FSH *(90–91)*. Whereas some studies using a polyclonal antibody to the α-subunit have failed to show a change in serum inhibin concentrations associated with the monotropic rise in FSH *(87,92,93)*, decreased secretion of inhibin-B has been shown to be associated with this elevation in FSH *(94)*. Thus, decreased inhibin-B may reflect diminished function of the granulosa cells of older women and play a role in the regulation of FSH during the perimenopause *(95)*.

In summary, the earliest endocrinologic evidence of diminished ovarian reserve may be diminished inhibin-B secretion and the monotropic rise in FSH. This may occur in the presence of elevated circulating levels of estradiol. These changes form the basis for the endocrine tests for ovarian reserve discussed below.

Endocrine Tests for Diminished Ovarian Reserve

Many endocrinologic tests have been proposed to be useful predictors of diminished ovarian reserve, particularly in the setting of infertility treatment (Table 2). Many involve the measurement of FSH, either under basal conditions (typically on d 3) or in response to a clomiphene citrate or GnRH challenge. Others have used FSH:LH ratios to predict poor response to exogenous gonadotropin stimulation. Recently, measurements of d 3 levels of estradiol and inhibin-B have also been used as predictors of ovarian reserve.

Basal FSH Levels

The use of basal FSH to predict ovarian response to gonadotropin stimulation and outcome during in vitro fertilization was first described in 1988 by Muasher and col-

Table 2
Endocrine Tests for Detecting Diminished Ovarian Reserve

Basal Tests (Measured on Day 3 of the Menstrual Cycle)
• Follicle Stimulating Hormone (FSH) Level
• Estradiol Level
• Inhibin-B Level
• Follicle Stimulating Hormone: Luteinizing Hormone (LH:FSH) Ratio
Stimulated Tests
• Clomiphene Citrate Challenge Test
• GnRH (Gonadotropin Releasing Hormone) Stimulation Test

leagues (96). A subsequent study of 758 IVF cycles (22) showed that women with low basal (d 3) FSH levels had significantly greater number of follicles per retrieval, increased recovery of preovulatory oocytes and higher peak estradiol levels than women with elevated d 3 FSH levels. Furthermore, the pregnancy rates were 4–5 times greater in the women with low basal FSH (<15 mIU/mL) as compared to women with elevated d 3 FSH levels (>25 mIU/mL). Additional studies (9,97) have confirmed that basal FSH levels were more useful for predicting performance in IVF cycles than patient age. Combining basal FSH determination with patient age further improves prognostic accuracy. It is important to realize, however, that the variation in normal basal FSH levels is considerable among individual labs. Therefore, each institution needs to establish guidelines for normal and elevated basal FSH levels based on their individual laboratory results. Although most studies describe measurement of FSH on d 3 of the cycle, serum FSH concentrations are similar on ds 2–5 (93,98).

Some women display significant intercycle variability in basal FSH levels (99,100). Scott and colleagues noted that the intercycle variability was greater in women who had elevated basal FSH levels than in those with normal basal FSH levels. Furthermore, women who have had an elevated FSH in any prior cycle respond poorly in IVF cycles, even if their basal FSH is normal in the current cycle (99,100). Thus, many clinicians recommend that women with elevated basal FSH levels be discouraged from pursuing further IVF cycles, regardless of whether it is persistently or variably elevated.

On average, women who have undergone unilateral oophorectomy have elevated d 3 FSH levels as compared to women with two ovaries. However, in individual women with one ovary, the basal FSH levels retain their prognostic accuracy. It appears that the same threshold values for predicting poor outcome in IVF can be used in these women (101).

Demonstration of an elevated basal FSH is highly predictive of poor responsiveness in IVF cycles. However, a normal d 3 FSH level does not exclude patients who will be low responders to ovulation induction in preparation for IVF. Thus, other tests that demonstrate more sensitivity have been sought.

Clomiphene Citrate Challenge Test

The clomiphene citrate challenge test was introduced in 1987 as a means of assessing ovarian reserve by Navot and others (19). The test consists of measuring FSH levels on cycle ds 3 and 10 with the administration of 100 mg of clomiphene citrate on ds 5–9 of the cycle. An abnormal result is defined as elevation of either the d 3 and/or d 10 FSH level. It is theorized that normal recruitment of a cohort of follicles leads to increased feedback on the hypothalamic–pituitary axis to suppress FSH levels by d 10. Recent evidence suggests that this normal feedback mechanism may be mediated by inhibin-B *(102)*. An abnormal test occurs when the ovary, because of diminished ovarian reserve, is unable to respond to the elevated FSH induced by clomiphene citrate. Thus, the clomiphene citrate challenge test represents a provocative test used to improve detection of diminished ovarian reserve in women with a normal basal FSH.

The clomiphene challenge test has been used most extensively in patients undergoing ovulation induction and ARTs. In the original study by Navot et al. *(19)*, women with diminished ovarian reserve, as defined by an abnormal d 10 FSH during the clomiphene citrate test, had a 6% pregnancy rate during their 1–2 yr period of treatment. In contrast, women with a normal clomiphene citrate challenge test experienced a 42% pregnancy rate over this period. It is important to note that all of these women were demographically similar and had normal basal FSH levels.

The validity of this test for prediction of outcomes in ART protocols has been confirmed by several subsequent studies *(103–106)*. The specificity of this test is high, where a 100% positive predictive value for failure to achieve pregnancy is typically found *(104,106)*. The clomiphene citrate challenge test identifies about twice as many patients with diminished ovarian reserve as compared to the basal FSH level alone *(106)*.

Recently, use of the clomiphene citrate challenge test has been described in the evaluation of the general infertility population *(107)*. Abnormal clomiphene citrate challenge tests were found in about 10% of this population. The incidence of an abnormal test increased with increasing age, from 7% in women less than age 30 to 26% in women older than age 39. As described in ART patients, an abnormal result predicted significantly lower pregnancy rates (9%) than did a normal result (43%). Interestingly, the incidence of unexplained infertility was higher (52% vs 9%) in patients with an abnormal vs normal clomiphene citrate challenge test. Thus, diminished ovarian reserve may be a distinct etiology of infertility in some patients previously labeled with unexplained infertility. It is important to remember that while an abnormal clomiphene citrate challenge test predicts poor pregnancy rates independent of age, patients of advancing age with a normal clomiphene citrate challenge test still experience decreased pregnancy rates as compared to their younger counterparts *(108)*. In other words, the clomiphene citrate challenge test has a high positive predictive value, but the negative predictive value remains suboptimal for detecting diminished ovarian reserve.

GnRH Stimulation Test

The GnRH agonist stimulation test (GAST) has been proposed as a more quantitative alternative to the clomiphene citrate challenge test *(109)*. The test consists of administration of 1 mg of leuprolide acetate on cycle d 2 followed by analysis of the change in estradiol levels over the subsequent d. The peak estradiol levels after this stimulation were reported to correlate with number of mature oocytes, number of embryos attained and pregnancy rates better than either basal FSH levels or age.

In contrast, a recent study *(110)* using a similar protocol of GnRH agonist treatment during the early follicular phase was unable to demonstrate changes in inhibin or estradiol levels during a 2-h sampling period. The percent change in LH and FSH above baseline, which occurred at 30 min after GnRH stimulation, was significantly diminished in older vs younger women. However, no correlation was found between the gonadotropin response during the stimulation test and the clinical response to exogenous gonadotropins during ovulation induction in the small sample of infertility patients studied.

Thus, larger studies are necessary before the usefulness of the GAST to predict ovarian reserve in ART patients can be determined. If it is established as a screening test for diminished ovarian reserve in this setting, it usefulness in screening the general infertility population will need to be addressed.

Basal FSH:LH Ratios

Other efforts to increase sensitivity for detecting diminished ovarian reserve over that provided by the basal FSH level have included measurement of FSH:LH ratios (96,111). Muasher's group first described diminished estradiol response, oocyte recovery and pregnancy rates in women in an IVF program who had elevated FSH:LH ratios on cycle d 3. Mukherjee also reported on the predictive value of d 3 FSH:LH ratios in 74 women undergoing IVF who had normal d 3 FSH levels. An FSH:LH ratio of 3.6 was predictive of a poor response to ovarian stimulation, as evidenced by lower estradiol levels and dramatically decreased numbers of large follicles (>15 mm) recruited (1.3 vs 17.1 follicles in women with FSH:LH ratios 3.6 vs <3.6). Twelve of the 14 women with FSH:LH 3.6 were canceled for low estradiol levels or less than four mature follicles on d 12. There were no pregnancies in this group. In contrast, only 3% of cycles were canceled in women with FSH:LH <3.6. This group had a pregnancy rate of 25%. Thus, the FSH:LH ratio may predict ovarian reserve in women with a normal d 3 FSH. Further studies are necessary to confirm the clinical usefulness of this test.

Day 3 Estradiol and Inhibin-B Levels

Two other endocrine tests, which have been proposed as predictors of ovarian reserve, are d 3 levels of estradiol and inhibin-B. Early studies failed to show any advantage of basal estradiol levels over d 3 FSH levels in the prediction of ovarian reserve (22). More recent examination of the usefulness of basal estradiol levels has yielded different results. Smotrich and colleagues (112) demonstrated that patients with elevated d 3 estradiol (80 pg/mL) had a higher cancellation rate (18.5% vs 0.4%) and lower pregnancy rate (14.8% vs 37%) than women with basal estradiol levels <80 pg/mL. This association was independent of the FSH level. Licciardi et al. (113) also showed that elevated d 3 estradiol levels were associated with a poor response and pregnancy rate in ART cycles. The association was not independent of basal FSH levels in this latter study. However, prediction of ART performance was improved by using the d 3 estradiol and FSH level together compared to using the basal FSH level alone. Thus, elevated estradiol levels at d 3 may be associated with diminished ovarian reserve. However, determining the value of the basal estradiol level, alone, or in combination with basal FSH, as a prognostic test for ovarian reserve requires further study.

Given that inhibin-B has been implicated as a possible regulator of the monotropic rise in FSH that occurs in the perimenopause, it is logical to suspect that inhibin-B might be a useful predictor of ovarian reserve. It has recently been demonstrated that women with d 3 serum inhibin-B levels <45 pg/mL perform poorly in ART cycles (95). The prognostic value of the d 3 inhibin-B level for the number of oocytes retrieved and clinical pregnancy rate was independent of age as well as basal FSH and estradiol levels. The odds ratio of clinical pregnancy was 6.8 for those women with inhibin-B levels 45 pg/mL as compared to those with inhibin-B levels <45 pg/mL. Thus, with further clinical studies measurement of serum inhibin-B levels may be useful for assessing ovarian reserve before ovulation induction protocols are initiated.

DEPLETION OF FOLLICULAR STORES AND MENOPAUSE

Menopause is generally thought to result from depletion of the oocyte-follicle pool. The maximal number of oocytes, 6–7 million, is found at about 16–20 wk of fetal life *(114)*. The pool of follicles is gradually depleted over a woman's lifetime by follicular growth and atresia, which occur regardless of physiologic state. These processes are not interrupted in childhood, pregnancy or periods of anovulation. Therefore, the number of follicles in the human ovaries continuously declines from fetal life through the perimenopausal period *(115)*. This decline was initially described to occur in an exponential fashion *(116)*. Recent evidence suggests that there is a more rapid disappearance rate of follicles in aging women because of increased recruitment into the growing follicle pool *(117)*. This dramatic decline in follicle numbers in the later reproductive years with age is best described as biexponential *(118,119)* in mathematical models.

Although primordial follicles have been described qualitatively in the postmenopausal human ovary *(120)*, a more recent quantitative study of human ovaries during the perimenopausal transition has emerged *(121)*. The women in this study, aged 45–55, were divided into three groups based on their recent menstrual history: regular menses, irregular menses characteristic of perimenopause, or postmenopausal (>1 yr since last menses). Although the mean ages were similar among the three groups, the number of primordial follicles were ten times greater in the regularly menstruating women (about 1400/ovary) as compared to the perimenopause women (about 140/ovary). Furthermore, only one follicle was found in all four postmenopausal ovaries examined. Thus, this study supports the theory that accelerated follicular depletion to near exhaustion occurs as menopause approaches.

Recently, apoptosis has been identified as the principal mechanism responsible for prenatal loss of the oogonia as well as prenatal and postnatal follicular atresia *(122)*. Apoptosis is characterized by condensation and fragmentation of DNA by endonucleases, followed by phagocytosis. Thus, increasing apoptosis in oocytes or granulosa cells may herald menopause.

Determining follicular numbers in vivo and assessing the incidence of apoptosis in oocytes or granulosa cells may useful anatomic predictors of ovarian reserve and/or onset of menopause *(123)*. Because natural menopause is associated with oocyte depletion, it seems logical that surgical depletion of the follicular pool via ovarian reductive surgery during the earlier reproductive years might also be an anatomic determinant of menopausal age.

Quantitative Assessment of the Follicular Pool

Changes in follicle numbers during women's lifetime, as reviewed above, have been established histologically using postmortem and surgical specimens. Recently, in vivo assessment of the follicular pool has been described, using transvaginal ultrasonography *(124,125)*. The latter study showed that the number antral of follicles of 2 mm decreased by 60% between the ages of 22 and 42 yr, although significant variability was seen within age groups. Perhaps, this individual variation might be useful in predicting reproductive function. To address this hypothesis, Tomas et al. *(126)* reported on the use of transvaginal ultrasound measurement of 2–5 mm follicles to predict oocyte recovery following gonadotropin stimulation in an IVF protocol. The number of follicles seen after GnRH down-regulation and before gonadotropin stimulation, correlated significantly with the number of oocytes recovered for IVF. Follicular number correlated with oocyte recovery more strongly than either age or ovarian volume. Twice as many oocytes were recovered from women with >15 follicles (10.5 oocytes) as compared to those with <5 follicles (5.4 oocytes). Thus, the authors concluded that pretreatment transvaginal ultrasound may be a useful tool for predicting ovarian reserve and IVF outcome. However, the relationship between the number of antral follicles measured by transvaginal ultrasonography and the total number of remaining follicles in various stages of the ovarian functioning needs to be clarified. Some data suggest that this relationship is constant through the menopausal transition *(127)*, whereas other studies suggest that the fraction of follicles in the antral stages increases as the total number of remaining follicles decreases *(128)*.

Highly accurate mathematical models have been developed to predict the age of onset of menopause by using number of remaining follicles *(118,119)*. Clinical use of these models is currently limited by an inability to reliably detect the total number of remaining follicles in the ovary in a noninvasive or minimally invasive manner. Transvaginal ultrasonography may be useful for this purpose if the relationship between early antral follicle numbers and total remaining follicle numbers were clearly defined.

Apoptosis and Ovarian Reserve

In addition to the decline in follicular numbers that is manifested initially by low ovarian reserve and ultimately by menopause, qualitative changes occur in the granulosa cells of these follicles. Women with diminished ovarian reserve, as reflected by d 3 FSH 10 mIU/mL, have preovulatory follicles that contain fewer granulosa cells than those from women with normal basal FSH levels *(123)*. Furthermore, the percentage of granulosa cells undergoing apoptosis was fourfold greater in the women with elevated d 3 FSH *(123)*. Thus, these data suggest that, in addition to *quantitative* changes in the follicular pool, there are *qualitative* changes that occur in the follicles of women with diminished ovarian reserve.

Nakahara and colleagues *(129,130)* have recently correlated the rates of apoptosis in granulosa cells to predict IVF outcome. An increase in apoptotic bodies in granulosa cells from pooled follicular aspirates was associated with significantly diminished oocyte recovery and decreased pregnancy rates *(129)*. Further studies of individual follicles showed a higher incidence of apoptosis in granulosa cells from follicles containing poor quality oocytes *(130)*. The fertilization rates of these oocytes were significantly diminished compared to those from follicles that showed a lower incidence of apoptosis in the granulosa cells. Further studies are needed to define the value of granulosa cell apoptotic rate as a predictor of ovarian reserve in individual women or as a predictor of oocyte quality in individual follicles.

Ovarian Reductive Surgery

Compensatory hypertrophy of the remaining ovary after unilateral oophorectomy has been demonstrated in many animal models *(131,132)*. It appears that a similar compensatory response occurs in women with one ovary. The evidence includes several studies that demonstrate that the number of follicles detected after gonadotropin stimulation during IVF did not differ between women with one or two ovaries *(133–135)*. It seems logical that excision of half of the follicular pool followed by a compensatory response in the remaining ovary might lead to premature depletion of follicles, and thus earlier menopause, in unilateral oophorectomized women.

Several studies have indeed shown an earlier age of menopause in women who have undergone various ovarian reductive surgeries: oophorectomy, ovarian cystectomy, or ovarian wedge resection *(136,137)*. The latter study showed significant earlier age of menopause in women who had undergone unilateral oophorectomy (43.5 yr) or bilateral ovarian wedge resection (40.3 yr) before the age of 30 as compared to control women (50.1 yr). Menopausal age was also significantly earlier in women who had these procedures performed after age 30, but the magnitude of the effect was less. Interestingly, women under 30 yr with intrinsic ovarian pathology such as polycystic ovarian syndrome experienced menopause much earlier (40.3 yr) after ovarian wedge resections than women who had unilateral oophorectomy for ectopic pregnancy (44.6 yr). Whether this difference represents an underlying effect of the polycystic ovarian disease process on follicular depletion or a more damaging effect of wedge resection on the remaining ovarian tissue requires more study.

SUMMARY

The transition into menopause probably represents a continuum that begins with diminished ovarian reserve, is followed by menstrual irregularity of the perimenopause, and culminates with cessation of menses. Some believe the "pacemaker" for the onset and progression of reproductive senescence in women is the granulosa cell *(138)*. Thus, the perimenopausal transition may involve attrition of follicular numbers in the ovary as well as qualitative changes in granulosa cell function *(138)*.

The temporal relationship between detection of diminished ovarian reserve and onset of menopause has not been well defined. It is important to determine whether women who display diminished ovarian reserve in their 30s undergo menopause at an earlier age. Alternatively, these women may experience a longer perimenopausal transition with normal timing of the onset of the last menses. Thus, it remains to be clarified how useful predictors of diminished ovarian reserve are for predicting the onset of menopause.

Predicting ovarian reserve and onset of menopause has become increasingly important as women delay childbearing and the menopausal segment of our population continues to grow. Accurate prediction of these processes would allow us to predict age-related infertility and responsiveness to fertility therapy, as well as appropriately timing initiation of hormone replacement therapy and assessing risks of chronic diseases.

Based on epidemiologic evidence, the onset of menopause appears to be earlier in smokers and later in parous women. Age of maternal menopause is predictive of the timing of menopause in daughters. In contrast to earlier beliefs, age of menarche and use of oral contraceptives have not been shown in recent studies to be related to age of menopause. A history of ovarian reductive surgery appears to hasten the onset of menopause by 5–10 yr, depending on the procedure and the presence of intrinsic ovarian pathology. The role of nutritional factors and prior toxic exposures, including DES, in determining menopausal age remains unclear.

Clinically useful predictors of ovarian reserve include the basal FSH and clomiphene citrate challenge test. Despite high positive predictive values, use of these tests is still limited by their relatively low sensitivity and interlaboratory variation in normal values. We anxiously await further study of the clinical usefulness of other endocrine tests for ovarian reserve, such as basal inhibin-B levels.

The possibility of determining ovarian reserve and predicting the onset of menopause in individual women by assessing the store of follicles in their ovaries is exciting. The limiting factor is optimizing a noninvasive or minimally invasive means to determine total follicular pool. Further studies of the use of transvaginal ultrasound for this purpose are necessary.

Research efforts in this area should address the physiologic basis of the menopausal transition, as well as seek clinical predictors of the decline in ovarian function. Advances in this area of reproductive medicine could impact the health and well being of large numbers of women.

REFERENCES

1. Hill K. The demography of menopause. Maturitas 1996;23:113–127.
2. Khaw KT. Epidemiology of the menopause. Br Med Bull 1992;48:249–261.
3. McKinlay SM, Brambilla DJ, Posner JG. The normal menopause transition. Am J Hum Biol 1992;4:37–46.
4. Fonteyn VJ, Isada NB. Nongenetic implications of childbearing after age thirty-five. Obstet Gynecol Surv 1988;43:709–720.
5. Mosher W, Pratt W. Fecundity and infertility in the United States, 1965–88. Adv Data 1990;192:1–12.
6. Federation CECOS, Schwartz D, Mayaux MJ. Female fecundity as a function of age: results of artificial insemination in 2193 multiparous women with azoospermic husbands. N Engl J Med 1982;306:404–406.
7. Society for Assisted Reproductive Technology and The American Society for Reproductive Medicine. Assisted reproductive technology in the United States and Canada: 1994 results generated from the American Society for Reproductive Medicine/Society for Assisted Reproductive Technology Registry. Fertil Steril 1996;66:697–705.
8. Sowers MR, La Pietra MT. Menopause: its epidemiology and potential association with chronic diseases. Epidemiol Rev 1995;17:287–302.
9. Toner JP, Philput CB, Jones GS, Muasher SJ. Basal follicle-stimulating hormone level is a better predictor of in vitro fertilization performance than age. Fertil Steril 1991;55:784–791.
10. Jacobs SL, Metzger DA, Dodson WC, Haney AF. Effect of age on response to human menopausal gonadotropin stimulation. J Clin Endocrinol Metab 1990;71:1525–1530.
11. Roest J, van Heusden AM, Mous H, Zeilmaker GH, Verhoeff A. The ovarian response as a predictor for successful in vitro fertilization treatment after the age of 40 years. Fertil Steril 1996;66:969–973.
12. Piette C, de Mouzon J, Bachelot A, Spira A. In vitro fertilization: influence of woman's age on pregnancy rates. Hum Reprod 1990;5:56–59.
13. Sharma V, Riddle A, Mason BA, Pampiglione J, Campbell S. An analysis of factors influencing the establishment of a clinical pregnancy in an ultrasound-based ambulatory in vitro fertilization program. Fertil Steril 1988;49:468–478.
14. Corson SL, Dickey RP, Gocial B, Batzer FR, Eisenberg E, Huppert L, Maislin G. Outcome in 242 in vitro fertilization-embryo replacement or gamete intrafallopian transfer-induced pregnancies. Fertil Steril 1989;51:644–650.
15. Craft I, Al-Shawaf T, Lewis P, Serhal P, Simons E, Ah-Moye M, Fiamanya W, Robertson D, Shrivastav P, Brinsden P. Analysis of 1071 GIFT procedures—the case for a flexible approach to treatment. Lancet 1988;1:1094–1098.
16. Hughes EG, King C, Wood EC. A prospective study of prognostic factors in in vitro fertilization and embryo transfer. Fertil Steril 1989;51:838–844.
17. Padilla SL, Garcia JE. Effect of maternal age and number of in vitro fertilization procedures on pregnancy outcome. Fertil Steril 1989;52:270–273.
18. Penzias AS, Thompson IE, Alper MM, Oskowitz SP, Berger MJ. Successful use of gamete intrafallopian transfer does not reverse the decline in fertility in women over 40 years of age. Obstet Gynecol 1991;77:37–39.
19. Navot D, Rosenwaks Z, Margalioth EJ. Prognostic assessment of female fecundity. Lancet 1987;2:645–647.
20. Scott RT, Jr., Hofmann GE. Prognostic assessment of ovarian reserve. Fertil Steril 1995;63:1–11.
21. Pearlstone AC, Fournet N, Gambone JC, Pang SC, Buyalos RP. Ovulation induction in women age 40 and older: the importance of basal follicle-stimulating hormone level and chronological age. Fertil Steril 1992;58:674–679.
22. Scott RT, Toner JP, Muasher SJ, Oehninger S, Robinson S, Rosenwaks Z. Follicle-stimulating hormone levels on cycle day 3 are predictive of in vitro fertilization outcome. Fertil Steril 1989;51:651–654.

23. World Health Organization Scientific Group. Research on the Menopause, WHO Tech Rep Ser 670. 1981; World Health Organization, Geneva, Switzerland.

24. Brambilla DJ, McKinlay SM. A prospective study of factors affecting age at menopause. J Clin Epidemiol. 1989;42:1031–1039.

25. Bromberger JT, Matthews KA, Kullerm LH, Wingm RR, Meilahnm EN, Plantinga P. Prospective study of the determinants of age at menopause. Am J Epidemiol 1997;145:124–133.

26. Jick H, Porter J. Relation between smoking and age of natural menopause. Report from the Boston Collaborative Drug Surveillance Program, Boston University Medical Center. Lancet 1977;1:1354–1355.

27. Lindquist O, Bengtsson C. The effect of smoking on menopausal age. Maturitas 1979;1:171–173.

28. Adena MA, Gallagher HG. Cigarette smoking and the age at menopause. Ann Hum Biol 1982;9:121–130.

29. Willett W, Stampfer MJ, Bain C, Lipnick R, Speizer FE, Rosner B, Cramer D, Hennekens CH. Cigarette smoking, relative weight, and menopause. Am J Epidemiol 1983;117:651–658.

30. McKinlay SM, Bifano NL, McKinlay JB. Smoking and age at menopause in women. Ann Int Med 1985;103:350–356.

31. Parazzini F, Negri E, La Vecchia C. Reproductive and general lifestyle determinants of age at menopause. Maturitas 1992;15:141–149.

32. Torgerson DJ, Avenell A, Russell IT, Reid DM. Factors associated with onset of menopause in women aged 45–49. Maturitas 1994;19:83–92.

33. van Noord PAH, Dubas JS, Dorland M, Boersma H, te Velde E. Age at natural menopause in a population-based screening cohort: the role of menarche, fecundity, and lifestyle factors. Fertil Steril 1997;68:95–102.

34. Howe G, Westhoff C, Vessey M, Yeates D. Effects of age, cigarette smoking and other factors on fertility: findings in a large prospective study. Br Med J 1985;290:1697–1700.

35. Hughes EG, Brennan BG. Does cigarette smoking impair natural or assisted fecundity? Fertil Steril 1996;66:679–689.

36. Harrison KL, Breen TM, Hennessey JF. The effect of patient smoking habit on the outcome of IVF and GIFT treatment. Austr NZ J Obstet Gynaecol 1990;30:340–342.

37. Elenbogen A, Lipitz S, Mashiach S, Dor J, Levran D, Ben-Rafael Z. The effect of smoking on the outcome of in-vitro fertilization- embryo-transfer. Hum Reprod 1991;6:242–244.

38. Trapp M, Kemeter P, Feichtinger W. Smoking and in-vitro fertilization. Hum Reprod 1986;1:357–358.

39. Hughes EG, Yeo J, Claman P, YoungLai EV, Sagle MA, Daya S, Collins JA. Cigarette smoking and the outcomes of in vitro fertilization: measurement of effect size and levels of action. Fertil Steril 1994;62:807–814.

40. Sterzik K, Strehler E, De Santo M, Trumpp N, Abt M, Rosenbusch B, Schneider A. Influence of smoking on fertility in women attending an in vitro fertilization program. Fertil Steril 1996;65:810–814.

41. Cramer DW, Barbieri RL, Xu H, Reichardt JKV. Determinants of basal follicle-stimulating hormone levels in premenopausal women. J Clin Endocrinol Metab 1994;79:1105–1109.

42. Sharara FI, Beatse SN, Leonardi MR, Navot D, Scott RT, Jr. Cigarette smoking accelerates the development of diminished ovarian reserve as evidenced by the clomiphene citrate challenge test. Fertil Steril 1994;62:257–262.

43. Van Voorhis J, Syrop CH, Hammitt DG, Dunn MS, Snyder GD. Effects of smoking on ovulation induction for assisted reproductive techniques. Fertil Steril 1992;58:981–985.

44. Barbieri RL, McShane PM, Ryan KJ. Constituents of cigarette smoke inhibit human granulosa cell aromatase. Fertil Steril 1986;46:232–236.

45. Michnovicz JJ, Hershcopf RJ, Naganuma H, Bradlow HL, Fishman J. Increased 2-hydroxylation of estradiol as a possible mechanism for the anti-estrogenic effect of cigarette smoking. N Engl J Med 1986;315:1305–1309.

46. Longcope C, Johnston CC, Jr. Androgen and estrogen dynamics in pre- and postmenopausal women: a comparison between smokers and nonsmokers. J Clin Endocrinol Metab 1988;67:379–383.

47. Mattison DR. The effects of smoking on fertility from gametogenesis to implantation. Environ Res 1982;28:410–433.

48. Mattison DR, Plowchalk DR, Meadows MJ, Miller MM, Malek A, London S. The effect of smoking on oogenesis, fertilization and implantation. Semin Reprod Endocrinol 1989;7:291–304.

49. Van Keep PA, Brand PC, Lehert P. Factors affecting the age at menopause. J Biosoc Sci (suppl) 1979;6:37–55.

50. Stanford JL, Hartge P, Brinton LA, Hoover RN, Brookmeyer R. Factors influencing the age at natural menopause. J Chron Dis 1987;40:995–1002.

51. Whelan EA, Sandler DP, McConnaughey DR, Weinberg CR. Menstrual and reproductive characteristics and age at natural menopause. Am J Epidemiol 1990;131:625–632.
52. Frisch RE. Population, food intake and fertility. Science 1978;199:22–30.
53. Frisch RE. Body fat, menarche, fitness and fertility. Hum Reprod 1987;2:521–533.
54. Ernster VL, Petrakis NL. Effect of hormonal events in earlier life and socioeconomic status on age at menopause. Am J Obstet Gynecol 1981;140:471–472.
55. Cramer DW, Xu H, Harlow BL. Family history as a predictor of early menopause. Fertil Steril 1995;64:740–745.
56. Torgerson DJ, Thomas RE, Campbell MK, Reid DM. Alcohol consumption and age of maternal menopause are associated with menopause onset. Maturitas 1997;26:21–25.
57. Torgerson DJ, Thomas RE, Reid DM. Mother and daughters menopausal ages: is there a link? Eur J Obstet Gynecol Reprod Biol 1997;74:63–66.
58. Krauss CM, Turksoy RN, Atkins L, McLaughlin C, Brown LG, Page DC. Familial premature ovarian failure due to interstitial deletion of the long arm of the X chromosome. N Engl J Med 1987;317:125–131.
59. Veneman TF, Beverstock GC, Exalto N, Mollevanger P. Premature menopause because of inherited deletion in the long arm of the X-chromosome. Fertil Steril 1991;55:631–633.
60. Kaufert PA, Gilbert P, Tate R. Defining menopausal status: the impact of longitudinal data. Maturitas 1987;9:217–226.
61. Scragg RFR. Menopause and reproductive span in rural Niuguini. In: Papua New Guinea Medical Society, ed. Proceedings of the Annual Symposium of the Papua New Guinea Medical Society. Port Moresby, New Guinea, 1973, pp. 126–144.
62. Beser E, Aydemir V, Bozkaya H. Body mass index and age at natural menopause. Gynecol Obstet Invest 1994;37:40–42.
63. MacMahon B, Worcester J. Age at menopause: United States 1960–1962. In: US Vital and Health Statistics, Series 11, No. 19. U.S. Government Printing Office, Washington, D.C., 1966, pp. 1–20.
64. Sherman B, Wallace R, Bean J, Schlabaugh L. Relationship of body weight to menarcheal and menopausal age: implications for breast cancer risk. J Clin Endocrinol Metab 1981;52:488–493.
65. Garrido-Latorre F, Lazcano-Ponce EC, Lopez-Carrillo L, Hernandez-Avila C. Age of natural menopause among women in Mexico City. Int J Gynecol Obstet 1996;53:159–166.
66. Ash P. The influence of radiation on fertility in man. Br J Radiol 1980;53:271–278.
67. Gradishar WJ, Schilsky RL. Ovarian function following radiation and chemotherapy for cancer. Semin Oncol 1989;16:425–436.
68. Bibbo M, Gill WB, Azizi F, Blough R, Fang VS, Rosenfield RL, Schumacher CFB, Sleeper K, Sonek MG, Wied GL. Follow-up study of male and female offspring of DES-exposed mothers. Obstet Gynecol 1977;49:1–8.
69. Herbst AL, Hubby MM, Blough RR, Azizi F. A comparison of pregnancy experience in DES-exposed and DES-unexposed daughters. J Reprod Med. 1980;24:62–69.
70. Herbst AL, Hubby MM, Azizi F, Makii MM. Reproductive and gynecologic surgical experience in diethylstilbestrol-exposed daughters. Am J Obstet Gynecol 1981;141:1019–1028.
71. Senekjian EK, Potkul RK, Frey K, Herbst AL. Infertility among daughters either exposed or not exposed to diethylstilbestrol. Am J Obstet Gynecol 1988;158:493–498.
72. Haney AF, Newbold RR, McLachlan JA. Prenatal diethylstilbestrol exposure in the mouse: effects on ovarian histology and steroidogenesis in vitro. Biol Reprod 1984;30:471–478.
73. McLachlan JA, Newbold RR, Shah HC, Hogan MD, Dixon RL. Reduced fertility in female mice exposed transplacentally to diethylstilbestrol (DES). Fertil Steril 1982;38:364–371.
74. Hornsby PP, Wilcox AJ, Herbst AL. Onset of menopause in women exposed to diethylstilbestrol in utero. Am J Obstet Gynecol 1995;172:92–95.
75. Ying S. Inhibins, activins and follistatins: gonadal proteins modulating the secretion of follicle-stimulating hormone. Endocr Rev 1988;9:267–293.
76. Groome NP, Illingworth PJ, O'Brien M, Cooke I, Ganesan TS, Baird DT, McNeilly AS. Detection of dimeric inhibin throughout the human menstrual cycle by two-site enzyme immunoassay. Clin Endocrinol 1994;40:717–723.
77. Groome NP, Illingworth PJ, O'Brien M, Pai R, Rodger FE, Mather JP, McNeilly AS. Measurement of dimeric inhibin B throughout the human menstrual cycle. J Clin Endocrinol Metab 1996;81:1401–1405.
78. Sherman BM, Korenman SG. Hormonal characteristics of the human menstrual cycle throughout reproductive life. J Clin Invest 1975;55:699–706.
79. Sherman BM, West JH, Korenman SG. The menopausal transition: analysis of LH, FSH, estradiol and progesterone concentrations during menstrual cycles of older women. J Clin Endocrinol Metab 1976;42:629–636.

80. Reyes FI, Winter JSD, Faiman C. Pituitary-ovarian relationships preceding the menopause. I. A cross-sectional study of serum follicle-stimulating hormone, luteinizing hormone, prolactin, estradiol and progesterone levels. Am J Obstet Gynecol 1977;129:557–564.
81. Lee SJ, Lenton EA, Sexton L, Cooke ID. The effect of age on the cyclical patterns of plasma LH, FSH, oestradiol and progesterone in women with regular menstrual cycles. Hum Reprod 1988;3:851–855.
82. Lenton EA, Sexton L, Lee S, Cooke ID. Progressive changes in LH and FSH and LH:FSH ratio in women throughout reproductive life. Maturitas 1988;10:35–43.
83. Hee J, MacNaughton J, Bangah M, Burger HG. Perimenopausal patterns of gonadotrophins, immunoreactive inhibin, oestradiol and progesterone. Maturitas 1993;18:9–20.
84. Burger HG, Dudley EC, Hopper JL, Shelley JM, Green A, Smith A, Dennerstein L, Morse C. The endocrinology of the menopausal transition: a cross-sectional study of a population-based sample. J Clin Endocrinol Metab 1995;80:3537–3545.
85. Buckler HM, Evans CA, Mamtora H, Burger HG, Anderson DC. Gonadotropin, steroid, and inhibin levels in women with incipient ovarian failure during anovulatory and ovulatory rebound cycles. J Clin Endocrinol Metab 1991;72:116–124.
86. Batista MC, Cartledge TP, Zellmer AW, Merino MJ, Axiotis C, Bremner WJ, Nieman LK. Effects of aging on menstrual cycle hormones and endometrial maturation. Fertil Steril 1995;64:492–499.
87. Klein NA, Battaglia DE, Miller PB, Branigan EF, Guidice LC, Soules MR. Ovarian follicular development and the follicular fluid hormones and growth factors in normal women of advanced reproductive age. J Clin Endocrinol Metab 1996;81:1946–1951.
88. Santoro N, Brown JR, Adel T, Skurnick JH. Characterization of reproductive hormonal dynamics in the perimenopause. J Clin Endocrinol Metab 1996;81:1495–1501.
89. Blake EJ, Adel T, Santoro NS. Relationships between insulin-like growth hormone factor-1 and estradiol in reproductive aging. Fertil Steril 1997;67:697–701.
90. Pellicer A, Simon C, Remohi J. Effects of aging on the female reproductive system. Hum Reprod 1995;10:77–83.
91. Seifer DB, Gardiner AC, Lambert-Messerlian G, Schneyer AL. Differential secretion of dimeric inhibin in cultured luteinized granulosa cells as a function of ovarian reserve. J Clin Endocrinol Metab 1996;81:736–739.
92. Lenton LA, De Kretser DM, Woodward AJ, Robertson DM. Inhibin concentrations throughout the menstrual cycles of normal, infertile, and older women compared with those during spontaneous conception cycles. J Clin Endocrinol Metab 1991;73:1180–1190.
93. Klein NA, Battaglia DE, Fujimoto VY, Davis GS, Bremner WJ, Soules MR. Reproductive aging: accelerated ovarian follicular development associated with a monotropic follicle-stimulating hormone rise in normal older women. J Clin Endocrinol Metab 1996;81:1038–1045.
94. Klein NA, Illingworth PJ, Groome NP, McNeilly AS, Battaglia DE, Soules MR. Decreased inhibin B secretion is associated with the monotropic FSH rise in older, ovulatory women: a study of serum and follicular fluid levels of dimeric inhibin A and B in spontaneous menstrual cycles. J Clin Endocrinol Metab 1996;81:2742–2745.
95. Seifer DB, Lambert-Messerlian G, Hogan JW, Gardiner AC, Blazar AS, Berk CA. Day 3 serum inhibin-B is predictive of assisted reproductive technologies outcome. Fertil Steril 1997;67:110–114.
96. Muasher SJ, Oehninger S, Simonetti S, Matta J, Ellis LM, Liu H-C, Jones GS, Rosenwaks Z. The value of basal and/or stimulated serum gonadotropin levels in prediction of stimulation response and in vitro fertilization outcome. Fertil Steril 1988;50:298–307.
97. Cahill DJ, Prosser CJ, Wardle PG, Ford WCL, Hull MGR. Relative influence of serum follicle stimulating hormone, age and other factors on ovarian response to gonadotrophin stimulation. Br J Obstet Gynaecol 1994;101:999–1002.
98. Hansen LM, Batzer FR, Gutmann JN, Corson SL, Kelly MP, Gocial B. Evaluating ovarian reserve: follicle stimulating hormone and oestradiol variability during cycle days 2–5. Hum Reprod 1996;3:486–489.
99. Scott RT, Hofmann GE, Oehninger S, Muasher SJ. Intercycle variability of day 3 follicle-stimulating hormone levels and its effect on stimulation quality in in vitro fertilization. Fertil Steril 1990;54:297–302.
100. Martin JSB, Nisker JA, Tummon IS, Daniel SAJ, Auckland JL, Feyles V. Future in vitro fertilization pregnancy potential of women with variably elevated day 3 follicle-stimulating hormone levels. Fertil Steril 1996;65:1238–1240.
101. Khalifa E, Toner JP, Muasher SJ, Acosta AA. Significance of basal follicle-stimulating hormone levels in women with one ovary in a program of in vitro fertilization. Fertil Steril 1992;57:835–839.
102. Hofmann GE, Danforth D, Seifer DB. Inhibin-B: the physiologic basis of the clomiphene citrate challenge test for ovarian reserve screening. Fertil Steril 1998;69:474–477.

103. Tanbo T, Dale PO, Abyholm T, Stokke KT. Follicle-stimulating hormone as a prognostic indicator in clomiphene citrate/human menopausal gonadotrophin-stimulated cycles for in-vitro fertilization. Hum Reprod 1989;6:647–650.

104. Loumaye E, Billion JM, Mine JM, Psalti I, Pensis M, Thomas K. Prediction of individual response to controlled ovarian hyperstimulation by means of a clomiphene citrate challenge test. Fertil Steril 1990;53:295–301.

105. Nader S, Berkowitz AS. Use of the hormonal response to clomiphene citrate as an endocrinological indicator of ovarian aging. Hum Reprod 1991;6:931–933.

106. Tanbo T, Dale PO, Lunde O, Norman N, Abyholm T. Prediction of response to controlled ovarian hyperstimulation: a comparison of basal and clomiphene citrate-stimulated follicle stimulating hormone levels. Fertil Steril 1992;57:819–824.

107. Scott RT, Leonardi MR, Hofmann GE, Illions EH, Neal GS, Navot D. A prospective evaluation of clomiphene citrate challenge test screening of the general infertility population. Obstet Gynecol 1993;82:539–544.

108. Scott RT, Opsahl MS, Leonardi MR, Neall GS, Illions EH, Navot D. Life table analysis of pregnancy rates in a general infertility population relative to ovarian reserve and patient age. Hum Reprod 1995;10:1706–1710.

109. Winslow KL, Toner JP, Brzyski RG, Oehninger SC, Acosta AA, Muasher SJ. The gonadotropin-releasing hormone agonist stimulation test—a sensitive predictor of performance in the flare-up in vitro fertilization cycle. Fertil Steril 1991;56:711–717.

110. Fujimoto VY, Klein NA, Battaglia DE, Bremner WJ, Soules MR. The anterior pituitary response to a gonadotropin-releasing hormone challenge test in normal older reproductive-age women. Fertil Steril 1996;65:539–544.

111. Mukherjee T, Copperman AB, Lapinski R, Sandler B, Bustillo M, Grunfeld L. An elevated day three follicle-stimulating hormone:luteinizing hormone ratio (FSH:LH) in the presence of a normal day 3 FSH predicts a poor response to controlled ovarian hyperstimulation. Fertil Steril 1996;65:588–593.

112. Smotrich DB, Widra EA, Gindoff PR, Levy MJ, Hall JL, Stillman RJ. Prognostic value of day 3 estradiol on in vitro fertilization outcome. Fertil Steril 1995;64:1136–1140.

113. Licciardi FL, Liu HC, Rosenwaks Z. Day 3 estradiol serum concentrations as prognosticators of ovarian stimulation response and pregnancy outcome in patients undergoing in vitro fertilization. Fertil Steril 1995;64:991–994.

114. Baker TG. A quantitative and cytological study of germ cells in the human ovaries. Proc Royal Soc London 1963;158:417–433.

115. Block E. Quantitative morphological investigation of the follicular system in women. Acta Anat 1952;14:18–123.

116. Thomford PJ, Jelovsek FR, Mattison DR. Effect of oocyte number and rate of atresia on the age of menopause. Reprod Toxicol 1987;1:41–51.

117. Gougeon A, Ecochard R, Thalabard JC. Age-related changes of the population of human ovarian follicles: increase in the disappearance rate of non-growing and early-growing follicles in aging women. Biol Reprod 1994;50:653–663.

118. Faddy MJ, Gosden RG, Gougeon A, Richardson SJ, Nelson JF. Accelerated disappearance of ovarian follicles in mid-life: implications for forecasting menopause. Hum Reprod 1992;7:1342–1346.

119. Faddy MJ, Gosden RG. A model conforming the decline in follicle numbers to the age of menopause in women. Hum Reprod 1996;11:1484–1486.

120. Costoff A, Mahesh VB. Primordial follicles with normal oocytes in the ovaries of postmenopausal women. J Am Geriatr Soc 1975;23:193–196.

121. Richardson SJ, Senikas V, Nelson JF. Follicular depletion during the menopausal transition: evidence for accelerated loss and ultimate exhaustion. J Clin Endocrinol Metab 1987;65:1231–1237.

122. Tilly JL. Apoptosis and ovarian function. Rev Reprod 1996;1:162–172.

123. Seifer DB, Gardiner AC, Ferreira KA, Peluso JJ. Apoptosis as a function of ovarian reserve in women undergoing in vitro fertilization. Fertil Steril 1996;66:593–598.

124. Pache TD, Wladimiroff JW, de Jong FH, Hop WC, Fauser BCJM. Growth patterns of nondominant ovarian follicles during the normal menstrual cycle. Fertil Steril 1990;54:638–642.

125. Reuss ML, Kline J, Santos R, Levin B, Timor-Tritsch I. Age and the ovarian follicle pool assessed with transvaginal ultrasonography. Am J Obstet Gynecol 1996;174:624–627.

126. Tomas C, Nuojua-Huttunen S, Martikainen H. Pretreatment transvaginal ultrasound examination predicts ovarian responsiveness to gonadotrophins in in-vitro fertilization. Hum Reprod 1997;12:220–223.

127. Cran DG, Moor RM. The development of oocytes and ovarian follicles of mammals. Sci Prog 1980;66:371–383.
128. Gougeon A, Chainy GBN. Morphometric studies of small follicles in ovaries of women at different ages. J Reprod Fertil 1987;81:433–442.
129. Nakahara K, Saito H, Saito T, Ito M, Ohta N, Sakai N, Tezuka N, Hiroi M, Watanabe H. Incidence of apoptotic bodies in membrana granulosa of the patients participating in an in vitro fertilization program. Fertil Steril 1997;67:302–308.
130. Nakahara K, Saito H, Saito T, Ito M, Ohta N, Takahashi T, Hiroi M. Incidence of apoptotic bodies in membrana granulosa can predict prognosis of ova from patients participating in in vitro fertilization programs. Fertil Steril 1997;68:312–317.
131. Biggers JD, Finn CA, McLaren A. Long-term reproductive performance of female mice. I. Effect of removing one ovary. J Reprod Fertil 1962;3:303–312.
132. Fleming MW, Rhodes RC, Dailey RA. Compensatory response after unilateral ovariectomy in rabbits. Biol Reprod 1984;30:82–86.
133. Diamond MP, Wentz AC, Herbert CM, Pittaway DE, Maxson WS, Daniell JF. One ovary or two: differences in ovulation induction, estradiol levels, and follicular development in a program for in vitro fertilization. Fertil Steril 1984;41:524–529.
134. Alper MM, Seibel MM, Oskowitz SP, Smith BD, Ransil BJ, Taymor ML. Comparison of follicular response in patients with one or two ovaries in a program of in vitro fertilization. Fertil Steril 1985;44:652–655.
135. Dodds WG, Chin N, Awadalla S, Miller F, Friedman C, Kim M. In vitro fertilization and embryo transfer in patients with one ovary. Fertil Steril 1987;48:249–253.
136. Rozewicki K, Rzepka I, Rozewicki S, Strzelecki E. Premature menopause after unilateral ovariectomy. Ginekologia Polska (suppl) 1979;130–132.
137. Melica F, Chiodi S, Cristoforoni PM, Ravera GB. Reductive surgery and ovarian function in the human—can reductive ovarian surgery in reproductive age negatively influence fertility and age at onset of menopause? Int J Fertil 1995;40:79–85.
138. Seifer DB, Naftolin F. Moving toward an earlier and better understanding of the perimenopause. Fertil Steril 1998;69:387–388.

2

Endocrinology of the Climacteric

Nanette Santoro, MD *and Drew V. Tortoriello,* MD

Contents

DEFINITIONS AND EPIDEMIOLOGY

Menopause is that point of time in a woman's life when there occurs the permanent cessation of menstrual activity. Although this itself is a discrete milestone on whose basis we very often classify women for health and social issues, the event itself is merely the manifest culmination of an altered endocrinological milieu, the origins of which usually precede the menopause by more than a decade. It was not until after 1900 that the average life expectancy of a woman actually exceeded the time at which most women would naturally encounter the menopause *(1)*. Therefore the study of the menopausal transition is still in its early stages. However, as the world's population continues to expand *(2)*, and as the projected life expectancy of women approaches the mid-80s, it becomes critical to better understand the physiology of the menopause. Therein lies the ability to improve the quality and duration of the mature woman's life.

The regularity and length of the menstrual cycle shows variation among different women and also across the reproductive life span of any individual woman. The 7-yr intervals immediately following menarche and preceding menopause are marked by the greatest amount of cycle variability. The intermenstrual interval is at its lowest between the ages of 36 and 40 *(3)*. Thereafter, marked variation in the length of menstrual cycles occur. The perimenopausal onset is clinically defined by the first break in cyclicity a previously regularly cycling woman experiences *(4)*. The median age of onset for these symptoms is 47.5 yr *(5)*. This definition will likely expand to include younger women as our knowledge of the process of reproductive senescence becomes more sophisticated. More than 90% of women over age 45 who have experienced one year of amenorrhea will

From: *Contemporary Endocrinology: Menopause: Endocrinology and Management*
Edited by: D. B. Seifer and E. A. Kennard © Humana Press Inc., Totowa, NJ

not menstruate again, and it is even more unlikely that they will conceive *(6)*. The median age of the menopause has been estimated by the Women's Massachusetts Health Study at approximately age 51.3 yr. Only 10% of the women studied however, had an abrupt and permanent cessation of monthly menses *(5)*. The term "climacteric" refers to the time frame encompassing both the peri- and postmenopausal periods of life. The majority of a woman's life may be spent in this state.

Unlike the age at menarche, which has been getting progressively younger throughout the 20th century, the age at menopause has not been observed to change. The main forces underlying the onset of menopause in chromosomally normal women are probably genetically multifactorial; however, some environmental factors may contribute independently to its earlier occurrence. A profound predictor of an earlier menopause is cigarette smoking, which in a dose-response fashion advances the process by a mean of 2 yr *(7,8)*. Familial features, such as the age of menopause in close female relatives, also appear to be major predictors *(9)*. Factors which may also predispose women to an inappropriately early menopause include pelvic adhesions, living at high altitudes, and endometriosis *(10)*. Prior pelvic surgery, even minimally traumatic procedures such as ovarian cystectomies, is associated with diminished patient responsiveness to controlled ovarian hyperstimulation and significantly higher follicle-stimulating hormone (FSH) levels *(11–13)*. Whether this will hasten the onset of menopause remains to be seen. Approximately 1% of the female population will experience menopause before the age of 40, or premature ovarian failure *(14)*. Its basis is largely idiopathic, but there is a strong association in some subsets of patients with coexisting autoimmune disease or deletions of the distal arm of the X chromosome *(15,16)*.

The process of menopause occurs in tandem with the aging process. The extent to which reproductive aging interacts with somatic aging is poorly understood. Indeed, reproductive aging is often a confounding variable in studies of somatic aging in women. This chapter will review the current state of knowledge of the impact of aging on endocrine systems both reproductive and nonreproductive.

THE HYPOTHALAMUS

In middle-aged animals, clear-cut changes in hypothalamic-pituitary feedback sensitivity to sex steroids have been described *(17–19)*. Whether similar changes occur in humans is controversial. Several studies have compared older-reproductive-aged women to midreproductive-aged women using frequent blood sampling techniques to detect the frequency and amplitude of pulsatile gonadotropin secretion. Accelerated luteal phase luteinizing hormone (LH) pulsations in older women *(20)*, unchanged early follicular phase LH pulsatile patterns *(21,22)* and a decreased mid-to-late follicular phase frequency of LH pulsation *(23)* have all been observed in association with reproductive aging. These findings suggest that alterations in hypothalamic gonadotropin releasing hormone (GnRH) secretion are subtle, at least in the cycle stages that have been studied to date. Dynamic testing of the hypothalamic-pituitary axis in women in their mid-40s has suggested that women with dysfunctional uterine bleeding and ovulatory abnormalities have a decreased ability to respond to an estradiol challenge with an LH surge *(24,25)*. However, such studies were based upon relatively small groups of women who were selected by symptomatology. The clinical relevance of altered hypothalamic-pituitary feedback in middle age is potentially large as dysfunctional bleeding complaints, endometrial curettages, and hysterectomies are all common in women in their mid-40s *(26–28)*.

THE PITUITARY

Pituitary physiology may also be altered in the late reproductive years. Despite increased estrogen, older women (age 42–47) demonstrated lower growth hormone (GH) and insulin-like growth factor-1 (IGF-1) as compared to normal midreproductive-aged women *(21)*. The effect of these alterations on a perimenopausal woman's physiology is not yet understood. These events begin prior to the appearance of any overt menstrual cycle disturbances. Because growth hormone and the insulin-like growth factors may play a synergistic role with gonadotropins in ovarian stimulation, this age-related loss may be a clinically meaningful one. It appears, however, that the sudden hypoestrogenemia associated with the menopause may facilitate this age-related GH decrease, as well as blunt the ability of the pituitary somatotroph cells to respond to GH-releasing hormone. This effect is partially reversed with estrogen replacement therapy *(29)*.

Thyroid regulation may also change in mid and later life. The prevalence of antithyroid antibodies and hypothyroidism is believed to increase with aging *(30)*. Thyrotropin (TSH) and prolactin levels were not found to be different between younger and older postmenopausal women, however there was a significant decline in the triiodothyronine (T3) concentration. The finding that the TSH and prolactin levels were strongly positively correlated over time despite a dramatic decrease in T3 levels led the researchers to surmise a preserved episodic pulsatility of TSH and prolactin but an impaired negative feedback on the hypothalamic-pituitary unit in the elderly menopausal patient *(31)*.

The menstrual cycle changes prior to the menopause are marked by elevated FSH levels, decreased levels of inhibin, and normal levels of estradiol *(32–37)*. Recently, it has come to light that subtle increases in LH may also occur in the older reproductive aged woman, earlier than previously believed *(38)*. A large body of literature has correlated these elevations in FSH with a poor fertility prognosis in patients undergoing treatment for infertility *(11,39)*. Normal populations of women appear to demonstrate similar, age-related increases in FSH, particularly in the early follicular phase of the menstrual cycle.

The very elevated levels of gonadotropins seen in the menopause are because of an increase in the magnitude, but not frequency, of their pituitary pulsatile secretion, without a concomitant increase in their metabolism. The increased amplitude has been attributed to diminished follicular inhibin production and a heightened sensitivity of pituitary gonadotroph cells to GnRH in the hypoestrogenic postmenopausal environment. Eventually, a 10–20-fold increase in FSH and a threefold increase in LH occur, reaching a maximum level 1–3 yr after menopause. There may be a gradual, but slight, decline in gonadotropin levels thereafter. FSH levels are higher than LH levels simply on the basis of clearance; the circulating half-life of LH is only 30 min, whereas that of FSH is nearly 4 h. Elevated levels of both FSH and LH are indirect evidence of ovarian failure.

THE OVARY

Perimenopause

The locus of reproductive aging is the ovary. It is here that the seeds of menopause are sown, because the ovary contains a finite number of irreplaceable primordial follicles. The perimenopausal years are marked by their accelerated attrition. As the number of follicles dwindles, elaboration of ovarian hormones appears to change somewhat unpredictably. The menstrual regularity a woman experiences during the perimenopausal years appears to be more related to her remaining primordial follicle number than to her age

(40). As the number diminishes, irregular bleeding can occur after an estradiol peak without subsequent ovulation or corpus luteum formation. Both normal *(36,41)* and inadequate *(38,42)* corpus luteum secretion of progesterone have been described in perimenopausal women. Because all groups studied to date have been rather small, it is probably necessary to study a larger group of women to determine the consistency of these findings.

Follicular growth appears to be accelerated in perimenopausal cycles, with a mean decrease in follicular phase length of about 3 d *(22,38,43)*. Recent studies have compared the architecture and endocrinology of menstrual cycles in healthy, regularly menstruating women of younger (age 20–25) and older (age 40–45) reproductive years. They suggest the monotropic rise in FSH is responsible for the accelerated recruitment and ovulation of a dominant follicle that is seen in the older women. There is some controversy, however, as to whether or not the monotropic rise in FSH represents a primary central event that induces an accelerated consumption of ovarian follicles, or instead is merely a reflection of the naturally occurring decrease in follicle number after years of ovulation. The inverse relationship between FSH and inhibin suggests inhibin to be a more sensitive marker of ovarian follicular competence whereas FSH measurement is more a clinical assessment of inhibin. Indeed, a recent study has demonstrated menstrual cycle d 3 levels of inhibin B to be a more sensitive indicator of response to exogenous gonadotropin therapy for in vitro fertilization than d 3 FSH levels *(44)*. Although elevated FSH levels do herald the menopause, they poorly predict as to when the final menses will occur *(39)*. Estrogen replacement therapy during menopause, in the context of absent inhibin, will not completely suppress the elevated gonadotropin levels normally encountered. Therefore, FSH levels can neither be used to clinically forecast the timing of the menopause nor to titrate the estrogen replacement dosage.

Coordinately, early follicular phase estradiol concentrations are elevated in perimenopausal women compared with midreproductive-aged women *(21,32,38,45,46)*. In two small studies of women aged 43 and older who were still cycling, ovulatory cycles with high estrogen production were observed *(38,46)*, suggesting that this accelerated folliculogenesis could be exuberant throughout (Fig. 1). In other words, the ovary, less responsive to FSH, requires greater circulating quantities of FSH to initiate folliculogenesis. Once started, the FSH induces an "overshoot" of estradiol and hyperestrogenemia occurs. These elevations in estrogen may be a feature of the early perimenopause, with reduced estrogen accounting for the immediately premenopausal cycles. It is clinically important to understand how commonly diminished progesterone secretion might be coupled with hyperestrogenic cycles, since this combination predisposes women to menorrhagia, endometrial hyperplasia, dysfunctional uterine bleeding, and even endometrial cancer.

The follicular fluid progesterone concentration and estrogen to androgen ratio in normal older cycling females are high, suggesting healthy follicles *(45)*. However, there is a large body of information accumulating from in vitro fertilization studies that suggest otherwise *(47)*. The perimenopausal decreased fecundability, and perhaps to some extent the increased rate of spontaneous abortion seen in women of advanced reproductive age, is presumably secondary to an age-related decline in the functional integrity of the follicle and a concomitant decline in the structural integrity of the oocyte. Follicles which have been aspirated from older reproductive aged women demonstrate abnormalities of oocyte spindle formation *(48)*. Furthermore, cleavage stage aneuploidy in

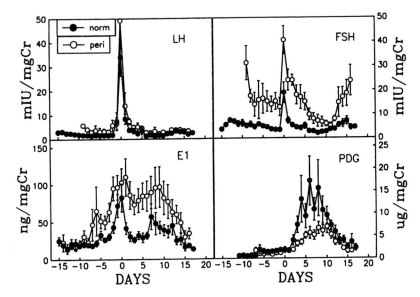

Fig. 1. Mean +/- SEM daily urinary gonadotropin and sex steroid excretion patterns in 11 perimenopausal women, aged 43–52 yr (open circles) compared to those in 11 midreproductive-aged women (closed circles). Data are standardized to d 0, the day of ovulation. E1 = estrone conjugates, PDG = pregnanediol glucuronide. (Reprinted with permission, from ref. *38*).

morphologically and developmentally normal human embryos has been shown to significantly increase with maternal age *(49)*. It is difficult to discern whether age itself or the hormonal changes that accompany it underlie these aberrations.

Glycoprotein hormones elaborated by the granulosa cell include inhibin, a disulfide linked heterodimer, which has been shown to decrease over the perimenopausal transition *(34,39)*. A decrease in inhibin secretion by the granulosa cells begins at approximately age 35, but accelerates dramatically after age 40. The decline in inhibin, which probably reflects both lesser follicular competence and a smaller ovarian follicular pool, is believed to facilitate the early follicular phase rise in FSH. Activin, a homodimer of the inhibin β-subunit, may be increased locally in the perimenopausal ovary, since inhibin α-subunit is declining at this time of life *(34)*. This increase in activin may further increase circulating FSH, and, at least in an animal model, has been shown to lead to hyperestrogenic superovulation *(50)*.

Thus, the early perimenopause is heralded by the appearance of elevated FSH, possible elevations in estrogen, and decreased progesterone secretion. The hormonal milieu is one of relatively unopposed estrogen, and this may promote the growth of uterine leiomyomata and a variety of disconcerting bleeding problems. The perimenopausal reproductive hormonal environment should not be regarded as a simple waning of ovarian function over time. It is a waxing and waning process, at times more like a "roller coaster" in its hormonal dynamics. It is critical that the clinician takes these features into account when attempting to diagnose or treat the perimenopausal woman.

Menopause

At the time of menopause, the ovary is nearly devoid of primordial follicles *(51)*. Granulosa cell estrogen production is essentially nonexistent. The circulating level of estrogen in women shows a very steep decline over the first 12 mo after the menopause, with only a very slight further decline in the years thereafter (52,53). The daily production rate of estrogen falls nearly eightfold to a level of approx 48 µg per 24 h. Essentially, all estrogen in the postmenopausal woman is derived from the peripheral conversion of androstenedione. Indeed, postmenopausal women who have undergone bilateral oophorectomies for endometrial cancer show no significant reduction in their circulating levels or urinary excretion rates of estrogen (54–56). Glucocorticoid suppression, however, dramatically reduces the circulating level of estrogen (54,57), whereas adrenalectomy effectively eliminates measurable estrogens from the urine (55). The circulating level of estrone in postmenopausal women is approx 30–70 pg/mL. The circulating level of estradiol is even lower, approx 10–20 pg/mL, as most is derived from the peripheral conversion of estrone (53,58,59). Estrone sulfate is an inactive metabolite of both estradiol and estrone, which diminishes in a similar manner postmenopausally. However, it still is present in higher concentrations than its precursors in both plasma and breast tumor tissue. It may have significant biological effects as culture studies with rat mammary tumor cell lines show nearly complete desulfation of the hormone and tumor colony proliferation (60). Sporadic and transient increases in estradiol concentrations, neither accompanied nor followed by elevations in progesterone, have been noted in some postmenopausal women (61). Such instances may represent residual follicular activity without subsequent ovulation, or perhaps are associated with stromal hyperplasia.

A limited capacity of the ovarian stroma to aromatize androgens and therefore to more directly contribute to the circulating pool of estrogen was first postulated by Wotiz et al. in 1956 (62). They reported the in vitro conversion of testosterone to estrogen by slices of ovarian stroma obtained from women at least 20 yr into their climacteric phase. In a similar experiment, Dennefors et al. demonstrated androstenedione and estradiol production, with a notably larger production of both from tissue consistent with stromal hyperplasia (63). The majority of such studies, however, have not been able to demonstrate any significant direct production of estrogen (64–66). Lending additional credence to Dennefors' data is the existence of an estrogen concentration gradient noted by selective venous sampling, in which estradiol and estrone levels in the ovarian vein have been shown to be approximately twice those in the peripheral circulation (58,67). Immunohistochemical examination of ovarian stromal cells has also recently demonstrated the presence of aromatase cytochrome P-450 in both pre and postmenopausal ovaries (68). Whatever ability to aromatize androgens the postmenopausal ovary may possess in vivo, it is generally agreed to be at most quite limited. This may be because of a disproportionately lower concentration of FSH as compared to LH receptors in the ovarian stromal cells.

Androgen Production

As women traverse the menopause, ovarian androgen secretion declines (52,69). Midcycle testosterone and androstenedione have been reported to be decreased at midcycle in women in their mid-40s who are still having regular menstrual periods, when compared to younger, midreproductive-aged women (70). This aside, a solid foundation of evidence exists that demonstrates the postmenopausal ovary to remain a highly functional androgen-secreting organ. Histologic examination reveals the stromal cell of the ovarian cortex and the hilar cell of the ovarian medulla to be responsible for this production.

In vitro studies using tritium-labeled pregnenolone have demonstrated the ability of the ovarian cortical stroma to produce progesterone, dehydroepiandrosterone, and testosterone *(67)*. Measurable amounts of both androstenedione and progesterone have been noted in other in vitro experiments *(65)*. These cells also retain their ability to respond to gonadotropins; studies have demonstrated their increased cyclic AMP formation in the presence of human chorionic gonadotropin *(71)*. Pharmacologic suppression of gonadotropins results in a significant decrease in circulating levels of testosterone, further illustrating this relationship *(72,73)*. Infrequently, the elevated gonadotropins of the climacteric can stimulate the ovarian stroma until significant hyperplasia develops. The hyperplastic cells resemble theca interna cells, hence, the term stromal hyperthecosis. This condition, when severe, can produce enlarged ovaries and virilizing levels of androstenedione and testosterone *(68,74,75)*. The larger portion of the climacteric ovary is the medulla, primarily consisting of corpora albicantia and sclerotic blood vessels. The medullary hilar cell, sometimes called the adneural interstitial cell because of its proximity to bundles of nonmyelinated nerve fibers, is homologous to the interstitial cells of Leydig in the testes. These cells retain a prodigious steroidogenic capability in the postmenopausal state, as well as the ability to respond to gonadotropin stimulation. In fact, the hilar cells secrete substantially more androgen in vitro than their cortical stromal cell counterparts and probably are responsible for the bulk of the circulating androgens in the postmenopausal woman *(71)*. Rarely these hilar cells form functional tumors and they usually present with signs and symptoms of virilization, but can potentially precipitate hyperestrogenic symptoms such as dysfunctional uterine bleeding if significant peripheral aromatization occurs.

Analysis of peripheral and ovarian venous effluents indicate that the climacteric ovary secretes mainly androstenedione and testosterone. There is approximately a fivefold greater concentration for both androgens in the climacteric ovarian vein *(76)*. However, the ovarian production of androstenedione is still only one-half that seen prior to the menopause *(55)*, and there is no appreciable lowering of the circulating testosterone levels. The postmenopausal ovary maintains or exceeds the amount of testosterone it secreted prior to the menopause. The overall direct and indirect contribution to the testosterone level by the climacteric ovary is significant. Bilateral oophorectomies result in a 50% decrease in circulating levels postmenopausally *(77)*. Because of the more marked decline in estrogen, the androgen to estrogen ratio changes dramatically after the menopause. This shift may cause increased bioavailable testosterone secondary to decreased hepatic production of sex hormone binding globulin in the face of lower estrogen levels. As a consequence, a new onset of mild hirsutism in the immediate postmenopause is not uncommon.

Studies have therefore demonstrated the climacteric ovary to be far from a defunct endocrine organ. Autoradiography has demonstrated binding sites for both LH and FSH in the cortical stroma and hilar area *(78,79)*. Culture studies have demonstrated increased cyclic AMP levels produced by hyperplastic stromal cells in the presence of hCG. In vivo studies in which hCG was administered to climacteric women resulted in elevated peripheral testosterone levels, hyperplasia of the ovarian hilus, and histochemical analysis consistent with active steroidogenesis *(80,81)*. This portrait depicts the climacteric ovary as gonadotropin receptive and steroidogenically responsive.

THE ADRENAL GLAND

There is a slight age-related decrease in the amount of androstenedione produced by the adrenal gland of approximately 20%. The climacteric ovary, however, demonstrates a 50% decrease in its rate of androstenedione production. As a result, the circulating level of androstenedione is about one-half that seen previously, but the contribution of the adrenal gland to the entire circulating pool of androstenedione rises from 50% to nearly 80% after the menopause. Studies reflecting this dominant adrenal influence point out that corticotropin and not hCG will increase androstenedione levels in the postmenopausal patient, whereas dexamethasone administration significantly lowers it (60,82). Moreover, the androstenedione levels of the postmenopausal patient demonstrate a diurnal pattern, consistent with an adrenal secretory pattern (60). The overall production rate of testosterone decreases by approximately 28% during the climacteric, largely because of a decreased adrenal contribution. This age-related decline in adrenal androgen secretion does not appear to be affected by the process of menopause. Consequences of the gradual reductions in androgen secretion in women from both ovarian and adrenal sources have not been clearly identified. The adrenal production of dehydroepiandrosterone (DHEA), and its sulfated form (DHEAS), which is the most abundant hormone in the body, selectively decrease with age in both sexes. A gradual decrease in DHEA levels appears to begin at approximately the beginning of the third decade of life and continues thereafter until levels plateau near age 70. With aging, DHEAS secretion diminishes dramatically until elderly levels are only 10% of youthful concentrations (83). The menopause has no bearing on this decline in women. Recently, Liu et al. investigated the age-related disparity between adrenal DHEA secretion and cortisol secretion. The notably lower DHEA levels in postmenopausal women as compared to younger cycling women seemed because of an attenuation of both ultradian and circadian pulse amplitude. In addition, postmenopausal women demonstrated blunted DHEA and DHEAS, but not cortisol, responses to an 8-h human corticotropin releasing factor infusion as compared to controls. An age-related event limiting 17,20-desmolase activity was postulated as the etiology (84). In contrast to the adrenal androgen pattern, glucocorticoid secretion is preserved and even enhanced with aging. Challenge testing of the adrenal axis results in greater response in older compared to younger subjects. The 24-h patterns of cortisol secretion demonstrate a loss of the late night/early morning nadir in cortisol in older persons (85), possibly exacting a toll upon their quality of sleep. The role of glucocorticoid abnormalities in perimenopausal morbidity such as hot flashes and sleep disturbances remains to be elucidated. Oral melatonin therapy has been shown to augment daytime cortisol levels in postmenopausal women, but not in younger women, suggesting an age-related alteration of adrenal function (86). One study has shown a minimal decrease in the circadian amplitude of aldosterone secretion in menopausal women (87). At the present time, a significant intrinsic menopause-related effect upon the circulating levels of either cortisol or aldosterone has not been shown.

THE ENDOMETRIUM

Endometrial physiology in the perimenopausal woman is an area deserving of further study. Many conditions involving abnormal endometrial function in the perimenopause culminate in hysterectomy or at least curettage procedures. The fifth decade of life is responsible for the most intensive utilization of these procedures (26,28). Methods targeted towards understanding endometrial physiology and managing it medically would likely result in fewer hysterectomies for benign disease.

It is unclear why menstrual bleeding problems are so common in the premenopausal years. Perhaps some hormonal predisposition (hyperestrogenemia) occurs along with an as yet undescribed intrinsic, age-related local change. Currently, the approach to the perimenopausal woman complaining of excessive menstrual bleeding is either symptomatic or hormonal. Prior to prescribing therapy, anatomic evaluation is warranted, and should consist of an office endometrial sampling as a minimum. In the majority of instances, the endometrial pathology will prove benign. Approximately 15% of biopsies will demonstrate hyperplasia, which necessitates progestational therapy (88). Women suspected of having intrauterine lesions such as leiomyomata should be evaluated further as needed (89). In the face of benign endometrial sampling and an absence of anatomic lesions, several lines of therapy can be pursued. So-called dysfunctional uterine bleeding can be managed with nonsteroidal antiinflammatory agents. Additionally, tranexamic acid is used frequently in Europe with a minimum of adversity (90). Hormonal therapy should be targeted towards achieving cycle control. Oral contraceptive pills, especially low-dose formulations, will minimize endometrial growth and result in reduction of menstrual blood loss. Progestin-impregnated IUDs have also been documented to be effective, as have medroxy-progesterone acetate depot and more expensive agents such as danocrine. Note that liberal use of progestins is advocated in all of the hormonal regimens. Flexibility in modality and careful targeting of therapy to the patient's chief complaints may help prevent surgical intervention in many cases.

The postmenopausal endometrium, in the absence of HRT, is atrophic and very thin. Surprisingly, the sporadic elevations of estradiol that may occur in the postmenopausal state from halting follicular activity or stromal hyperthecosis are very infrequently accompanied by endometrial withdrawal bleeding. It has been suggested that the endometrial sensitivity to estrogenic stimulation may diminish postmenopausally (63). The lack of an age-associated effect on uterine preparation with exogenous estrogen prior to embryo transfer bespeaks otherwise, but larger studies examining postmenopausal recipients need to be done (91). Noci et al. demonstrated an equal presence of both estrogen and progesterone receptors, as well as cellular proliferation indices, in both atrophic and hyperplastic postmenopausal endometrium (92). This portrays the postmenopausal endometrium to be more quiescent than atrophic. Although atrophic spotting is the most common etiology of postmenopausal vaginal bleeding, all bleeding in this context should be evaluated to rule out the rare, but possible, malignancy. Relative hyperestrogenemia in the postmenopausal patient may occur secondary to extraglandular conversion of androgen, especially with obese patients. Other causes include steroid-producing tumors of the ovary, ovarian stromal hyperthecosis, and liver disease with its concomitant decreased level of sex hormone binding globulin production. A more difficult clinical situation occurs in the postmenopausal patient on hormone replacement therapy who experiences abnormal bleeding. Generally, a predictable bleeding pattern occurs in those patients on cyclic regimens and little breakthrough bleeding is expected in those patients on continuous regimens. However, whenever the issue is in doubt, a work-up is mandatory. Approximately 2% of postmenopausal endometrial biopsies will demonstrate carcinoma (88). Newer techniques for minimizing instrumentation of the postmenopausal patient include vaginal ultrasound measurement of endometrial thickness. The risk of malignancy when the endometrium measures less than 4 mm is reportedly very low (93). Saline infusion sonography is another modality that is quite sensitive in demonstrating intracavitary abnormalities (94). In the event of equivocal findings or persistent bleeding, tissue sampling or hysteroscopic evaluation of the uterine cavity can be considered.

ADIPOSE TISSUE

In general, the metabolism of hormones does not appear to be affected by the menopausal transition. A notable exception appears to be a significantly greater peripheral aromatization of androstenedione and testosterone in postmenopausal women as compared to younger women *(94)*. This increase is not related to time from last menses, and may therefore have begun in an independent fashion prior to menopause. Through peripheral conversion of androgens, estrogen in the postmenopausal woman can reach biologically significant levels despite a virtual absence of estrogen production by the ovaries. The clinical impact of this estrogen will vary among women according to the levels achieved and a variety of individual factors. There is an increased production of estrogen from androstenedione with increasing body weight, and this is probably because of the ability of adipose tissue to aromatize androgens *(96–98)*. The levels obtained, however, will usually prove inadequate to prevent atrophic degeneration of the female secondary sexual tissues and bone demineralization. Adipose tissue exclusively expresses leptin, the protein product of the OB gene, which has a prominent role in satiety and energy metabolism. Recently, a significant inverse relationship between age and serum leptin concentration has been demonstrated in a cohort of female athletes ranging in ages from 18 to 69. This effect was uncovered after controlling for percent body fat, which is the most influential determinant of leptin levels *(99)*. The role of the menopause in this age-related effect is unknown.

CONCLUSION

The menopausal transition implies the end of female reproductive capability. As clinical and basic research proceed, it becomes more evident that the process has remote origins and is sublimely subtle in its development. Indeed, some would say the process of reproductive senescence begins *in utero*.

With time, ovarian primordial follicles and inhibin levels diminish. Consequently, elevations in pituitary gonadotropins occur. Steroid hormones are mildly affected prior to menopause, but thereafter, significant drops in their production, especially of estrogen and progesterone, occur. The adrenal gland shows a marked age-related decline in production of androgens, but retains nearly unchanged ability to respond to stress with the manufacture of glucocorticoids and mineralocorticoids. The postmenopausal ovary also retains a significant ability to synthesize androgens.

The hypothalamus, pituitary, and thyroid may all show some alteration of function with aging. These changes, however, appear small in extent compared to those of the reproductive axis. Their relationship to the climacteric appears for the most part indirect.

REFERENCES

1. Cope E. Physical changes associated with the post-menopausal years. In: Campbell S, ed. The Management of the Menopause and Post-Menopausal Years, University Park Press, Baltimore, MD, 1976, p. 33.
2. U.S. Bureau of the Census, Projections of the population of the United States: 1977 to 2050, Current Population Reports, Series P-25, No. 704.
3. Treolar AE, Boynton RE, Borghild GB, Brown BW. Variation of the human menstrual cycle through reproductive life. Int J Fertil 1967;12:77.
4. Brambilla DJ, McKinlay SM. A prospective study of factors affecting age at menopause. J Clin Epidemiol 1989;42:1031.
5. McKinlay SM, McKinlay JB. The impact of menopause and social factors on health. In: Hammond CB, Haseltine FP, Schiff I, eds. Menopause: Evaluation, Treatment, and Health Concerns, Liss, New York, 1989, pp. 137–161.

6. Wallace RB, Sherman BM, Bean JA, et al. Probability of menopause with increasing duration of amenorrhea in middle-aged women. Am J Obstet Gynecol 1979;135:1021.

7. McKinlay SM, Bifano NL, McKinlay JB. Smoking and age at menopause in women. Ann Intern Med 1985;103:350.

8. Midgette AS, Baron JA. Cigarette smoking and the risk of the natural menopause. Epidemiology 1990;1:474.

9. Cramer DW, Zu H, Harlow BL. Family history as a predictor of early menopause. Fertil Steril 1995;64:740.

10. Nelson JF, Felicio LS, Reproductive aging the female: an aetiological perspective. Rev Biol Res Aging 1985;2:251.

11. Khalifa E, Toner JP, Muasher SJ, Acosta AA. Significance of basal follicle-stimulating hormone levels in women with one ovary in a program of in vitro fertilization. Fertil Steril 1992;57:835.

12. Siddle N, Sarrel P, Whitehead M. The effect of hysterectomy on the age at ovarian failure: identification of a subgroup of women with premature loss of ovarian function and literature review. Fertil Steril 1987;47:94.

13. Nargund G, Cheng WC, Parsons J. The impact of ovarian cystectomy on ovarian response to stimulation during in-vitro fertilization cycles. Hum Reprod 1996;11:81.

14. Coulam CB, Adamson SC, Annaegers JF. Incidence of premature ovarian failure. Obstet Gynecol 1986;67:604.

15. Krauss CM, Turksoy RN, Atkins L, McLaughlin C, Brown LG, Page DC. Familial premature ovarian failure due to an interstitial deletion of the long arm of the X chromosome. N Engl J Med 1987;16:125.

16. Ahmed-Ebbiary NA, Lenton EA, Cooke ID. Hypothalamic-pituitary aging: progressive increase in FSH and LH concentrations throughout the reproductive life in regularly menstruating women. Clin Endocrinol 1994;41:199.

17. Nash TE, LaPolt PS, Judd HL, Lu JKH. Alterations in ovarian steroid and gonadotropin secretion preceding the cessation of regular oestrous cycles in aging female rats. J Endocrinol 1984;100:43.

18. Scarbrough K, Wise PM. Age-related changes in pulsatile luteinizing hormone release precede the transition to estrous acyclicity and depend upon estrous cycle history. Endocrinology 1990;126:884.

19. Wise PM. Estradiol-induced daily luteinizing hormone and prolactin surges in young and middle-aged rats: correlations with age-related changes in pituitary responsiveness and catecholamine turnover rates in microdissected brain areas. Endocrinology 1984;115:801.

20. Reame NE, Kelch RP, Beitins IZ, Yu M-Y, Zawacki CM, Padmanabhan V. Age effects on follicle-stimulating hormone and pulsatile luteinizing hormone secretion across the menstrual cycle of premenopausal women. J Clin Endocrinol Metab 1996;81:1512.

21. Wilshire G, Loughlin JS, Brown JR, et al. Diminished function of the somatotropin axis in older reproductive-aged women. J Clin Endocrinol Metab 1995;80:608.

22. Klein NA, Battaglia DE, Fujimoto VY, Davis GS, Bremner WJ, Soules MR. Reproductive aging: accelerated ovarian follicular development associated with a monotropic follicle-stimulating hormone rise in normal older women. J Clin Endocrinol Metab 1996;81:1038–1045.

23. Matt DW, Veldhuis JD, Evans WS. Age-related alterations in LH secretory activity and half-life in premenopausal women. Proc 10th Int Congress Endocrinol. June 12–15, 1996, San Francisco, CA, #P3–398.

24. Fraser IS, Baird DT. Blood production and ovarian secretion rates of estradiol 17–beta and estrone in women with dysfunctional uterine bleeding. J Clin Endocrinol Metab 1974;39:564.

25. Van Look PFA, Lothian H, Hunter WM, et al. Hypothalamic-pituitary ovarian function in perimenopausal women. Clin Endocrinol 1977;7:13.

26. Rutkow IM. Obstetrics and gynecologic operations in the United States, 1979–1984. Obstet Gynecol 1996;67:755.

27. Unger JB, Meeks GR. Hysterectomy after endometrial ablation. Am J Obstet Gynecol 1996;175:1432.

28. Wilcox LS, Koonin LM, Pokras R, Strauss LT, Xia Z, Peterson HB. Hysterectomy in the United States, 1988–1990. Obstet Gynecol 1994;83:549.

29. DeLeo V, Lanzetta D, D'Antona D, Danero S. Growth hormone secretion in premenopausal women before and after ovariectomy: effect of hormone replacement therapy. Fertil Steril 1993;60:268.

30. Sawin CT, Castelli WP, Hershman JM, McNamara P, Bacharach P. The aging thyroid: thyroid deficiency in the Framingham study. Arch Intern Med 1985;145:1386.

31. Rossmanith WG, Szilagyi A, Scherbaum WA. Episodic thyrotropin (TSH) and prolactin (PRL) secretion during aging in postmenopausal women. Horm Metab Res 1992;24:185.

32. Klein NA, Illingworth PJ, Groome NP, McNeilly AS, Battaglia De, Soules MR. Decreased inhibin B secretion is associated with the monotropic FSH rise in older ovulatory women: a study of serum and follicular fluid levels of dimeric inhibin A & B in spontaneous menstrual cycles. J Clin Endocrinol Metab 1996;81:2742.

33. Seifer DB, Gardiner AC, Lambert-Messerlian G, Schneyer AL. Differential secretion of dimeric inhibin in cultured luteinized granulosa cells as a function of ovarian reserve. J Clin Endocrinol Metab 1996;81:736.

34. Buckler HM, Evans CA, Mamtora H, et al. Gonadotropin, steroid, and inhibin levels in women with incipient ovarian failure during anovulatory and ovulatory rebound cycles. J Clin Endocrinol Metab 1991;72:116.

35. Metcalf MG, Livesey JH. Gonadotropin excretion in fertile women: Effect of age and the onset of the menopausal transition. J Endocrinol 1985;105:357.

36. Sherman BM, West JH, Korenman SG. The menopausal transition: Analysis of LH, FSH, estradiol and progesterone concentrations during menstrual cycles of older women. J Clin Endocrinol Metab 1976;42:629.

37. McNaughton J, Bangah M, McCloud P, Hee J, Burger H. Age-related changes in follicle-stimulating hormone, luteinizing-hormone, oestradiol, and immunoreactive inhibin in women of reproductive age. Clin Endocrinol 1992;36:339.

38. Santoro N, Brown JR, Adel T, et al. Characterization of perimenopausal reproductive hormonal dynamics. J Clin Endocrinol Metab 1996;81:1495.

39. Burger HG. Diagnostic role of follicle-stimulating hormone (FSH) measurements during the menopausal transition-an analysis of FSH, oestradiol and inhibin. Eur J Endocr 1994;130:38.

40. Richardson SJ, Senikas V, Nelson JF. Follicular depletion during the menopausal transition: evidence for accelerated loss and ultimate exhaustion. J Clin Endocrinol Metab 1987;65:1231.

41. Lenton EA, Sexton L, Lee S, et al. Progressive changes in LH and FSH and LH:FSH ratios in women throughout reproductive life. Maturitas 1988;100:35.

42. Reyes FI, Winters JSD, Faiman C. Pituitary-ovarian relationship preceding the menopause: A cross-sectional study of serum follicle-stimulating hormone, luteinizing hormone, prolactin, estradiol, and progesterone levels. Am J Obstet Gynecol 1977;129:557.

43. Lenton EA, Landgren B-M, Sexton L, et al. Normal variation in the length of the follicular phase of the menstrual cycle: effect of chronological age. Br J Obstet Gynecol 1984;91:681.

44. Seifer DB, Lambert-Messerlian G, Hogan JW, Gardiner AC, Blazar AS, Berk CA. Day 3 serum inhibin-B is predictive of assisted reproductive technologies outcome. Fertil Steril 1997;67:110.

45. Klein NA, Battaglia DE, Miller PB, Branigan EF, Giudice LC, Soules MR. Ovarian follicular development and the follicular fluid hormones and growth factors in normal women of advanced reproductive age. J Clin Endocrinol Metab 1996;81:1946.

46. Shideler SE, DeVane GW, Kaira PS, et al. Ovarian-pituitary hormone interactions during the perimenopause. Maturitas 1989;11:331.

47. Navot D, Bergh PA, Williams MA, Garrisi GJ, Guzman I, Sandler B, Grunfeld L. Poor oocyte quality rather than implantation failure as a cause of age-related decline in female fertility. Lancet 1991;337:1375.

48. Battaglia DE. Influence of maternal age on meiotic spindle assembly in oocytes from naturally cycling women. Hum Reprod 1996;11:2217.

49. Munne S, Alikani M, Giles T, Grifo J, Cohen J. Embryo morphology, developmental rates, and maternal age are correlated with chromosomal abnormalities. Fertil Steril 1995;64:382.

50. Erickson, GF, Kokka S, Rivier C. Activin causes premature superovulation. Endocrinology 1995;136:4804.

51. Gosden RG. Follicular status at menopause. Hum Reprod 1987;2:617.

52. Longcope C, Franz C, Morello C, et al. Steroid and gonadotropin levels in women during the perimenopausal years. Maturitas 1986;8:189.

53. Meldrum DR, Davidson BJ, Tataryn IV, Judd HL. Changes in circulating steroids with aging in postmenopausal women. Obstet Gynecol 1981;57:624.

54. Procope BJ. Studies on urinary excretion, biological effects and origin of estrogens in postmenopausal women. Acta Endocrinol 1968;95(suppl):135.

55. Barlow JJ, Emerson J, Saxena BN. Estradiol production after ovariectomy for carcinoma of the breast. N Engl J Med 1969;280:633.

56. Bulbrook RD, Grenwood FC. Persistence of urinary oestrogen excretion after oophorectomy and adrenalectomy. Br Med J 1957;1:662.

57. Breuer H, Nocke W, Bayer JM. Effect of ACTH and cortisone on the urinary oestrogens in oophorectomized and postmenopausal women with mammary cancer. Acta Endocrinol 1958;38(suppl):69.
58. Judd HL, Judd GE, Lucas WE, Yen SSC. Endocrine function of the postmenopausal ovary; concentration of androgens and estrogens in ovarian and peripheral vein blood. J Clin Endocrinol Metab 1974;39:1020.
59. Judd HL, Shamonki IM, Frumar AM, Lagasse LD. Origin of serum estradiol in postmenopausal women. Obstet Gynecol 1982;59:680.
60. Santen RJ, Leszcynski D, Tilson-Mallet N, et al. Enzymatic control of estrogen production in breast cancer: relative significance of aromatase versus sulfatase pathways. Ann NY Acad Sci 1986;464:126.
61. Metcalf MG, Donald RA, Livesey JH. Pituitary-ovarian function before, during and after menopause: a longitudinal study. Clin Endocrinol 1982;17:489.
62. Wotiz HH, Davis JW, Lemon HM, Gut M. Studies in steroid metabolism. V. The conversion of testosterone-4-C^{14} to estrogens by human ovarian tissue. J Biol Chem 1956;222:487.
63. Dennefors BL, Janson PO, Knutson F, Hamberger L. Steroid production and responsiveness to gonadotropin in isolated stromal tissue of the postmenopausal ovaries. Am J Obstet Gynecol 1980;136:997.
64. Longcope C, Hunter R, Franz C. Steroid secretion by the postmenopausal ovary. Am J Obstet Gynecol 1980;138:564.
65. Mattingly RF, Huang WY. Steroidogenesis of the menopausal and postmenopausal ovary. Am J Obstet Gynecol 1969;103:679.
66. Nagamani M, Stuart CA, Doherty MG. Increased steroid production by the ovarian stromal tissue of postmenopausal women with endometrial cancer. J Clin Endocrinol Metab 1992;74:172.
67. Kobayashi M, Nakano R, Shima K. Immunohistochemical localization of pituitary gonadotropins and estrogen in human postmenopausal ovaries. Acta Obstet Gynecol Scand 1993;72:76.
68. Inkster SE, Brodie AMH. Expression of aromatase cytochrome P-450 in premenopausal and postmenopausal ovaries: an immunocytochemical study. J Clin Endocrinol Metab 1991;73:717.
69. Longcope C, Baker S. Androgen and estrogen dynamics: relationships with age, weight, and menopausal status. J Clin Endocrinol Metab 1993;76:601.
70. Mushayandebvu T, Adel TE, Gimpel T, et al. Evidence for diminished midcycle androgen production in older reproductive aged women. Fertil Steril 1996;65:721.
71. Dennefors BL, Janson PO, Hamberger L, Knutson F. Hilus cells from human postmenopausal ovaries: gonadotropin sensitivity, steroid and cyclic AMP production. Acta Obstet Gynecol Scand 1982;61:413.
72. Dowsett M, Cantwell B, Anshumala L, Jeffcoate SL, Harris SL. Suppression of postmenopausal ovarian steroidogenesis with the luteinizing hormone-releasing hormone agonist Goserelin. J Clin Endocrinol Metab 1988;66:672.
73. Andreyko JL, Monroe SE, Marshall LA, Fluker MR, Nerenberg CA, Jaffe RB. Concordant suppression of serum immunoreactive luteinizing hormone (LH), follicle-stimulating hormone, a subunit, bioactive LH, and testosterone in postmenopausal women by a potent gonadotropin releasing hormone antagonist (Detirelix). J Clin Endocrinol Metab 1992;74:399.
74. Marcus CC. Ovarian cortical stromal hyperplasia and cancer of the endometrium. Obstet Gynecol 1963;21:175.
75. Braithwaite SS, Erkman-Balis B, Avila TD. Postmenopausal virilization due to ovarian stromal hyperthecosis. J Clin Endocrinol Metab 1978;46:295.
76. Nagamani M, Hannigan EV, Dillard EA, Dinh TV. Ovarian steroid secretion in postmenopausal women with and without endometrial cancer. J Clin Endocrinol Metab 1986;62:508.
77. Judd HL, Lucas WE, Yen SSC. Effect of oophorectomy on circulating testosterone and androstenedione levels in patients with endometrial cancer. Am J Obstet Gynecol 1974;118:793.
78. Peluso JJ, Steger RW, Jaszczak S, Hafez ESE. Gonadotropin binding sites in human postmenopausal ovaries. Fertil Steril 1976;27:789.
79. Nakano R, Shima K, Yamoto M, Kobayashi M, Nishimori K, Hiraoka J. Binding sites for gonadotropins in human postmenopausal ovaries. Obstet Gynecol 1989;73:196.
80. Vermeulen A. The hormonal activity of the postmenopausal ovary. J Clin Endocrinol Metab 1976;42:247.
81. Poliak A, Jones GES, Goldberg B, Solomon D, Woodruff ID. Effect of human chorionic gonadotropin on postmenopausal women. Am J Obstet Gynecol 1968;101:731.
82. Maroulis GB, Abraham GE. Ovarian and adrenal contributions to peripheral steroid levels in postmenopausal women. Obstet Gynecol 1976;48:150.
83. Orentreich N, Brind JL, Rizer RL, et al. Age changes and sex difference in serum dehydroepiandrosterone sulfate concentrations throughout adulthood. J Clin Endocrinol Metab 1984;59:551.

84. Liu CH, Laughlin GA, Fischer UG, Yen SSC. Marked attenuation of ultradian and circadian rhythms of dehydroepiandrosterone in postmenopausal women: evidence for a reduced 17,20–desmolase enzymatic activity. J Clin Endocrinol Metab 1990;71:900.

85. Van Cauter E, Leproult R, Kupfer DJ. Effects of gender and age on the levels and circadian rhythmicity of plasma cortisol. J Clin Endocrinol Metab 81:2468, 1996.

86. Cagnacci A, Soldani R, Yen SSC. Melatonin enhances cortisol levels in aged but not young women. Eur J Endocrinol 1995;133:691.

87. Cugini P, Scavo D, Halberg F, Schramm A, Pusch HJ, Franke H. Methodologically critical interactions of circadian rhythm, sex, and aging characterize serum aldosterone and the female adrenopause. J Geront 1982;37:403.

88. Einerth Y. Vacuum curettage by the Vabra method. A simple procedure for endometrial diagnosis. Acta Obstet Gynecol Scand 1982;61:373.

89. Townsend DE, Fields G, McCausland, Kauffman K. Diagnostic and operative hysteroscopy in the managmenet of persistent postmenopausal bleeding. Obstet Gynecol 1993;82:419.

90. Bonnar J, Sheppard BL. Treatment of menorrhagia during menstruation: randomized controlled trial of ethamsylate, mefenamic acid, and tranexamic acid. Br Med J 1996;313:579.

91. Check JH, Askari HA, Fisher C, Vanaman L. The use of a shared donor oocyte program to evaluate the effect of uterine senescence. Fertil Steril 1994;61:252.

92. Noci I, Borri P, Scarselli G, Chieffi O, Bucciantini S, Biagiotti R, Paglierani M, Moncini D, Taddei G. Morphological and functional aspects of the endometrium of asymptomatic post-menopausal women: does the endometrium really age? Hum Reprod 1996;11:2246.

93. Smith P, Bakos O, Heimer G, Ulmsten U. Transvaginal ultrasound for identifying endometrial abnormality. Acta Obstet Gynecol Scand 1991;70:591.

94. Widrich T, Bradley LD, Mitchinson AR, Collins RL. Comparison of saline infusion sonography with office hysteroscopy for the evaluation of the endometrium. Am J Obstet Gynecol 1996;174:1327.

95. Hemsell DL, Grodin SM, Brenner PF, Siiteri PK, MacDonald PC. Plasma precursors of estrogen. II. Correlation of the extent of conversion of plasma androstenedione to estrone with age. J Clin Endocrinol Metab 1974;38:476.

96. Vermeulen A, Verdonck L. Sex hormone concentrations in post-menopausal women: relation to obesity, fat mass, age and years post-menopause. Clin Endocrinol 1978;9:59.

97. MacDonald PC, Edman CD, Hernsell DI, Porter JC, Siiteri PK. Effect of obesity on conversion of plasma androstenedione to estrone in post-menopausal women with and without endometrial cancer. Am J Obstet Gynecol 1978;130:448.

98. MacDonald PC, Siiteri PK. The relationship between the extraglandular production of estrogen and the occurrence of endometrial neoplasia. Gynecol Oncol 1974;2:259.

99. Ryan AS, Elahi D. The effects of acute hyperglycemia and hyperinsulinemia on plasma leptin levels: its relationships with body fat, visceral adiposity, and age in women. J Clin Endocrin Metab 1996;81:4433.

3

Cardiovascular Changes in Menopause

Anne W. Moulton, MD

INTRODUCTION

The decline in estrogen levels, which begins several years before menopause and is most pronounced with the cessation of menstrual periods, appears to predispose older women to an increasing risk of coronary disease. Coronary artery disease (CAD) is the leading cause of death in all United States women after the age of 40; but it is a disease of older women. CAD develops approx 10–15 yr later in life in women than in men, but by the age of 70, the male/female ratio for the incidence of coronary disease starts to approach one *(1)*.

Coronary atherosclerosis is a disease of older women and, thus, age is truly the greatest predictor of the development of CAD in women but the influence of age on the development of coronary disease is confounded by the effect of menopause. Because there is no direct evidence of this, epidemiologic studies suggest at least three lines of evidence to support this hypothesis. In premenopausal women, rates of CAD are substantially lower than in men of the same age. In the Framingham Study, for patients aged 50–59 even after controlling for other risk factors, men still have 3.5 times the risk of developing CAD compared with women, suggesting some residual advantage for women *(2)*. It is also known that women with premature menopause have an increased age-adjusted risk of coronary heart disease as compared to age-matched premenopausal women *(3)*. Finally, numerous epidemiologic studies of estrogen replacement therapy in postmenopausal women indicate a decrease risk of coronary heart disease in estrogen treated women

From: *Contemporary Endocrinology: Menopause: Endocrinology and Management*
Edited by: D. B. Seifer and E. A. Kennard © Humana Press Inc., Totowa, NJ

Table 1
Cardioprotective Effects of Estrogen

Effects on Vasculature
• Potentiation of endothelium-derived relaxing factor.
• Calcium channel antagonism.
• Inhibition of vascular constrictor factors.
• Inhibition of angiotensin II induced constrictor effects.
• Modulation of neurotransmitter release.
• Inhibition of smooth muscle cell biosynthesis.
• Inhibition of myointimal hyperplasia.
Effects on Cardiac Physiology
• Increase in plasma volume.
• Increase in stroke volume.
• Increase in cardiac output.
• Decrease in peripheral resistance.
Effects on Metabolism and Clotting
• Beneficial effect on lipids (decrease total cholesterol, LDL, and Lp[a]; increase
      HDL, etc.).
• Antioxidant effect (decrease LDL oxidation).
• Beneficial effect on clotting factors (decrease fibrinogen, platelet aggregation).
• Beneficial effect on fibrinolysis (decreases in PAI-1).

compared to controls. Since 1970, there have been at least 31 observational studies. Three meta-analyses (4–6) suggest a substantial reduction of risk of CAD in women who take hormone replacement therapy (HRT). One subsequent analysis that grouped the data by study design reported a summary risk estimate of 0.56 (95% CI 0.5–0.61) (7).

The mechanisms by which estrogen protects women from the development of CAD are not completely understood. The current hypothesized mechanisms are listed in Table 1. These have been proposed based on in vitro, animal studies and/or human studies. The earliest explanation was that there was a beneficial effect on lipid metabolism, however, multiple regression analysis suggest that only 25–50% of the risk reduction conferred by estrogen is attributable to its effects on lipids (8). Recent literature suggests several other beneficial effects of estrogen on vascular tone including hormone-induced release of endothelium-derived relaxing factors and calcium antagonism and suppression of constricting factors, as well as beneficial effects on clotting and thrombolysis. Thus, it is likely that the increase in incidence of atherosclerosis after the menopause is due not simply to changes in lipid metabolism but also to changes in coronary and peripheral vascular tone as a direct consequence of falling plasma concentrations of ovarian hormones.

GENDER DIFFERENCES IN THE EFFECT OF AGING ON THE HEART AND VASCULATURE

Research has been done to determine the effects of normal aging on the heart independent of the interaction between aging and disease. In women, it is essential to distinguish changes in the cardiovascular system, owing to healthy aging, from those owing to menopause, which are discussed later.

Cardiac afterload increases with aging because of several mechanisms including decreased vascular compliance and increased total peripheral resistance and blood pressure. There are several ways to measure afterload related to these components; an increase in arterial pulse wave velocity, a measure of compliance, is observed with aging. Changes in the compliance properties of the major arteries because of age are caused by alterations in the structure and composition of collagen, smooth muscle cells, and ground substances surrounding the blood vessel. The pulse wave travels in the central arterial path system towards the brain, arms, and feet much more rapidly in older than in younger individuals. Because the left ventricle is ejecting blood into a stiffer aorta, the systolic blood pressure tends to climb as patients age, even in the absence of disease. Studies suggest that systolic pressure in older individuals is even higher in the central aorta than it is in the periphery *(9)*. An age-associated left ventricular hypertrophy, which evolves secondary to the increase in left ventricular load, is more prominent in older females than older males. Analysis of some of the healthy Framingham patients suggests a slight age-related increase in LV mass in women and a slight decline in men. An increased prevalence of LVH corrected for body mass has also been noted in women with essential hypertension *(10)*.

There are some other gender differences in cardiovascular adaptations to aging. Males show an age-associated increase in left ventricular end-diastolic volume and end-systolic volume at rest and, therefore, little change in ejection fraction. In contrast, women show no increase in end-diastolic or end-systolic volume with age. During beta-adrenergic blockade, there are no major age differences at rest *(9)*. Maximal coronary vasodilating capacity and flow are unchanged with age. In fact, resting coronary blood flow may actually increase slightly with age probably because of mild cardiac hypertrophy. Endothelial dependent vasodilation is reduced with age but this decrease is noted in healthy men years before an age-related decline in women presumably secondary to menopause *(11)*. In contrast, the response to direct smooth muscle vasodilators is unchanged in both males and females.

In patients at rest, studies using both echocardiography and gated blood pool scans with and without beta-adrenergic blockade demonstrate a moderate increase in end-diastolic and end-systolic stroke volumes with age in males, but these volumes do not change with aging in females *(12)*. At rest, an increase in blood pressure is noted with increasing age in both sexes *(12)*. Whereas resting cardiac index and total systemic vascular resistance did not vary in men, in women, however, there was a decrease in cardiac index and a large increase in total systemic vascular resistance, which may be secondary to declining estrogen levels (*see* below). A prolonged relaxation of cardiac muscles is also demonstrated by many gated blood and echocardiographic parameters. For example, slowed early diastolic filling with age means a greater contribution of atrial contraction to diastolic filling and the appearance of a S-4 sound. Therefore, age-related increases in arterial stiffness and compensatory left ventricular hypertrophy preserve systolic function at the expense of diastolic function.

Exercise Performance in the Elderly

Changes with aging that effect hemodynamics include increased vascular stiffness with resultant left ventricular hypertrophy and a decrease in general beta-sympathetic response that causes decreased augmentation of heart rate and contractility and reduced arterial vasodilation *(9)*.

The age-associated decrease in beta-sympathetic response appears to contribute to several of the changes in the cardiovascular response to exercise including: a decrease in maximum heart rate, the increases in ventricular volume indices, and the decreased ejection fraction and left ventricular contractility. Of note, catecholamine levels are actually higher in older people than in young people with exercise and, thus, do not explain these differences *(9)*. With exercise, heart rate actually increases more in women than in men *(12)*, although women have a higher ejection fraction at rest than men. Across the life span, women also demonstrate a lesser augmentation of ejection fraction (EF) with exercise, which is important because this finding in men is considered an indication of the presence of CAD.

EFFECTS OF ESTROGEN AND ESTROGEN WITHDRAWAL ON THE PHYSIOLOGY OF THE HEART AND VASCULATURE

The addition of estrogen has been shown to increase cardiac output, arterial compliance, and myocardial perfusion, and to decrease vascular resistance and systolic and diastolic blood pressure both in animals and humans. The effect of the physiologic removal of estrogen with menopause on cardiovascular function is less clear.

Changes in Blood Flow

The endothelium plays a critical role in the control of blood flow in the interaction between the blood and the vessel wall. Endothelial function has been assessed in patients by measuring coronary hemodynamic response to intracoronary administration of an endothelium dependent vasodilator, acetylcholine. Coronaries with normally functioning endothelium exhibit acetylcholine-induced dilation, manifested by an increased epicardial cross-sectional area and coronary flow augmentation. In patients with atherosclerosis or dysfunctional endothelium, paradoxical acetylcholine-induced constriction is manifested by decreases both in area and blood flow. Of note, acetylcholine-induced changes in coronary tone mimic those to common vasomotor stimuli, such as exercise and mental stress and, thus, are useful in experimental settings. Endothelial dysfunction is increasingly recognized as an important factor in the progression of cardiovascular disease. Numerous studies suggest that estrogen has a beneficial effect on endothelial dysfunction and, thus, declining estrogen levels with menopause and the subsequent negative effect on vascular tone, could be an important mechanism by which atherosclerosis occurs in postmenopausal women. The clinical evidence and proposed mechanisms are summarized below.

Clinical Evidence: Effects of Estrogen on Vasculature

Most of the recent literature has focused on the effects (acute and chronic) of estrogen administration to postmenopausal women with atherosclerosis and impaired vascular tone. A few cross-sectional studies have looked at the direct effect of menopause (and, thus, estrogen withdrawal) on vascular tone. A group of investigators used high resolution ultrasound to evaluate endothelial responsiveness in the brachial artery (which has been shown to be an effective proxy for coronary endothelial function *(13)* in a large series of males and females) *(11)*. Flow-mediated dilation was preserved in young male subjects and then declined after 40 yr of age. In women, however, flow mediated dilation was maintained until the early 50s, and then declined significantly more than it did in men. Another recent study looked at both normotensive and hypertensive males and females and found that age-related endothelial dysfunction is attenuated in premenopausal women both with and without hypertension as compared to males. This gender difference was not seen postmenopausally *(14)*. The same authors who studied changes in forearm blood flow used brachial artery strain gauge plethysmography to measure the effect of surgical menopause on vascular tone in a small series of women who were scheduled to have TAH/BSO for uterine leiomyoma. In association with dramatic drops in estrogen levels these women had a significant reduction in acetylcholine-induced vasodilation compared to their presurgical baseline. These changes were significantly attenuated in a small subset of the women who received estrogen replacement over the next three months *(15)*.

There are data that both short- and long-term estrogen administration improves endothelial cell-mediated vasodilation in ovariectomized monkeys fed an atherogenic diet *(15,16,18)*. Recent studies looking at the effects of estrogen administration on vascular tone in postmenopausal women are summarized in Table 2. Most of these studies have looked at the acute effect of estrogen on vascular reactivity. As seen in Table 2, earlier studies used cardiac catheterization to measure coronary flow resistance in cross-sectional areas before and after intravenous estrogen. Later studies used brachial strain gauge plethysmography and brachial artery high-resolution ultrasound. There is limited data on the effects of long-term estrogen administration and coronary endothelial cell function. One study, in ovariectomized monkeys treated with hormonal replacement for 26 mo, has shown a beneficial effect *(17)*. A study by Lieberman *(22)*, treated 13 postmenopausal women with hormone replacement therapy in a double-blind placebo controlled crossover trial. Measurements of flow-mediated vasodilation of the brachial artery taken at the end of each 9-wk treatment suggested statistically significant changes in flow-mediated vasodilation in postmenopausal women on short-term hormone replacement therapy. In contrast, Gilligan *(24)* found no improvement after 3 wk of hormone replacement therapy in contrast to the effect of acute estrogen administration on flow mediated dilation using the same method. The recent study by McCrohon, which was a cross-sectional study comparing postmenopausal women who had taken HRT with age-matched controls (who had never taken HRT), demonstrated statistically significantly greater flow mediated dilation in women taking HRT, as measured by brachial artery high-resolution ultrasound *(26)*.

In summary, clinical studies suggest a role for acute estrogen in the improvement of endothelial-dependent flow-mediated vasodilation. The data for short-term or chronic hormone replacement therapy is less clear. There are a number of possible reasons for these differences. First, the plasma level of estradiol achieved by acute infusion, when measured in studies, was 3–4 times higher than what would be achieved by usual doses of hormone replacement therapy. It is also possible that chronic estrogen administration acts through different cellular mechanisms in regulating vascular tone. Finally, studies to date have been limited to small sample sizes, suggesting the possibility of a beta error (i.e., inability to detect a small benefit in vasomotor responsiveness in patients on chronic hormone replacement therapy).

Proposed Mechanisms

Hormone Receptors

Estrogen receptors are found in a number of tissues, including reproductive organs, breast, liver, and some vascular tissue. However, the expression of hormone receptors in vascular tissue has been somewhat controversial reflecting intervessel and/or species variability as well as limitations of the different technologies used to study the tissues *(27,28)*. Animal studies have demonstrated the specific binding of estrogen to vascular cells in canine vascular tissue, rat aorta, and the baboon cardiovascular system, among

Table 2
Estrogen Effects on Cardiovascular System in Postmenopausal Women[a]

Author	Estrogen	Dose	Duration	Assessment	Effect
Reis (19) (1994)	Ethinyl estradiol	35 mcg p.o.	Acute	Cardiac cath	Measured potentiation of endothelium-dependent vasodilation in athero-sclerotic coronary arteries.
Gilligan (20) (1994)	17-β estradiol	IV infusion	Acute	Cardiac cath	Measured potentiation of endothelium-dependent vasodilation in athero-sclerotic coronary arteries.
Gilligan (21) (1994)	17-β estradiol	IV infusion	Acute	Brachial strain gauge plethysmography	Measured potentiation of endothelium-dependent vasodilation in athero-sclerotic coronary arteries.
Lieberman (22) (1994)	17-β estradiol	1–2 mcg p.o.	8–9 wk	Brachial artery high-resolution ultrasound	Improves flow mediated endothelium-dependent vasodilation
Collins (23) (1994)	17-β estradiol	2.5 mcg IV infusion	Acute	Cardiac cath	Attenuates acetylcholine-induced coronary arterial constriction.
Gilligan (24) (1995)	Transdermal estrogen	0.1 mcg	Acute and 3 wk	Brachial strain gauge plethysmography	Acute estrogen effects flow mediated dilation, but not chronic.
Volterrani (25) (1995)	17-β estradiol	1 mcg sl	Acute	Venous occlusion plethysmography	Acute administration of estrogen affects blood flow in the peripheral vasculature
McCrohon (26) (1996)	HRT		2 yr	Brachial artery high-resolution ultrasound	Chronic HRT replacement is associated with improved flow-mediated dilatation

[a]Modified from Samaan (1995).

others. One in vitro study looking at vascular smooth muscle cells from surgical specimens of saphenous vein and mammary artery demonstrated that human vascular smooth muscle cells express estrogen receptor mRNA and protein suggesting that they are capable of estrogen-dependent gene activation *(29)*. There are conflicting data on the presence of estrogen receptors in the female coronary arteries. One study done on surgical specimens from pre- and postmenopausal women with and without significant atherosclerosis demonstrated differential estrogen receptor expression *(28)*. There was a statistically significant inverse relationship between the amount of atherosclerosis in the vessel and the amount of estrogen receptor staining. In postmenopausal women there was no statistically significant relationship, perhaps reflecting an estrogen deficient state *(28)*. In contrast, another postmortem study using a different assay did not demonstrate the presence of estrogen receptors in either the endothelial layer or the vascular smooth muscle layer in women or men, although the age of the women was not specified *(30)*.

Evidence from animal studies suggests that estrogen receptor levels within the vasculature may be closely related to the hormonal milieu and may require a period of estrogen priming *(27,31)*. Therefore, both the time since menopause and duration of chronic estrogen exposure may play a role in regulating receptor density or response to exogenous estrogen administration. In summary, the identification of estrogen receptors in female coronary arteries is somewhat controversial. Some of estrogen's acute effect on the vasculature may be independent of the estrogen receptor.

Endothelium Dependent Vasodilation

The endothelium consists of a monolayer of cells that lines the intimal surface of the entire cardiovascular system. It plays a major role in regulating vascular tone through the release of dilator and constrictor substances that act upon vascular smooth muscle. There is accumulating evidence that impairment of endothelium-mediated vasodilation is an important early feature in the development of vascular disease not only in patients with known atherosclerosis but also with patients with hypertension, hypercholesterolemia, smoking, and diabetes *(32–37)*.

Nitric Oxide

Endothelium dependent vasodilators, such as acetylcholine stimulate the endothelium to produce endothelial-derived relaxing factor (EDRF), which is nitric oxide (NO). Nitric oxide is released by normal vascular endothelium in response to many types of clinical and physical stimuli, including neurotransmitters (acetylcholine), catecholamines, platelet products (serotonin), shear stress and changes in oxygen tension. NO causes vasodilation in endothelium intact coronary arteries and is a product of the conversion of L-arginine by nitric oxide synthetase (NOS) to NO and citrulline. NO is released in response to many factors, including acetylcholine, causing a subsequent relaxation of the blood vessel. In arteries damaged by atherosclerosis, however, acetylcholine causes constriction suggesting that atheroma impairs endothelium mediated dilation of the coronary arteries. Patients with central hypertension also have impaired endothelium dependent vasodilation. At least one study has demonstrated that abnormal endothelial function of patients with central hypertension is related to a defect in the endothelium-derived nitric oxide system, because of reduced synthesis, release, or diffusion of nitric oxide to vascular smooth muscle *(38)*.

NO has several actions that are cardioprotective including vasodilation, inhibition of platelet adhesion and aggregation, and inhibition of smooth muscle cell proliferation and migration. NOS can be divided into two functional groups based on their calcium sensitivity *(39)*. Estrogen can induce calcium dependent NOS, thus enhancing the amount of available NOS in a cell. NO has also been observed to slow the development of atheroma by inhibiting smooth cell proliferation or stimulating proliferation of endothelial cells. Estrogen is also a potent antioxidant of lipids and oxidized lipids inhibit NO. Estrogen may, therefore, protect the vascular tone by enhancing and/or prolonging the half-life of released NO. The time course for this effect is unknown and effects may only be seen with long-term estrogen therapy. In one study of HRT in postmenopausal women, researchers measured NO_2 and NO_3 levels as markers for NOS synthase activity and found an increase in women who were on estrogen alone *(40)*. One study in guinea pigs has suggested that long-term administration of estrogen up-regulates the transcription of nitric oxide synthase. A recent study in humans has demonstrated variations in expired NO production with cyclical hormone changes in premenopausal women. NO levels peak at the middle of the menstrual cycle suggesting an influence of hormones on the synthesis and release of NO in humans *(41)*.

Calcium Antagonism

Vascular smooth muscle (VSM) contraction is enhanced by intravascular calcium. Substances that block the flow of calcium into cells cause VSM relaxation and decreased vascular tone. It has been hypothesized, based on animal models, that some of the cardiovascular benefit of estrogen replacement therapy may be because of a calcium antagonistic effect of estrogen *(43)*. These properties have been demonstrated in several animal models. 17-β Estradiol was shown to have a negative inotropic effect on single-isolated guinea pig ventricular myocytes by inhibiting inward calcium currents and so reducing intracellular free calcium *(42)*.

Prostaglandins

Prostacyclin is a prostaglandin produced by endothelial cells. Its synthesis is thought to be coupled to NO release. It has been shown to induce vasodilation and inhibition of platelet activation in animal models. Evidence in humans is scant, but there is an indication that estrogen may effect coagulation and vasodilatation by its effects on prostacyclin *(39)*.

Inhibition of Constrictor Factors

Animal studies suggest that estrogen inhibits the release of or response to vascular constrictor factors. Vasoconstrictors include endothelin and fibronectin. There is a correlation between high endothelin levels and the development of atherosclerosis in humans *(44)*. One study demonstrated that plasma endothelin levels tend to be higher in men than women and lower still in pregnant women *(45)*. As a corollary, the same authors demonstrated in transsexuals that sex hormones may modulate endothelin levels, with male hormones increasing and female hormones decreasing the level. The effect of declining levels of estrogen with menopause on vascular constrictor factors is still unclear.

Estrogen also inhibits angiotensin II-induced constrictor effects in animal studies suggesting an inhibitory effect on the renin-angiotensin system *(39)*. In males elevated activity of serum angiotensin-converting-enzyme (ACE) may be associated with an increased risk of developing CAD. To date, there are no studies looking at ACE levels in women pre- and postmenopausally and correlating them with increased risk of developing CAD. In one of postmenopausal women treated with 6 mo of hormone replacement therapy, ACE-activity was reduced by 20% in 28 treated women as compared with 16 untreated controls *(46)*.

Effects on Vasoactive Neurotransmitters

Epinephrine and norepinephrine are released from sympathetic and parasympathetic nerve endings in the arterial wall and, thus, can cause vasoconstriction and vasodilation, playing an important role in the maintenance of vascular tone. Estrogens and progestins are thought to influence the release of these neurotransmitters by several mechanisms *(47)*. Of note, vasomotor instability (VMI) the hallmark of estrogen deficiency, occurs with rapid fluctuations in serum epinephrine and norepinephrine concentrations. Medications that decrease central noradrenergic activity, such as clonidine, have been shown to successfully treat hot flashes. The decline of estrogen levels that is seen with menopause is also associated with a relative increase in catecholamine release associated with physical and mental stress *(48)*.

Effects on Vascular Wall Composition

Animal studies have shown that vascular smooth muscle hyperplasia and collagen biosynthesis are reduced by estrogen administration *(49)*. In one clinical study, postmenopausal estrogen use was associated with significant borderline reductions in measured common carotid artery wall intimal medial thickness even after controlling for other risk factors such age, smoking, lipids, etc. *(50)*.

In a subanalysis of the Asymptomatic Carotid Atherosclerosis Progression Study (ACAPS), women who used ERT (preparation and dose not specified) were assessed for carotid artery wall intimal-medial thickness (IMT) by carotid ultrasonography. IMT, which is a marker for atherosclerosis, appeared to be retarded and to possibly reverse in women who took estrogen without receiving lipid-lowering therapy *(51)*.

Changes in Vascular Compliance and Blood Pressure

A newly recognized marker for hypertension and atherosclerosis is reduced vascular compliance. The latter describes the condition of the arterial wall that influences the relation between volume and pressure. In stiffer vessels, a smaller volume change will cause a greater pressure rise as compared to a normally compliant system. Vascular compliance is known to decrease with menopause.

One direct measure of vascular stiffness is the pulsatility index (PI). This represents the impedance to blood flow downstream from the point of measurement. An increase in PI is closely correlated with the time elapsed after the menopause. Decreases in arterial waveform pulsatility index in the uterine and carotid arteries have been demonstrated in postmenopausal women after chronic estrogen replacement suggesting an improvement in arterial compliance *(52)*. In another recent study, patients were treated with estrogen and progesterone for 1 yr and a significant decrease in PI was observed at 48 wk *(53)*. Arterial compliance is increased with pregnancy but returns to normal within 8 wk postpartum suggesting that these changes were not secondary to a change in vascular structure, but to a reduction in smooth muscle tone *(56)*.

Premenopausal women have lower systolic blood pressure than men of a similar age. After menopause, however, systolic blood pressure tends to be higher than in age-matched males. One study has also shown that an increase in pulsatile components of blood pressure is associated with higher cardiovascular risk in postmenopausal women *(55)*. The changes in blood pressure with menopause were explored in a study of both premenopausal and postmenopausal women who were compared with age-matched men *(56)*. Using ultrasound/Doppler to measure vascular flow, the authors found that premenopausal women had lower systolic blood pressure in their peripheral arteries, but not in their central (i.e., carotid) artery. Males had greater peripheral blood pressure that was attributed to amplification of blood pressure from central to peripheral arteries, which increased with body height and decreased with arterial distensibility. In contrast, in postmenopausal women, arterial distensibility was similar to that of age-matched men and no longer compensated for smaller body size, resulting in a persistent increased defect of wave reflections in central arteries, and greater peripheral blood pressure *(56)*.

In a related study, 18 women with essential hypertension were followed for 3 yr, during which time they went through menopause, to investigate whether a natural decrease in sex hormones in hypertensive women caused an increase in the stiffness of the aortic root *(57)*. The authors found that aortic root distensibility decreased significantly in women who had gone through menopause as compared with age-matched controls, suggesting an important role for declining estrogen levels in this process.

Changes in Cardiac Function

Estrogens effect hemodynamic parameters through several different mechanisms. There is less evidence about the effects of declining estrogen levels with menopause on hemodynamic function. In one study, which followed women through the menopause transition, no significant change in echocardiographic measurements of end-diastolic and end-systolic dimensions were found after menopause. However, significant decreases in rest Doppler measurements of left ventricular contractility appeared progressively over the years after menopause in women not treated with hormone replacement therapy *(58)*. These factors appeared to be modified with hormone replacement therapy suggesting a positive inotropic effect of estrogen *(59,60)*.

Changes in Exercise Tolerance

Exercise tolerance decreases in postmenopausal women for a variety of physiologic and sociologic reasons. However, to date, studies in healthy postmenopausal women have not suggested an improvement in exercise tolerance with HRT *(61,62)*. In contrast, one study of stress testing in women with known coronary artery disease, suggested that acute administration of estrogen prolonged exercise time to chest pain and electrocardiographic changes *(63)*. The effect of long-term estrogen administration on exercise tolerance in postmenopausal women with angina is unclear.

Metabolic Changes with Menopause

Changes in Lipid Metabolism

Several epidemiologic studies have suggested increases in levels of total cholesterol, low-density lipoproteins and triglyceride rich lipoproteins associated with menopause. In general, HDL levels are stable in the years after menopause, although there may be a small reduction in HDL_2 subfraction. Presumably, these changes with menopause are secondary to reduction in endogenous hormones. This is certainly supported by the beneficial effect of postmenopausal hormone therapy on lipoprotein metabolism in postmenopausal women. Studies suggest that estrogen use is associated with elevations in high-density lipoprotein (HDL) cholesterol, especially HDL_2 by as much as 20% and reductions in low-density lipoprotein (LDL) cholesterol by as much as 19%.

Lipoprotein(a) (Lp[a]) decreases by at least 13% and apolipoprotein (A1) increases by 13–22%. Finally, serum triglyceride levels are elevated by 16–42% (49).

An elevated Lp(a) level is independently associated with the development of CAD in women (64) as well as men. Lp(a) is a modified form of LDL to which an apolipoprotein is attached. Its genetic structure is similar to plasminogen and, thus, it interferes with the binding of plasminogen to sites of cells and molecules. Levels of Lp(a) are primarily determined by genetics and, as such, there are no abrupt changes in Lp(a) with menopause. However, estrogen therapy appears to reduce Lp(a) levels. An elevated plasma homocysteine level is an independent risk factor for CAD especially premature atherosclerosis. Levels are known to increase in both genders with age. After menopause, fasting homocysteine levels may increase or stay the same (65). Thus, the impact of declining estrogen levels on homocysteine levels is unclear.

In animal studies, estrogen appears to interfere with cholesterol deposition in the arterial wall (66) and in laboratory studies to reduce arterial smooth muscle cells proliferation (29). Oxidative modification of LDL cholesterol may be an important step in atherogenesis. In animal studies, the oxidized form of LDL appears to be more effective than inactive LDL in impairing endothelium-dependent vasodilation. One recent study suggests that endothelium mediated vasodilation is improved with lipid lowering drugs in patients with elevated cholesterol particularly if the lipid lowering therapy lowers rates of LDL oxidation (67). In vitro studies suggest that 17-β estradiol appears to inhibit LDL oxidation and reduce cholesterol ester formation (68). In one study, 17-β estradiol administration significantly reduced the oxidation of LDL cholesterol from postmenopausal women (69).

Changes in Clotting

Certain hemostatic variables change with menopause with a potential impact on both thrombosis and fibrinolysis. After menopause, fibrinogen levels increase as do levels of factor VII and antithrombin III. Higher levels of PAI-1 an antagonist of fibrinolysis in humans, have been noted in postmenopausal women in the Framingham Offspring Study (71). Studies of HRT in postmenopausal women suggest a decrease in fibrinogen (72), and a decrease in PAI-1 (73). Animal studies also suggest that estrogen inhibits platelet aggregation.

RELEVANT CLINICAL SYNDROMES

Symptoms of Vasomotor Instability

Symptoms of vasomotor instability include palpitations and, in a small percentage of women, symptoms of chest pressure. Although they occur most often in conjunction with hot flashes, an increase in palpitations can be seen in the absence of other symptoms. The severity of these cardiac symptoms appears to be related to the severity of the hot flashes (74). Vasomotor symptoms and associated cardiac symptoms are more severe in patients who experience a sudden drop in their estrogen level (e.g., surgical menopause). In one longitudinal study of 200 perimenopausal women from Scandinavia, palpitations figured prominently in the symptomatology in association with other vasomotor complaints (75). In another survey of 501 women, 12–20% of those who were postmenopausal noted pressure in chest and 36–47% noted a change in heart rate in association with their hot flashes (76).

Syndrome X

Syndrome X is a term applied to patients with angina-like chest pain who, despite a positive exercise stress test, have angiographically normal coronary arteries. This cardiac syndrome X must be distinguished from a metabolic Syndrome X discovered by Reaven in 1988. The latter, which predisposes to atherosclerosis, includes patients with insulin resistance, glucose intolerance, hyperinsulinemia, hyperlipidemia, and hypertension. There appears to be some overlap between the two syndromes in addition to the name. However, cardiac syndrome X is strictly defined as a history of typical angina, a positive exercise test with ST-segment depressions of greater than 1 mm during treadmill testing and normal coronary arteries at the time of coronary catheterization. Of note, in most case series of syndrome X, more than 50% of the patients are female. Syndrome X appears to be increased in other vasospastic disorders such as Raynaud's phenomenon and migraine. Studies suggest that microvascular endothelial dysfunction may contribute to the reduced vasodilator reserve in these patients *(77,78)*. The emergence of generalized vasospasm in a certain small percentage of women as they age appears to be related to the declining levels of estrogen *(79)*.

In one series of 134 patients with syndrome X, 107 patients were women, and of these, 95 were either peri- or postmenopausal *(80)*. Of note, two-thirds of the female patients who were postmenopausal had experienced a hysterectomy and the incidence of hysterectomy in this study population (40%) was actually four times greater than that of an age-matched population. There is limited data to suggest that estrogen replacement has a beneficial effect in syndrome X. In one small study, the application of transdermal 17-β-estradiol prior to stress testing in 15 postmenopausal women with syndrome X significantly reduced ST segment depression, increased time to angina, and increased exercise tolerance *(81)*.

In another study, 25 postmenopausal women with syndrome X completed a double-blind, placebo-controlled study of the effect of 17-β-estradiol (transdermal patch) on the frequency of chest pain and on exercise tolerance *(82)*. There was a significant reduction in the incidence of chest pain during the study period. In contrast to the previous study, there was no difference in exercise duration or ST segment depression. In summary, syndrome X is more common in postmenopausal women and estrogen replacement may be beneficial for the treatment of associated chest pain.

Approach to Menopausal Patients with Certain Risk Factors for CAD

The menopausal transition is an optimal time to address the prevention of CAD with patients in the office. Often, women who present with menopausal symptoms have not been routinely screened for risk factors for heart disease. A recent survey of a thousand women suggests that a substantial percentage (58%) of women believe they are as or more likely to die of breast cancer than heart disease *(83)*. More than 40% of women aged 45–59 had never been "counselled by a physician about how to reduce the risk of a heart attack." A similar percent did not know their own cholesterol values.

There are important interactions between known cardiovascular risk factors and the decline of estrogen with menopause in the development of atherosclerosis in postmenopausal women. Diabetes mellitus is a more important risk factor for CAD in women than it is in men *(84)*. Women with diabetes actually have a greater risk of CAD than men with diabetes and, thus, diabetes eliminates any female advantage in the development of heart disease. The Framingham Study suggests that abnormal glucose intolerance alone is a risk factor for CAD in women because of a relationship between poorer glucose control (as assessed by higher level of hemoglobin A_{1c}) and risk of cardiovascular disease *(85)*. There is limited data on changes in glucose tolerance in women with the menopausal transition. The PEPI Study looked at 869 women in the pretreatment stage, aged 45–65 and found a positive, graded and significant relation between age and plasma glucose. No significant association between age and serum insulin was found. Controlling for age, body mass index (BMI) and waist hip ratio (WHR) were the most important independent predictors of glucose intolerance *(86)*. The PEPI Trial, which randomized women to one of five HRT regimens, including placebo, demonstrated no significant differences in 2-h insulin levels, but significantly higher 2-h glucose levels after a low-dose glucose tolerance test in women on HRT. Fasting insulin and glucose levels decreased with HRT.

Diabetes appears to enhance the process of accelerated atherosclerosis through several mechanisms including other risk factors such as hyperlipidemia and hypertension. Diabetic patients have higher levels of triglycerides and higher levels of oxidized lipoproteins, (known to be cytotoxic to vascular endothelial cells and smooth muscle cells). Diabetes also appears to predispose patients to abnormalities in the various pathways involved in coagulation, hemostasis, and fibrinolysis *(84)*. Finally, diabetic patients appear to have abnormalities of vascular tone *(34)*. It is unclear what effect the menopausal transition has on the risk of developing CAD in diabetic women, but one could hypothesize that the process is accelerated and that HRT could be helpful. Ongoing studies will help to clarify this.

Hypertension is a powerful predictor of the development of cardiovascular disease in women, particularly because it is the most prevalent of the major risk factors ranging from 20 to 40% of women, with the highest proportion being among black women. The development of hypertension is due to changes in arterial tone presumed to be secondary to aging. The withdrawal of estrogen with menopause also causes an increasing stiffness of the arterial wall. Estrogen replacement does not appear to cause or worsen existing hypertension *(87,88)*. The risk of development of CAD also parallels the severity of hypertension. Hypertension is associated with endothelial dysfunction and there is some controversy about the efficacy of blood pressure treatment on this particular dysfunction *(38,89)*. Evidence from the Nurses Health Study suggest that patients with hypertension treated with HRT appear to have a reduction in their risk of CAD *(90)*.

The changes in lipids with menopause are summarized previously as are the effects of HRT on lipids. Hormone replacement does not fully restore a premenopausal lipoprotein profile but numerous studies suggest a beneficial effect on lipids overall *(72)*. Some authors recommend HRT for first line treatment of hypercholesterolemia in women especially if the patient has other indications for HRT.

Smoking is an important risk factor for the development of coronary artery disease, especially in young women, even among those women who continue to smoke only small amounts (one to four cigarettes per d) *(91)*. Smoking is thought to have antiestrogen effects causing menopause in women who smoke an average of 2 yr earlier. Cigarette smokers also have lower levels of HDL cholesterol and lower levels of plasminogen. One study suggests that smoking causes endothelial dysfunction in asymptomatic young smokers and this effect is reversed with smoking cessation *(92)*. Of all behavior interventions, smoking cessation offers the most substantial (50–70% within 5 yr) benefit.

Obesity is a significant independent risk factor for the development of CAD in females only. This relationship is independent of other risk factors. A truncal distribution of adipose distribution (i.e., increased waist/hip circumference) appears to increase the risk of CAD in women. Most women experience about a 5–10-lb weight gain with menopause. One study suggested that menopause was associated with a significant increase in the proportion of android fat (increased WHR ratio) and a significant reduction in proportion of gynecoid fat *(93)*. Women who are less than 20% above their ideal body weight (IBW) appear to have a 35–55% lower risk of CAD compared to women who weigh more than 20% of their IBW.

There is limited data on psychosocial factors for the development of heart disease. Studies suggest that cardiovascular and neuroendocrine responses to mental stress may be influenced by reproductive hormone status. Postmenopausal women have larger increases in heart rate, systolic blood pressure, and plasma epinephrine levels during public speaking than their age-matched premenopausal counterparts *(94)*. Another study found that relative to premenopausal women, both men and postmenopausal women have higher ambulatory diastolic blood pressure levels throughout the workday even after controlling for BMI, baseline blood pressure, and age *(95)*. These findings suggest that postmenopausal women are more reactive to the stress of their work experience than premenopausal women. The etiology of this is unclear, but these effects may contribute to an increased risk of cardiovascular morbidity and mortality after menopause. Programs in stress reduction and regular exercise may be beneficial although there is no definite data to suggest this.

SUMMARY

Research in the last decade has contributed much to the understanding of the cardiovascular effects of menopause. Additional prospective long-term studies following women through the menopausal transition are needed to clarify the mechanisms for the development of cardiovascular disease in women and the relationship to changes in hormones. These studies will need to include not only detailed assessment of risk factor status, but also repeated measurements of cardiac function using the latest technology in order to ascertain the development of subclinical heart disease.

REFERENCES

1. Lerner DJ, Kannell WB. Patterns of coronary heart disease morbidity and mortality in the sexes. A 26–year follow up of the Framingham population. Am Heart J 1986;111:383–390.
2. Eaker ED, Packard B, Thom TJ. Epidemiology and risk factors for coronary heart disease in women. In: Douglas PS, ed. Heart Disease in Women. FA Davis, Philadelphia, 1989.
3. Kannel WB, Hjortland MC, McNamara PM, et al. Menopause and risk of cardiovascular disease. The Framingham Study. Ann Intern Med 1976;85:447–452.
4. Grady D, Rubin SM, Petitti DB. Hormone therapy to prevent disease and prolong life in postmenopausal women. Ann Intern Med 1992;117(12):1016–1037.
5. Bush TL. Extraskeletal effects of estrogen and the prevention of atherosclerosis. Osteopor Int 1991;2:5–11.
6. Stampfer MJ, Colditz GA. Estrogen replacement and coronary heart disease: a quantitative assessment of the epidemiologic evidence. Prev Med 1991;20:47–63.
7. Psaty BM, Heckbert SR, Atkins D. A review of the association of estrogens and progestins with cardiovascular disease in postmenopausal women. Arch Intern Med 1993;153:1421–1427.
8. Barrett-Connor E, Bush TL. Estrogen and coronary heart disease in women. JAMA 1991;256:1861–1867.
9. Klapholz M, Buttrick P. Myocardial Function and Cardiomyopathy. In: Douglas PS, ed. Heart Disease in Women. FA Davis, Philadelphia, 1989, pp. 105–115.

10. Lakata EG, Gerstenblith G, Weisfeldth ML. The aging heart: structure, function, and disease. In: Braunwald EG. The Heart. W. B. Saunders, Philadelphia, PA, 1996, pp. 1687–1703.
11. Celermajer DS, Sorensen KE, Spiegelhalter DJ, et al. Aging is associated with endothelial dysfunction in healthy men years before the age-related decline in women. J Am Coll Cardiol 1994;24:471–476.
12. Fleg JL, O'Connor F, Gerstenblith G, et al. Impact of age on the cardiovascular response to dynamic upright exercise in healthy men and women. J Appl Physiol 1995;78:890.
13. Anderson TJ, Uehata A, Gerhard MD, et al. Close relation of endothelial function in the human coronary and peripheral circulations. J Am Coll Cardiol 1995;26:1235–1241.
14. Taddei S, Virdis A, Ghiadoni L, et al. Menopause is associated with endothelial dysfunction in women. Hypertension 1996;28:576–582.
15. Pinto S, Virdis A, Ghiadoni L, Bernini G, et al. Endogenous estrogen and acetylcholine- induced vasodilation in normotensive women. Hypertension 1997;29(2):268–273.
16. Adams MR, Kaplan JR, Manuck SB, et al. Inhibition of coronary artery atherosclerosis by 17-β-estradiol in ovariectomized monkeys: lack of an effect of added progesterone. Arteriosclerosis 1990;10:1051–1057.
17. Williams JK, Adams MR, Klopfenstein S. Estrogen modulates responses of atherosclerotic coronary arteries. Circulation 1990;81:1680–1687.
18. Williams JK, Adams MR, Herrington DM, et al. Short-term administration of estrogen and vascular responses of atherosclerotic coronary arteries. J Am Coll Cardiol 1992;20:452–457.
19. Reis SE, Gloth ST, Blumenthal RS, et al. Ethinyl estradiol acutely attenuates abnormal coronary vasomotor responses to acetylcholine in postmenopausal women. Circulation 1994;89:52–60.
20. Gilligan DM, Badar DM, Panza JA, et al. Acute vascular effects of estrogen in postmenopausal women. Circulation 1994;90:786–791.
21. Gilligan DM, Quyyumi AR, Cannon RO, et al. Effects of physiological levels of estrogen on coronary vasomotor function in postmenopausal women. Circulation 1994;89:2545–2521.
22. Lieberman EH, Gerhard MD, Uehata A, Walsh BW, et al. Estrogen improves endothelium- dependent, flow-mediated vasodilation in postmenopausal women. Ann Intern Med 1994;121:936–941.
23. Collins P, Rosano G, Sarrel PM, et al. 17ß-estradiol attenuates acetylcholine-induced coronary arterial constriction in women but not men with coronary heart disease. Circulation 1995;92:24–30.
24. Gilligan DM, Badar DM, Panza JA, et al. Effects of estrogen replacement therapy on peripheral vasomotor function in postmenopausal women. Am J Cardiol 1995;75:264–268.
25. Volterrani M, Rosano G, Coats A, et al. Estrogen acutely increases peripheral blood flow in postmeno-pausal women. Am J Med 1995;99:119–122.
26. McCrohon JA, Adams MR, McCredie RJ, et al. Hormone replacement therapy is associated with improved arterial physiology in healthy post-menopausal women. Clin Endocrinol 1996;45:435–441.
27. White MM, Zamudio S, Stevens T, et al. Estrogen, progesterone, and vascular reactivity: potential cellular mechanisms. Endocrine Rev 1995;16(6):739–751.
28. Losordo DW, Kearney M, Kim EA, et al. Variable expression of the estrogen receptor in normal and atherosclerotic coronary arteries of premenopausal women. Circulation 1994;89:1501–1510.
29. Karas RH, Patterson BL, Mendelsohn ME. Human vascular smooth muscle cells contain functional estrogen receptor. Circulation 1994;89:1943–1950.
30. Collins P, Sheppard M, Beale CM, et al. The classical estrogen receptor is not found in human coronary arteries. Circulation 1995;92 supp 1(8):1–37.
31. Weiner CP, Lizasoain I, Baylis SA, et al. Induction of calcium-dependent nitric oxide synthases by sex hormones. Proc Natl Acad Sci 1994;91:5212–5216.
32. Zeiher AM, Drexler H, Wollschlager H, et al. Modulation of coronary vasomotor tone in humans. Progressive endothelial dysfunction with different early stages of coronary atherosclerosis. Circulation 1991;83:391–401.
33. McVeigh GE, Brennan GM, Johnston GD, et al. Impaired endothelium-dependent and independent vasodilation in patients with Type 2 (non-insulin-dependent) diabetes mellitus. Diabetologia 1992;35:771–776.
34. Johnstone MT, Creager SJ, Scales KM, et al. Impaired endothelium-dependent vasodilation in patients with insulin-dependent diabetes mellitus. Circulation 1993;88:2510–2516.
35. Calver A, Collier J, Vallance P. Inhibition and stimulation of nitric oxide synthesis in the human forearm arterial bed of patients with insulin-dependent diabetes. J Clin Invest 1992;90:2548–2554.
36. Creager MA, Cooke JP, Mendelsohn ME et al. Impaired vasodilation of forearm resistance vessels in hypercholesterolemic humans. J Clin Invest 1990;86:228–234.

37. Creager MA, Gallagher SJ, Girerd XJ, et al. $_L$-Arginine improves endothelium-dependent vasodilation in hypercholesterolemic humans. J Clin Invest 1992;90:1248–1253.

38. Panza JA, Quyyumi AA, Callahan TS, et al. Effect of antihypertensive treatment on endothelium-dependent vascular relaxation in patients with essential hypertension. J Am Coll Cardiol 1993;21:1145–1151.

39. Beale C, Collins P. Estrogen and cardiovascular dynamics. Seminars in Reproductive Endocrinology 1996;14(1):71–77.

40. Roselli M, Imthurn B, Keller PJ. Circulating nitric oxide levels in postmenopausal women substituted with 17-β estradiol and norethisterone acetate: A two-year follow-up study. Hypertension 1995;25:848–853.

41. Kharitonov SA. Longan-Sinclair RB, Busset CM, et al. Peak expiratory nitric oxide differences in men and women: relation to the menstrual cycle. Br Heart J 1994;72:243–245.

42. Jiang C, Poole-Wilson PA, Sarrell PM, et al. Effect of 17-β-oestradiol on contraction, calcium current and intracellular free calcium in guinea-pig isolated cardiac myocytes. Br J Pharmacol 1992;106:739–745.

43. Collins P, Rosano G, Jiang C, et al. Cardiovascular protection by oestrogen—a calcium antagonist effect? Lancet 1993;341:1264–1265.

44. Lerman A, Edwards BF, and Hallett JW, et al. Circulating and tissue endothelin immuno-1. reactivity in advanced atherosclerosis. N Engl J Med 1991;325:997–1001

45. Polderman KR, Stenhouwer DA, van Kamp GJ, et al. Influence of sex hormones on plasma endothelin levels. Ann Intern Med 1993;118:429–432.

46. Proudher AJ, Ahmed AIH, Crook D, et al. Hormone replacement therapy and serum angiotensin-converting-enzyme activity in postmenopausal women. Lancet 1995; 346:89–90.

47. Sarrel PM. Blood flow. In: Lobo RA, ed. Treatment of the Postmenopausal Woman. Raven, New York, 1994, pp. 251–262.

48. Matthews KA, Wing RR, Kuller LH, et al. Influence of the perimenopause on cardiovascular risk factors and symptoms of middle-aged healthy women. Arch Intern Med 1994;154:2349–2355.

49. Samaan SA, Crawford MH. Estrogen and cardiovascular function after menopause. J Am Coll Cardiol 1995; 26:1403–1410.

50. Manolio TA, Furburg CD, Shemanski L, et al. Associations of postmenopausal estrogen use with cardiovascular disease and its risk factors in older women. Circulation 1993;88:1113–1117.

51. Espeland MA, Applegate W, Furberg CD, et al. Estrogen replacement therapy and progression of intimal-medial thickness in the carotid arteries of postmenopausal women. Am J Epidemiol 1995;142:1011–1019.

52. Gangar KF, Vyas S, Whitehead M, et al. Pulsatility index in internal carotid artery in relation to transdermal oestradiol and time since menopause. Lancet 1991;338:839–842.

53. Penotti M, Farina Massimiliano, Sironi L, et al. Long-term effects of postmenopausal hormone replacement therapy on pulsatilty index of internal carotid and middle cerebral arteries. Menopause: J North Am Menopause Soc 1997; 4(2):101–104.

54. Poppas A, Shroff SG, Korcarz CE, et al. Serial assessment of the cardiovascular system in normal pregnancy. Role of arterial compliance and pulsatile arterial load. Circulation 1997;95:2407–2415.

55. Darne B, Girerd X, Safar M, et al. Pulsatile versus steady component of blood pressure: a cross-sectional analysis on cardiovascular mortality. Hypertension 1989;13(4):392–400.

56. London GM, Guerin AP, Pannier B, et al. Influence of sex on arterial hemodynamics and blood pressure. Role of body height. Hypertension 1995;26:514–519.

57. Karpanou EA, Vyssoulis GP, Papakyriakou SA, et al. Effects of menopause on aortic root function in hypertensive women. J Am Coll Cardiol 1996;28:1562–1566.

58. Pines A, Fisman EZ, Drory Y, et al. Menopause-induced changes in doppler-derived parameters of aortic flow in healthy women. Am J Cardiol 1992;69:1104–1106.

59. Pines A, Fisman EZ, Levo Y, et al. The effects of hormone replacement therapy in normal postmenopausal women: Measurements of doppler-derived parameters of aortic flow. Am J Obstet Gynecol 1991;164:806–812.

60. Pines A, Fisman EZ, Ayalon D, et al. Long-term effects of hormone replacement therapy on doppler-derived parameters of aortic flow in postmenopausal women. Chest 1992; 102:1496–1498.

61. Lindheim SR, Notelovitz M, Feldman EB, et al. The independent effects of exercise and estrogen on lipids and lipoproteins in postmenopausal women. Obstet Gynecol 1994;83:167–172.

62. Snabes MC, Herd JA, Schuyler N, et al. In normal postmenopausal women physiologic estrogen replacement therapy fails to improve exercise tolerance: A randomized, double- blind, placebo-controlled, crossover trial. Am J Obstet Gynecol 1996;175:110–114.

63. Rosano GMC, Sarrel PM, Poole-Wilson PA. Beneficial effect of oestrogen on exercise- induced myocardial ischaemia in women with coronary artery disease. Lancet 1993;342:133–136.
64. Bostom AG, Gagnon DR, Cupples LA, et al. A prospective investigation of elevated lipoprotein(a) detected by electrophoresis and cardiovascular disease in women: The Framingham Heart Study. Circulation 1994;90:1688–1695.
65. Mayer EL, Jacobsen DW, Robinson K. Homocysteine and coronary atherosclerosis. J Am Coll Cardiol 1996;27:517–527.
66. Adams MR, Washburn SA, Wagner JD, et al. Arterial changes. Estrogen deficiency and effects of hormone replacement. In: Lobo RA, ed. Treatment of the Postmenopausal Woman. Raven, New York, 1994, pp. 243–250.
67. Anderson TJ, Meredith IT, Charbonneau F, et al. Endothelium-dependent coronary vasomotion relates to the susceptibility of LDL to oxidation in humans. Circulation 1996;93:1647–1650.
68. Rifici VA, Khachadurian AK. The inhibition of low-density lipoprotein oxidation by 17-β estradiol. Metabolism 1992;41(10):1110–1114.
69. Sack MN, Rader DJ, Cannon RO. Oestrogen and inhibition of oxidation of low-density lipoproteins in postmenopausal women. Lancet 1994;343:269–270.
70. Meilahn EN, Kuller LH, Matthews KA, et al. Hemostatic factors according to menopausal status and use of hormone replacement therapy. Ann Epidermiol 1992;2:445–455.
71. Gebara O, Mittleman MA, Suterland P, Lipinska I, et al. Association between increased estrogen status and increased fibrinolytic potential in the Framingham Offspring Study. Circulation 1995;91:1952–1958.
72. The Writing Group for the PEPI Trial. Effects of estrogen or estrogen/progestin regimens on heart disease risk factors in postmenopausal women. JAMA 1995;273(3):199–207.
73. Koh KK, Mincemoyer R, Bui M, et al. Effects of hormone-replacement therapy on fibrinolysis in postmenopausal women. N Engl J Med 1997;336:683–690.
74. Who Technical Report Series. Research on the Menopause in the 1990's. Report of a WHO Scientific Group. 1994: Geneva, Switzerland.
75. Holte A. Influences of natural menopause on health complaints: a prospective study of healthy Norwegian women. Maturitas 1992;14:127–141.
76. Kronenberg F. Hot flashes: epidemiology and physiology. Ann NY Acad Sci 1990;592–586.
77. Quyyumi AA, Cannon RO, Panza JA, et al. Endothelial dysfunction in patients with chest pain and normal coronary arteries. Circulation 1992;86:1864–1871.
78. Egashira K, Inou T, Hirooka Y, et al. Evidence of impaired endothelium-dependent coronary vasodilatation in patients with angina pectoris and normal coronary angiograms. N Engl J Med 1993;328:1659–1664.
79. Collins P. Vascular aspects of oestrogen. Maturitas 1996; 23:217–226.
80. Rosano GM, Collins P, Kaski JC, et al. Syndrome X in women is associated with oestrogen deficiency. Eur Heart J 1995;16(5):610–614.
81. Albertsson PA, Emanuelsson H, Milsom I. Beneficial effect of treatment with transdermal estradiol-17–$_\beta$ on exercise-induced angina and ST segment depression in syndrome X. Intern J Cardiol 1996;54:13–20.
82. Collins P. Hormone replacement therapy and syndrome X. Br J Obstet Gynaecol 1996;103(13):68–72.
83. Legato MJ, Padus E, Slaughter E. Women's perceptions of their general health, with special reference to their risk of coronary artery disease: results of a national telephone survey. Journal of Women's Health 1997;6(2):189–198.
84. Ramen M, Nesto RW. Heart disease in diabetes mellitus. Endocrinol Metab Clinics North Am 1996;25:425–438.
85. Singer DE, Nathan DM, Anderson KM, et al. Association of HbA_{1c} with prevalent cardiovascular disease in the original cohort of the Framingham Heart Study. Diabetes 1992; 41:202–208.
86. Barrett-Connor E, Schrott HG, Greendale G, et al. Factors associated with glucose and insulin levels in healthy postmenopausal women. Diabetes Care 1996;19(4):333–340.
87. Lip GYH, Beevers M, Churchill, et al. Hormone replacement therapy and blood pressure in hypertensive women. J Hum Hypert 1994;8:491–494.
88. Sands RH, Studd JWW, Crook D, et al. The effect of estrogen on blood pressure in hypertensive postmenopausal women. Menopause: J North Am Menopause Soc 1997; 4(2):115–119.
89. Panza JA, Casino PR, Kilcoyne CM, et al. Role of endothelium-derived nitric oxide in the abnormal endothelium-dependent vascular relaxation of patients with essential hypertension. Circulation 1993;87:1468–1774.
90. Grodstein F, Stampfer MJ, Manson JE. Postmenopausal estrogen and progestin use and the risk of cardiovascular disease. N Engl J Med 1996;335:453–461.

91. Willett WC, Green A, Stampfer MJ, et al. Relative and absoulut excess risks of coronary heart disease among women who smoke cigarettes. N Engl J Med 1987;317:1303–1309.
92. Celermajer DS, Sorensen KE, Georgakopoulos D, Bull C, et al. Cigarette smoking is associated with dose-related and potentially reversible impairment of endothelium-dependent dilation in health young adults. Circulation 1993;88(part 1):2149–2155.
93. Ley CJ, Lees B, Stevenson JC. Sex-and-menopause associated changes in body fat distribution. Am J Clin Nutr 1992;55:950–954.
94. Saab PG, Matthews KA, Stoney CM, et al. Premenopausal and postmenopausal women differ in their cardiovascular and neuroendocrine responses to behavioral stressors. Psychophysiology 1989;26:270–280.
95. Owens JF, Stoney CM, Matthews KA. Menopausal status influences ambulatory blood pressure levels and blood pressure changes during mental stress. Circulation 1993;88:2794–2082.

4

Postmenopausal Osteoporosis
Pathogenesis, Diagnosis, and Treatment

Rebecca D. Jackson, MD

INTRODUCTION

Osteoporosis is the most common generalized disease of the skeleton. It is characterized by a reduction in bone mass with impairments in microarchitecture leading to enhanced bony fragility and ultimately an increase in fractures (*1*). In osteoporosis, there is a normal ratio of mineral to matrix. This distinguishes it from osteomalacia, which is characterized by a relative deficiency of mineral. Up to 20% of elderly patients have concurrent osteomalacia and osteoporosis.

As 75–85% of the variance in bone strength is because of bone density (*2*), measurements of bone mineral density (BMD) by absorptiometric techniques have provided the operational diagnosis of osteoporosis. An expert panel convened by the World Health Organization (WHO) has developed a definition of osteoporosis, based upon the variance of a specific individuals' bone mass in comparison to the mean for a reference population (Table 1) (*3*). This value, termed the T score, is calculated from the individual's deviation from the average result for a young normal (30 year old) reference population divided by the standard deviation of the measurement for the reference population (*4*). A woman with a bone mass less than 2.5 standard deviations (T < –2.5) is termed osteoporotic. This level of bone mass captures most patients with osteoporotic fractures. If the woman also has one or more fractures, this is then termed established osteoporosis. If the T score is

From: *Contemporary Endocrinology: Menopause: Endocrinology and Management*
Edited by: D. B. Seifer and E. A. Kennard © Humana Press Inc., Totowa, NJ

Table 1
World Health Organization Criteria for Osteoporosis

T Score	Definition	Frequency in postmenopausal women >65 yr old (%)
>−1.0	Normal	16
−1.0 to −2.5	Osteopenia	54
<−2.5	Osteoporosis	30

not more than one standard deviation below the young adult mean, the bone mass is considered normal. Osteopenia, or low bone mass, is defined as a value between −1.0 and −2.5 standard deviations below a normal young adult. The limitations of these criteria include the fact that there are no normative data relative to fracture risks defined for men, ethnic populations, or certain secondary causes of osteoporosis. Thus, these criteria may not be applicable to specific situations.

CLINICAL MANIFESTATIONS

The surrogate use of BMD to define osteoporosis has important clinical utility as bone mass loss may occur over many years prior to the first clinical manifestation. The hallmark of osteoporosis is the fracture. The classical fractures associated with osteoporosis occur at the vertebrae (anterior wedge, end plate, or crush fracture), distal forearm, and hip. However, in the elderly, almost any fracture may be due, in part, to low BMD. Complications of fractures also contribute to the morbidity of osteoporosis and these are specific to the site of fracture. For vertebral fractures, this may include kyphosis, decreased height, and chronic back pain (5). As kyphosis becomes more severe, it may lead to restrictive lung disease, early satiety, and constipation. Additional morbidity is associated with hip fractures, including diminished activities of daily living independence, changes in gait (6), and an increased risk of death. Up to 12–20% of persons who have a hip fracture die within one year of fracture (7) primarily because of the medical health and nutritional state of the individual who fractures (8). For those patients who survive the fracture, only 33–51% are restored to their prefracture state (9,10). Therefore, the manifestations of osteoporosis are significant and only through early intervention can the morbidity and mortality of this disease be reduced.

PREVALENCE

Based on WHO criteria, it has been estimated that 30% of postmenopausal white women in the United States will have osteoporosis at one or more skeletal sites and an additional 54% will have low bone mass or osteopenia (11). Thus, more than 26 million white women are at risk for fracture and may benefit from primary or secondary prevention. Ethnic minority women may further increase this estimate. Data from the Third National Health and Nutrition Examination Survey (NHANES III) have demonstrated that 10% of postmenopausal African-American women and 16% of postmenopausal Mexican-American women have a hip T score that is <-2.5 (12).

Osteoporosis is responsible for an incidence of 1.3 million fractures annually. This includes vertebral fractures (530,000), radial fractures (172,000) and more than 250,000 hip fractures per year. A 50-year-old white woman has a 14% lifetime probability of a hip

Table 2

Health Care Expenditures for Postmenopausal Osteoporosis (1995 Dollars)[a]

	White		Nonwhite		Total cost[b]
	Hip	Other	Hip	Other	
Hospital					6.805
No. discharges	178,096	141,328	13,006	8,761	
Days	2,076,056	985,072	162,185	64,105	
Nursing Home					3.252
No. residents	96,110	39,970	6,360	1,469	
Days	23,589,045	11,89079	1,561,066	360,625	
Outpatient[c]					1.007
Services	2,008,887	5,928782	251,333	445,781	

[a]Adapted with permission from Ray NF, Chan JK, Thamer M, Melton LJ, III. Medical expenditures for the treatment of osteoporotic fractures in the United States in 1995: report from the National Osteoporosis Foundation. J Bone Miner Res 1997;12:24–35.

[b]Health care expenditures in millions.

[c]Including physicians visits, emergency room encounters, out-patient hospital encounters, physical therapy, diagnostic radiology, medications, home health care visits, ambulance encounters and orthopedic, and other supplies.

fracture *(13,14)*. Also, as the incidence of this fracture increases with advancing age, it ranges from a 5-yr risk of hip fracture at the age of 50 of 2.3%, up to a 7.19% probability at the age of 85 *(14)*. Taking all fractures into account, more than 50% of all white women will suffer at least one osteoporosis-associated fracture during their lifetime.

The excess fractures associated with osteoporosis contribute to a significant economic burden (Table 2) *(15)*. There are more than 400,000 excess hospitalizations, averaging 9.6 d in length, because of osteoporosis. Although 57% of these hospitalizations are attributable to hip fractures, significant health care utilization is also attributed to other skeletal sites (spine [6.8%], forearm [3.1%], and other sites [33%]). In addition, the presence of an osteoporotic fracture as a secondary diagnosis also significantly increases the length of the hospital stay (4.4 d) in comparison to patients with no fractures, but a similar primary diagnosis. Osteoporosis also impacts the health care system by resulting in ~180,000 excess nursing home stays and 3.4 million outpatient visits per year.

The total health care expenditure for osteoporosis, expressed in 1995 dollars, is estimated at $13.76 billion, of which more than $11 billion was spent on the management of osteoporosis in women. Although the majority of costs were for treatment of white women, one-fourth of the total cost of osteoporosis was associated with fractures in men (19.6%) and nonwhite women (5.3%). These economic data, taken together with prevalence data from NHANES III, suggest that preventive efforts to reduce the incidence of osteoporosis and osteoporotic fracture should be addressed toward all members of the aging population and not just the white female population.

PATHOPHYSIOLOGY

The skeleton is comprised of compact and cancellous bone that is constantly undergoing a dynamic process of self-repair and renewal defined as bone turnover or remodeling *(16)*. This remodeling occurs at discrete foci on bone surfaces termed the bone modeling unit (BMU). Because there is a higher surface-to-volume ratio at cancellous sites, the extent of cancellous bone available for remodeling is much greater than that of cortical bone. This results in the potential for greater early losses in bone mass and a resultant earlier risk for fractures at skeletal sites containing the highest percentages of cancellous bone.

In the mature adult skeleton, remodeling occurs in approx 15% of the bone surfaces at any one time *(17)*. When bone remodeling is activated, a coordinated coupled sequence of events is initiated *(18)*. First, osteoclasts are activated and begin the process of bone resorption to create a resorption cavity. Once the erosion is complete, the osteoclasts leave the surface and are replaced by preosteoblasts. These differentiate into mature osteoblasts and begin the slower process of bone formation. This is followed by mineralization. A complete remodeling cycle takes from 3–6 mo to complete.

At skeletal maturity, the amount of bone formed is equal to the amount of bone resorbed, and bone mass is stable. However, any disruption of the remodeling cycle (increased or decreased activation of the BMU, enhanced resorption, or diminished bone formation) can lead to a net loss of bone. Thus, histologically, osteoporosis is a heterogeneous disorder.

The process of remodeling is affected by both menopause and aging. As estrogen levels fall with menopause, there is an increase in the release of interleukin-1 (IL-1) and tumor necrosis factor (TNF) from peripheral blood mononuclear cells and the release of IL-6, granulocyte-colony stimulating factor (GM-CSF), and macrophage CSF (M-CSF) from osteoblast and stromal cells *(19)*. The cytokines IL-1 and TNF stimulate bone resorption through inhibition of osteoclastic apoptosis, stimulation of proosteoclastogenic activity of stromal cells (with release of IL-6, GM-CSF, and M-CSF) and activation of mature osteoclasts indirectly through effects on the osteoblast. This leads to an increase in activation frequency and an increase in resorptive activity resulting in penetration into the trabecular plate and perforation. Further accentuating the net loss of bone is an uncoupling of bone resorption from formation that may also be mediated by both IL-1 and TNF.

This model is supported by in vitro studies *(20,21)*. and in vivo evidence is beginning to emerge to support the role of cytokine-mediated resorption in postmenopausal osteoporosis. Systemic levels of IL-1 (measured by bioassay) *(22)* and IL-1, TNF, and IL-6 messenger RNA in bone *(23)* is expressed at much higher levels in untreated women with postmenopausal osteoporosis than in women who are on hormone replacement therapy (HRT). However, when IL-1 is measured by immunoradiometric assays, no direct relationship between IL-1 and bone mass is noted. This has caused some authors to suggest that the impact of IL-1 on bone turnover may reflect the balance between IL-1 and IL-1 receptor antagonist *(24)*, although in vivo studies to confirm of this hypothesis studies have yielded conflicting results *(25)*. In addition, there appears to be a host of other local and systemic factors that may regulate the local bone milieu.

There are also physiologic changes with aging that result in bone loss in the elderly. There is evidence that the extent and depth of the resorption cavity increases with aging leading to cortical thinning and increased porosity of bone. There is also evidence of decreased osteoblastic recruitment with a reduction in the quantity of bone formed per remodeling cycle. This can result in progressive loss of bone mass even when the activation frequency is not increased or, in fact, when activation may be diminished.

Local changes in remodeling can have a profound effect upon calcium balance. This also differs between early menopause and the elderly. In early menopause, the accelerated bone resorption results in a transient increase in the serum calcium, which subse-

Table 3
Classification of Involutional Osteoporosis

	Type I	Type II
Name	Postmenopausal	Senile
Age	50–74	>75
Type of bone loss	Cancellous	Cancellous and cortical
Fractures	Vertebrate, radius	Hip, long bones
PTH	Decreased	Increased

quent suppresses parathyroid hormone (PTH) release. As PTH is the regulator of 1-alpha hydroxylase activity, this results in a decrease in circulating 1,25 dihydroxy vitamin D $(1,25(OH)_2D)$ resulting in decreased enteral calcium absorption and increased urinary calcium losses.

In contrast, with advancing age, declines in renal function lead to an inability to adequately form $1,25(OH)_2D$. This results in a decrease in enteral calcium absorption and a compensatory increase in PTH. This secondary hyperparathyroidism then stimulates bone remodeling by increasing osteoclastic activation and further contributes to the development of osteoporosis by increasing the remodeling rate in the setting of low bone formation.

As a result of these changes in bone remodeling, there is a net loss of bone mass *(26)*. Cross-sectional studies suggest that bone loss can begin as early as 10–15 yr prior to menopause. Significant apparent decreases in bone mass of 7–10% have been detected at cancellous bone sites only (lateral spine and Ward's triangle). As estrogen levels fall at menopause, bone loss is accentuated at all skeletal sites. This rapid decrease in bone mass within the first 10 yr of menopause is followed by a slower phase of loss over the next 10–15 yr. In the elderly (more than 25 yr postmenopause), the rate of loss increases again, potentially reflecting the impact of age-related secondary hyperparathyroidism on bone loss.

As a result of these changes in bone mass, the fracture incidence increases. The distribution of fractures reflects the preferential loss of cancellous bone in early menopause. This is demonstrated by the increased incidence of wrist fractures at the age of 50 followed by an increased incidence of vertebral fractures in the 60s. In contrast, hip fractures, a site containing larger amounts of cortical bone, are not seen until well into the 70s *(27)*.

When looking at the development of osteoporosis in a postmenopausal woman, it is important to be aware of the unique impact that both menopause and aging can have on bone loss. This can be conceptually stratified into two types of involutional osteoporosis based upon the pathophysiologic and clinical presentation (Table 3).

RISK FACTORS

Many factors have been described that may impact on the increased bony fragility and fractures characteristic of osteoporosis. These can be divided into factors that affect bone mineral density, microarchitecture, bone geometry, and the risk for falls.

Low bone mass, itself an independent risk factor for fracture *(28–33)*, is multifactorial *(34–36)*. Traditional lists of risk factors that affect BMD can be divided into those factors that are modifiable and nonmodifiable (Table 4). Determinants of BMD are principally

Table 4
Risk Factors for Low Bone Mass

Nonmodifiable	Modifiable
• Advancing age	• Negative calcium balance (nutrition)
• Body habitus	— inadequate calcium intake
— low body weight	— increased protein intake
• Genetic Predisposition	— increased sodium intake
— female gender	— increase caffeine intake
— white or Asian	• Gonadal steroid deficiency
— familial prevalence	— premature menopause
• Allelic polymorphism	— late menarche
— vitamin D receptor	— 1° or 2° amenorrhea
— estrogen receptor	anorexia
— apolipoprotein E	exercise-induced
— type 1 collagen a1	• Lifestyle
	— cigarettes
	— alcohol
	— reduced physical activity

genetic. Heritability account for up to 46–62% of the variance in BMD even after adjustment for age, weight, height, and lifestyle (35,37,38). Studies in twins, relatives of individuals with osteoporosis, adult children and parents, and growing children with parents and grandparents have all confirmed this observation (37,39,40). This genetic impact appears to affect acquisition of bone mass as serum osteocalcin, a marker of osteoblast function, is strongly dependent on genetically determined factors where as markers of bone resorption and rates of bone loss appear to have little genetic effect (41).

There have been intense research efforts directed at elucidating specific genetic polymorphisms or gene mutations that might play a role in stratifying at-risk individuals. Morrison et al. first reported several common restriction fragment length polymorphisms (RFLP) for the vitamin D receptor gene associated with BMD and bone loss (42). Not all subsequent studies have confirmed these results (43,52). A recent meta-analysis of 16 studies involving approx 3600 subjects confirmed that the *BsmI* BB genotype is associated with a 2.4% lower BMD at the hip and a 2.5% lower BMD at the spine when compared to individuals with the bb genotype (53). As estrogen plays a major role in the regulation of bone turnover, it has also been examined closely. A specific dinucleotide repeat polymorphism (12 TA repeats) located 1174 base pairs upstream of exon-I in the human estrogen receptor gene (ER) has been reported to be associated with significantly lower lumbar spine and whole body Z scores and higher markers of bone turnover (osteocalcin, pyridinoline, and deoxypyridinoline) when compared to women without this allele (54). In addition, a specific combination allele of a RFLP at a Pvu-II and Xba-I site, between intron-I and exon-II of the ER gene (PPxx) is also associated with low bone mass (55). Recently, allelic variation of the apolipoprotein E (ApoE) gene has been associated with low BMD in Japanese women who have at least 1 ApoE4 allele (56). All of these observations require additional confirmation in large population studies to determine their potential clinical significance.

Genetic polymorphism has also been associated with a lower bone mass and a greater incidence of fractures. Polymorphism at a recognition site for the transcription factor SP₁ in the type-I collagen gene is associated with lower BMD and a higher risk of vertebral fractures in comparison to controls *(57)*. The range of genes identified in these preliminary studies and the large number of other candidate genes that are being investigated at this time suggest that it is unlikely that a single gene will contribute more than a small part to the variance of this multifactorial disease *(19)*.

Body weight is the next greatest determinant of bone mass in adults and accounts for 15–20% of variance in BMD *(35,36,58,59)*. Only 3% of women greater than 70 kg will have osteoporosis. Although debate has raged over the relative impact of percent body fat versus lean body mass, data suggest that percent fat may play a greater role for the prevention of osteoporosis as it can contribute to higher estrone values and thus, slower rates of bone loss.

A reduction in estrogen levels, such as occurs at menopause, can result in an increased rate of bone loss. Premature menopause causes bone loss to occur at an earlier chronologic age, extending the length of time in life a woman may have significant osteopenia or osteoporosis *(60)*. Secondary amenorrhea in adolescents and young women can occur with anorexia nervosa or excessive exercise and causes bone loss during a time of life when bone mass should be reaching its peak. In contrast, the use of oral contraceptives may slightly increase bone mass. Parity and lactation appear to have no significant impact on BMD *(61)*.

The mechanism of the negative effects of smoking *(62,63)* and alcohol *(64)* have not been entirely elucidated. Women who smoke become menopausal at a younger age and smoking appears to increase the metabolism of estrogens. In fact, a previous study on HRT and hip fracture incidence showed no reduction in hip fractures in women who use HRT, but continue to smoke. Alcohol is directly toxic to the osteoblast and increases urinary calcium losses. The threshold at which alcohol is deleterious has not been defined.

Reduced physical activity, as seen with bed rest or neurologic injury, can dramatically decrease bone mass, but even a lack of regular exercise can contribute to a reduction in bone mass. This may be most important during the acquisition of peak bone mass in adolescence *(65,66)*. Mechanical strain, increased by physical activity, modulates the osteoblastic response. This follows the principles of Wolfe's law, which states that both mass and distribution of mass (structure) will be modified in response to the perceived loads imposed on it.

Nutrition plays a major role in the pathogenesis of osteoporosis through impacting calcium balance. Calcium is the principal cation in bone and serves as the reserve of calcium utilized to meet calcium requirements when either calcium intake is low or enhanced calcium losses result in a negative calcium balance. Low calcium intake in childhood is associated with an increased risk of osteoporosis later in life and an increased risk of fractures as early as the adolescent years *(67,68)*. Epidemiologic studies have confirmed that lifelong calcium intake is correlated with BMD at all ages *(69)*. Factors that adversely affect calcium balance can also increase the risk for low BMD. In addition to low calcium intake, excessively high protein or sodium intake can all lead to an increased risk for low BMD because of an increase in calciuria.

Bone geometry has a significant impact on fracture risk. A short hip-axis length (defined as the distance from the lateral surface of the trochanter to the inner surface of the pelvis over the axis of the femoral neck) results in a geometrically stronger structure for a given bone density *(70)*. This may be a plausible explanation for the low incidence of hip fractures in Oriental women compared to Caucasians despite equivalent BMD

Table 5
Risk Factors for Fracture Independent of BMD

	Prevalence	Relative Risk[a]
Family history fracture[b]	0.07	1.30
Current smoker	0.10	1.50
Prior history fracture[c]	0.37	1.40
Thin (<57.8 kg)	0.25	1.20

[a]RR if have factors vs if do not have factors adjusted for hip BMD and age.
[b]Fracture in first degree relative after age 50 of wrist, spine or hip.
[c]Any fracture after age 40.

values. Large vertebral end plates result in lower spine pressures and may be associated with a decrease in the risk for spine fracture (71). Finally, the correlation of height on osteoporotic fracture can be explained, in part, by geometric properties as the force sustained by bone during a fall is a function of height.

As the risk of fracture is a function of both the strength of bone and the force applied to bone, factors that increase the risk of falling also contribute to the risk of osteoporotic fracture (72–74). Generalized weakness, poor visual function (decreased depth perception), and certain medications (long-acting benzodiazepines and anticonvulsants) increase the risk of a significant fall, both by increasing the probability of the fall and decreasing the ability of the individual to use protective reflexes. Cigarettes may also increase the risk of fractures because smokers have poorer neuromuscular function (72,75). Studies have also shown that the direction of fall (to the side) may increase the risk of fracture, independent of BMD.

Combinations of risk factors (excluding genetics), however, account for only 20–40% of the variability in bone-mass risk factor assessment and have limited clinical utility in predicting who has osteopenia or osteoporosis (35,59,76–79). It is, therefore, best used to serve as a segue to initiate counseling as a critical part of preventive care. Recently, 16 specific risk factors have been identified that independently increase the risk for fractures in addition to low BMD (14,80). Fout specific risk factors have been utilized by the National Osteoporosis Foundation (NOF) that may help to further define an at-risk population for fracture (Table 5) (14). Women who have had a previous vertebral or nonvertebral fracture are at increased risk for a subsequent fracture independent of bone density (72,81,82). A history of fracture is defined as any fracture occurring since age 40. Low body weight, defined as a weight 57.8 kg (127 lbs), is predictive of bone mass and hip fracture (83,84). Weight loss is also associated with an increased risk of fracture (85). Cigarette smokers have increased rates of bone loss and a greater risk for fracture than nonsmokers or past smokers (59,72,86–88). Finally, as more than half of the variability in bone mass and potential fracture is because of genetic factors (35,37). a family history of a fracture at the wrist, spine, or hip in a first-degree relative after age 50 is also associated with an increased risk for fracture. These risk factors should be used in concert with BMD to help to determine the appropriate therapeutic intervention.

SECONDARY CAUSES

Although 80–85% of women with osteoporosis will have bone loss because of either menopause or age-related factors, there are many other medical conditions that can

Table 6
Secondary Causes of Osteoporosis

Endocrine
— Hyperparathyroidism
— Thyrotoxicosis
— Cushing's syndrome
— Type I diabetes
— Hyperprolactinemia
— Anorexia nervosa
— Acromegaly
Rheumatologic
— Rheumatoid arthritis
— Osteogenesis imperfecta
— Ehlers-Danlos syndrome
— Marfan syndrome
Gastroenterology
— Malabsorption syndrome
— Malnutrition
— Glucocorticoid
Hematologic
— Thalassemia
— Multiple myeloma
— Leukemia/lymphoma

Other
— Radiation
— Immobilization
— Systemic mastocytosis
— Renal tubular acidosis
— Hypoxemia
Drug
— Thyroid hormone
— Glucocorticoid
— Anticoagulants
— Chronic lithium
— GnRH agonists and antagonist
— Anticonvulsants
— Extended tetracycline
— Cyclosporine A

contribute to accentuated bone loss and the development of osteoporosis (Table 6). Most secondary causes of osteoporosis reflect an increased rate or amount of bone resorption, although several specific diseases (most notably Cushing's syndrome) are associated with diminished rates of bone formation. A number of medications have also been associated with osteoporosis. These include pharmacologic agents that contribute to enhanced urinary calcium losses (loop diuretics), increased vitamin D degradation (anticonvulsants), increased bone resorption (excessive thyroid hormone or cyclosporine A), diminished bone formation (glucocorticoids), or reset of the PTH set-point (lithium).

CLINICAL EVALUATION

A medical history and physical and gynecologic evaluation should be performed on each woman as part of her evaluation for the prevention and treatment of osteoporosis. The medical history should emphasize questions designed to assess factors that could affect the acquisition of peak bone mass, accelerate bone loss, or increase the risk of fractures independent of BMD. In addition, it should exclude the presence of diseases that can contribute to secondary osteoporosis.

The physical examination should focus on excluding secondary causes of osteoporosis and defining the extent of disease that is already present. As vertebral fractures are always associated with loss of height, measurement of height by means of a wall-mounted stadiometer should be performed annually. Thoracic vertebral fractures can result in increasing dorsal kyphosis whereas lumbar spine fractures result in flattening of the normal lumbar lordotic curve. With progressive osteoporotic deformity, the abdomen becomes more protuberant and eventually the ribs may rest on the iliac crest.

Unfortunately, most women at risk for osteoporosis will have no signs or symptoms suggestive of osteoporosis. Thus, diagnostic testing is necessary to determine the presence and extent of disease.

DIAGNOSTIC TESTING FOR OSTEOPOROSIS

Radiologic Studies

Osteoporosis can be detected with standard radiographs by using a number of specific features, but cannot be quantitated to use in the serial follow-up for progression of bone loss as the images are qualitative, not quantitative *(89)*. Trabecular bone resorption can lead to thinning and dissolution of transverse trabecula with relative preservation of trabecula oriented along the stress lines. This produces a striated appearance of bone on the X-ray. Loss of trabecular bone can also be seen as accentuation of cortical end plates with a relative increase in central lucency. In the appendicular skeleton, osteoporosis can be seen as thinning of the cortices with widening of the medullary cavity. The diagnosis of osteopenia is most commonly suggested by increased lucency of bone. This determination of osteopenia, however, is very insensitive as up to 20–30% of bone mass may be lost before a decrease in bone density is noted. As the degree of "demineralization" can be overestimated, it is also very inaccurate when the radiograph is overexposed.

Therefore, the role of X-rays in the diagnosis of osteoporosis is to assess the potential presence of a fracture or to exclude other etiologies for localized skeletal symptoms. The presence of one vertebral fracture increases the risk of a new vertebral fracture up to fivefold whereas two or more vertebral fractures increase the risk 12-fold.

The gold standard for the diagnosis of osteoporosis is the measurement of bone mineral density. BMD is both a surrogate for the definition of osteoporosis and an independent risk factor for fracture *(28–33,92–95)*. After adjusting for age, a one-standard deviation decrease in BMD at the lumbar spine, trochanter, or femoral neck is significantly related to the incidence of all fractures (relative risks of 1.4, 1.2, and 1.3, respectively) *(92)*. Although there is consensus about the utility of BMD in assessing the skeletal status, there is considerable debate about which measurement method, site and strategy should be used. Currently, available techniques vary in precision, accessibility, and discrimination (Table 7) *(4)*.

Radiographic absorptiometry (RA) was one of the first quantitative techniques to assess bone mass at sites containing mixed cortical and trabecular bone. In RA, hand radiographs are taken with an aluminum step wedge and BMD is calibrated relative to the aluminum wedge in arbitrary units *(96)*. The metacarpals or phalanges are typically measured. Used longitudinally, RA detects loss of bone in normal women age 22–79 comparable to that observed using spine and radial dual energy X-ray absorptiometry (DXA) *(97)*.

Single energy X-ray absorptiometry can make a quantitative assessment of bone mineral content (BMC) at peripheral sites of the distal or ultradistal radius or calcaneus *(98)*. A highly collimated beam from an X-ray tube is used to measure radiation attenuation across the specific skeletal site. Separation of trabecular and cortical bone is not possible with this technique. In an attempt to enhance discrimination of the impact of bone loss in cortical and trabecular bone, measurements of the radial shaft (95% cortical bone) and ultradistal radius (up to 45% trabecular bone) are often used.

Single energy measurements are not valid at sites with variable soft-tissue thickness. To assess bone loss at sites such as the spine and femur, which are the locations of the most

Table 7
Diagnostic Tests for Osteoporosis

Technique[a]	Site	Precision Error	Accuracy Error	Radiation (mrad)	% Loss bone/yr[b]
RA	Phalanx	1–2	5	5	0.51 ± .06
SXA	Radius, calcaneus	1–2	4–6	<1	—
DXA	Spine (PA)	1–15	4–10	~1	0.30 ± 0.03
	Spine (lat)	2–3	5–15	~3	0.58 ± 0.06
	Femur	1.5–3	6	~1	0.53 ~ 0.04c
QCT[d]	Spine	2–4	5–15	50	1.18 ± .06
QUS[e]	Calcaneus	1.3–3.8	?	0	0.52 ± 0.03

[a]RA, radioabsorptiometry; SXA, single energy X-ray absorptiometry; DXA, dual energy X-ray absorptiometry; QCT, quantitative computed tomography; QUS, quantitative ultrasound.

[b]Percent change in bone mass relative to predicted values at age 30. Data modified from Grampp S, Genant HK, Monthur A, et al. Comparisons of noninvasive bone mineral measurements in assessing age-related loss, fracture discrimination and diagnostic classification. J Bone Miner Res 1997;12:697–711.

[c]Femoral neck data only.

[d]QCT of trabecular bone of vertebrate.

[e]Broad-band ultrasound attenuation data only.

prevalent and clinically important fractures, dual energy X-ray absorptiometry (DXA) was developed (99). DXA uses two beams of distinct energy to correct for differential soft-tissue photon attenuation. DXA allows for measurement of bone mass in the axial skeleton, peripheral skeleton, or total body. The results are expressed in bone mineral content or areal BMD (gm/cm^2). It has excellent measurement precision and a low accuracy error that allows for serial follow-up for monitoring therapeutic efficacy. It has become the most widely used clinical technique for assessment of osteoporosis.

Quantitative computed tomography (QCT) is the only diagnostic method that can determine true volumetric density. In addition, it can isolate trabecular and cortical bone content. It has an in vivo precision error of 2–4% and an accuracy error of 5–15% that are much higher than the errors reported for DXA. However, its greater sensitivity in detecting trabecular bone loss has made it valuable as a research tool. Although it is potentially widely available as it can be performed on a standard clinical CT scanner, the high-radiation dose and cost have resulted in limited clinical use.

Recently, quantitative ultrasound (QUS) has been developed as a measure of bone quality. Measurements of ultrasound transmission velocity, the frequency dependency of alteration of ultrasound signal and Young's modulus are influenced by trabecular separation, connectivity, and elasticity, respectively. As osteoporosis is a disease characterized by both reduction in bone mass and changes in architecture, if studies continue to support the ability of QUS to discriminate structural properties in osteoporosis, it will be an important adjunct to the measure of BMD for the assessment of fracture risk. QUS also has widespread appeal as a potential screening device because of its low cost, ease of use, and lack of radiation exposure.

All the techniques described readily differentiate between premenopausal and postmenopausal subjects and reflect age and menopause-related bone loss (4). QCT appears to demonstrate the greatest sensitivity for discrimination between normal and osteoporotic women, followed by DXA of the lateral spine and DXA of the PA spine (97). In addition, multiple studies have shown that BMD at any specific site shows at least modest correlation with other skeletal sites *(98–101)*, which is not surprising given that osteoporosis is a generalized metabolic disease. In a study of postmenopausal women age 65 yr and older, these correlations ranged from 0.5 to 0.8 at the spine, regions of the hip, and forearm *(101)*. As rates of bone loss differ at different skeletal sites, however, the correlations decreased with advancing age.

Given the modest correlation of BMD measured by different techniques and at different sites, the diagnostic agreement of different measurements in classifying women as osteoporotic is poor *(97)*. Using measurements at the spine, hip, and forearm, each measure fails to detect 100% of the patients who meet a diagnosis of osteoporosis based on WHO criteria.

So, what site and what technique should be used to assess BMD? Clinically, it is known that, early in menopause, measurements at the spine will detect a greater number of women with postmenopausal osteoporosis than measurements at the hip. Later in life, the proportion of patients with osteoporosis detected by bone-mass measurements at the hip and the forearm is greater than the proportion identified by a posterior–anterior spine DXA. The BMD at this latter site can be falsely elevated with age because of degenerative bony changes in the spine or calcification of the aorta. In addition, there are abundant data that show that measurements of any skeletal site have some utility in predicting fractures. However, hip BMD is the best predictor of hip fracture and appears to predict all other types of fractures equally as well as measurements made at any other skeletal sites *(30)*. Therefore, BMD at the hip would be an adequate measurement for assessment of risk in postmenopausal women, although the addition of a measurement of spine BMD to assess the early cancellous bone loss in the perimenopause or early menopause may also be warranted.

BMD should be ordered to make an assessment of fracture risk and thus, risk for osteoporosis when the information obtained from the test will affect a treatment decision. Measurement of BMD can be especially helpful in the care of the perimenopausal woman to stratify her risk for osteoporosis and facilitate the decision of whether to begin hormone replacement therapy. DXA may also be indicated to diagnose osteoporosis in an individual in whom osteoporosis is suspected or in whom an atraumatic fracture is noted on radiograph. It can also be used to assess the course of metabolic diseases (e.g., hyperparathyroidism, Cushing's disease, chronic renal failure, etc.) or medications (chronic glucocorticoid therapy, thyroid hormone supplement) that can affect the skeleton.

Follow-up DXA can also be used to monitor the effectiveness of treatment in preventing further bone loss. Based on the precision error of DXA, a change in BMD of 5% must be seen to be considered as clinically significant. Except for cases where secondary osteoporosis results in very rapid losses of bone or in the very early part of menopause, a 5% change is generally not observed in less than 2 yr.

Recent studies have also suggested that measures of BMD have a significant impact on patient compliance with preventive and therapeutic regimens when used to facilitate the decision to prescribe a treatment course for osteoporosis at menopause *(102,103)*. However, knowledge of bone mass can also cause a woman to reduce her physical activity because of an increased fear of falling *(104)*. Appropriate counseling regarding the meaning of a BMD assessment is crucial in the care of women with osteopenia or osteoporosis. If DXA improves compliance, or if the unit course of the drug prescribed for the prevention or treatment osteoporosis is higher than that of hormone replacement, the use of DXA in the perimenopause to stratify which women should be treated has been shown to be cost-effective *(103)*.

Biochemical Assessment

Biochemical testing for renal and hepatic function, a complete blood count, electrolytes, and calcium, magnesium, and phosphorus should be obtained on patients before initiating therapy. In uncomplicated involutional osteoporosis, all of these laboratory studies will be normal. In addition, a urinalysis with specific attention to urine pH may help to exclude renal tubular acidosis. In individuals whose hip or wrist BMD is substantially lower than the spine BMD, measurement of an intact PTH would be appropriate. If accelerated bone loss relative to age-matched controls is noted (Z score on DXA <– 2.0), additional testing for secondary causes of osteoporosis as suggested by the history and physical examination should be performed.

It might be predicted that markers of bone turnover would be helpful for assessing osteoporosis as this heterogeneous disease reflects an imbalance between the rate of bone resorption and formation. Specific biomarkers of resorption (urinary N-telopeptide, pyridinoline, and deoxypyridinoline) and markers of formation (osteocalcin, bone-specific alkaline phosphatase) have been useful in research studies on metabolic bone disease *(105,106).* Theoretically, markers of bone resorption and formation should be useful to determine who should preferentially begin treatment when BMD is borderline and to choose between agents that are antiresorptive or stimulate bone formation. Unfortunately, however, markers of bone resorption have not been helpful in delineating who is likely to respond to treatment and to not correlate strongly with BMD response in an individual. Urinary markers of bone resorption have great day-to-day variability (up to 30%) and are affected by multiple factors including time of collection, season, diet, and exercise *(106,107).* Correction of the biomarkers to creatinine excretion and careful timing of the collection has improved the error.

The current use of biomarkers of resorption may be to monitor response to therapy. A decrease in bone resorption markers by 30% within 3 mo of initiating an antiresorptive treatment has been demonstrated to be related to improvements in BMD after 2 yr of treatment. This allows for potential adjustment in doses early in the treatment course long before such decisions can be made on the basis of BMD changes. More recently, preliminary data suggest that markers of bone resorption may predict risk of fracture-independent BMD *(108,109).* As more sensitive and specific tests of bone resorption are developed, and if subsequent studies confirm these initial observations, combining the measurement of BMD with bone resorption markers may help to improve the assessment of fracture risk in elderly women.

PRIMARY PREVENTION

The goal of primary prevention is to maximize attainment of peak bone mass and minimize rates of bone loss after menopause and with aging. Prevention strategies should include the avoidance of cigarettes and alcohol, minimizing the use of medications that contribute to accelerated bone loss or a negative calcium balance, assurance of an adequate calcium intake, and a regular exercise program. These recommendations are appropriate for all individuals throughout their lifespan.

Calcium and Vitamin D

An adequate calcium intake is necessary for the attainment of the genetic potential for peak bone mass and to decrease calcium deficiency-associated losses of bone. Calcium can suppress PTH-induced bone remodeling and is necessary for maintenance of an adequate ion product for mineralization of bone. Calcium supplements in children has a small impact on increasing bone mass *(110)*. However, when these supplements are discontinued, the apparent benefit is lost and within one year, the child's BMD is indistinguishable from their nonsupplemented peers *(111)*. When calcium supplements are used within the first 5 yr of menopause, it has no substantial impact on decreasing rates of bone loss *(112)*. This is probably because of the fact that bone loss in early menopause primarily reflects the effect of estrogen deficiency.

In elderly women, the pathophysiology of bone loss is due to different factors. Vitamin D deficiency, and thus, secondary hyperparathyroidism with accentuated loss of cortical bone is common in elderly women *(113,114)*. This may be because of, in part, a decreased milk intake and decreased sunlight exposure. In addition, vitamin D deficiency is further exacerbated during the winter months *(115)*. However, even without decreased calcidiol levels, mild increases in PTH are associated with an increase in hip fractures. In response to these changes, randomized prospective, controlled clinical trials of calcium, and vitamin D supplements in the elderly have shown that calcium is effective in decreasing rates of bone loss *(112,116–118)* and if given concurrently with vitamin D, it may also reduce the incidence of hip fractures by 25% *(119,120)* or overall fractures by 50% *(121)*.

The National Institutes of Health Consensus Conference recommended an optimal daily calcium intake of 1000 mg/d for postmenopausal women on HRT and 1500 mg/d of calcium for postmenopausal women not on HRT women *(122)*. As the average dietary calcium intake of an older U.S. citizen is 600 mg/d, the majority of these individuals do not meet these recommendations. Calcium is a threshold nutrient and at fully adequate intake, further increases in calcium will not result in additional skeletal benefit. The maximal tolerable level of calcium intake is 2.5 gm/d.

If modifications in the diet cannot successfully meet these recommended allowances, calcium supplements may be utilized. Calcium carbonate is the most commonly prescribed calcium source because of low cost and the high percentage of elemental calcium per pill. Since calcium carbonate is not effectively absorbed in individuals with achlorhydria, calcium citrate may be preferred in individuals who are medically treated for gastro-esophageal reflux or ulcers. Achlorhydria can occur in elderly individuals, and for women over the age of 70, calcium citrate might be preferred. Calcium supplements should be used in divided doses (<600 mg/dose) to enhance absorption or given at night to reduce the PTH-mediated calcium mobilization and excretion that occurs with fasting in a supine position. The most common side effect of calcium carbonate is constipation *(123)*. Although kidney stones and hypercalcemia are potential side effects of calcium supplementation, this is usually only seen in very high doses (>5 gm/d) or in persons with underlying disorders of calcium metabolism.

For women in early menopause, 400 U/d of vitamin D may help facilitate calcium absorption. If individuals increase their calcium intake through increased milk consumption, this will also increase their vitamin D intake by 100 IU/serving. In the elderly, there is some suggestion that the vitamin D requirement is higher and supplements of 800 IU/d may be appropriate. However, as some elderly individuals have a 1-alpha hydroxylase defect or end-organ resistance, calcitriol (0.25–0.50 μg/d) may be necessary.

Exercise

Increases in biomechanical strain can increase osteoblastic action and exercise in children can produce larger bones with a higher BMD *(124,125)*. The effect is greatest in young children and appears to be diminished by adolescence *(126)*. Sustained benefits of exercise-induced changes in children can be noted many years after exercise has been discontinued *(127,128)*. Cross-sectional studies have shown that athletes have greater bone mass than nonathletes with the greatest gain in bone mass seen at the skeletal sites that are affected by loading (e.g., greater BMC in the serving arm of professional tennis players) *(129)*. Prospective randomized exercise trials using strength and endurance activities have reported small, but significant, positive effects on lumbar spine BMD in young women *(130,131)* and in older men and women *(132–134)*. Walking, the most commonly recommended exercise for osteoporosis, has not been shown in prospective trials to decrease rates of bone loss *(135)*. Exercise benefits on BMD may be additive with antiresorptive regimens such as estrogen *(136)*.

As the gains in bone mass are, at most, modest, one of the primary benefits of exercise has been to decrease the risk of falls by improving neuromuscular function *(137)*. There are no definitive exercise trials to assess the impact of exercise on reducing fracture incidence. However, one small study comparing vertebral extension versus flexion exercises suggested that a higher incidence of osteoporosis compression fractures occur with flexion activities *(138)*.

The most effective exercise regimen for the prevention of bone loss has been high-load resistance training with a focus on exercises specifically targeting areas at risk for osteoporotic fracture. Other effective strategies include high-impact aerobics, walk-jog-dance regimens, and stationary cycling. Exercise must be performed for 30–60 min/d at least three times per week. However, since compliance with long-term exercise regimens is <50%, any increase in physical activity that will be done consistently should be encouraged. When exercise is discontinued, any gains in bone mass achieved with activity are quickly lost.

SECONDARY PREVENTION

The goal of secondary prevention is to prevent additional bone loss in an individual who already has evidence of early changes in bone mass. Treatment goals include elimination of iatrogenic and environmental factors that can accelerate bone loss; aggressive treatment of an underlying etiology, if one is detected, and the initiation of an appropriate pharmacologic intervention (*see* Table 8). Treatment choices for secondary prevention are often based upon the severity of osteoporosis, and the NOF guidelines utilize a combination of BMD and risk factors for recommendation regarding the initiation of specific pharmacologic agents.

Hormone Replacement Therapy

The gold standard for the treatment of postmenopausal osteoporosis is estrogen replacement therapy (ERT) *(139)*. Estrogen works as an antiresorptive compound *(140)* through modulating cytokine release. It decreases bone turnover *(141)* through decreasing osteoclast activation *(142)* and shortening the osteoclast life cycle *(143)*. It results in thickening of compact bone and reduction in intracortical porosity[144], but does not reverse the structural disruption that occurs prior to its initiation. Second, it corrects menopause-induced changes in calcium balance resulting in an increase in renal-tubular calcium reabsorption, enteral calcium absorption, and increases in 1,25 dihydroxy vitamin D *(145)*.

Table 8

Treatment Options for Postmenopausal Osteoporosis

Enhance Calcium Balance	Antiresorptive	Anabolic
Calcium	Estrogen	Exercise
Vitamin D	Calcitonin	Fluoride[b]
Calcitriol[a]	Alendronate	Growth
Thiazide	Etidronate	hormone
	Risedronate[b]	PTH
	Ibidronate[b]	
	Pamidronate	
	Tamoxifen	
	Raloxifene	

[a]Medication in italics are FDA-approved for some applications, but currently under study for osteoporosis.
[b]Under active investigation—not clinically available.

ERT can prevent bone loss *(146–150)* and reduce the incidence of vertebral and hip fractures by 70 and 50%, respectively *(151–154)*. Estrogen has traditionally been said to be most effective when started within the first several years of menopause. However, it may be possible to start later in life as recent data suggest no difference in BMD at the age of 70 between women who start HRT at menopause and those who start almost 10 yr later at age 60 *(155)*. Studies have shown that HRT is able to prevent bone loss even when started at the age of 65 *(156,157)*.

ERT may be utilized for either primary or secondary prevention of osteoporosis and a choice to initiate therapy may be based upon the initial bone mass and an assessment of the relative risk-to-benefit ratio for the individual *(158)*. Other potential benefits of HRT include a decrease in vasomotor symptoms, a reduction in genitourinary atrophy and a reduction in coronary heart disease incidence and mortality. There appears to be minimal attenuation of cardiovascular benefit with the addition of a progestin *(159)*.

Data for the PEPI trial *(160)* indicate that 98% of women who receive a dose of 0.625 mg of conjugated equine estrogen (CEE) or equivalent have vertebral bone loss of <1%/yr. When ERT is discontinued, there is an accelerated "catch-up" rate of bone loss and within 10 yr after discontinuation, the risk for hip fracture is identical to women who never used ERT *(146,161)*. Progesterone with either a cyclical or continuous regimen is utilized to reduce the incidence of endometrial cancer. BMD appears to increase to a slightly greater extent in women receiving continuous combined versus sequential therapy, and the compliance is somewhat greater *(162)*. In individuals who have undergone a hysterectomy, a progestin should not be added as there is no evidence that this results in an independent benefit on changes in bone mass or fracture risk.

Among the adverse effects associated with estrogen replacement is irregular vaginal bleeding, which can occur in women on the estrogen/progestin regimen. In addition, fluid retention, breast tenderness, abdominal pain, and headaches may occur. These symptoms are often associated with progesterone and may be improved by lowering the dosage. The greatest concern about long-term estrogen use continues to be regarding the relationship of estrogen and a possible increase in breast cancer risk. Although several studies have found no increase in breast cancer, long-term (>10 yr of estrogen) use appears to increase the risk of breast cancer by approx 36% *(158)*. The addition of progestin does not reduce the risk of breast cancer. The definitive answer regarding the risk-to-benefit ratio for HRT should be forthcoming from the results of the Women's Health Initiative (WHI).

ERT should be the first line agent for the prevention and treatment of osteoporosis. It is contraindicated in women who have postmenopausal bleeding of an unknown cause, an estrogen-dependent neoplasm (breast cancer, endometrial cancer, and malignant melanoma), or a history of thromboembolic disease.

The selective-estrogen-receptor modulators, tamoxifen and raloxifene, are likely to have a major impact on the prevention and treatment of osteoporosis. Tamoxifen given at doses of 20 mg/d can prevent bone loss at the lumbar spine and total body in the first year of treatment, but there was no further separation from the control group in the second year. In addition, there was no significant decline in the rate of bone loss noted at the proximal femur. Tamoxifen produced significant decreases in markers of bone resorption and formation consistent with an antiresorptive effect. It has been concluded that tamoxifen has a small protective effect on BMD comparable to the magnitude of calcium supplementation, but less than that of estrogen or the bisphosphonates. Its clinical utility is greatest for the prevention of osteoporosis in women with breast cancer requiring adjuvant therapy for secondary chemoprevention. Additional limitations to the long-term use of tamoxifen included an increased risk for the development of endometrial cancer and an increase in vasomotor symptoms.

The new selective-estrogen-receptor modulator, raloxifene, has tissue-specific estrogen agonist effects that result in a decrease in the rate of bone loss and improvements in lipid status with estrogen antagonistic effects at the breast and uterus. In clinical trials. raloxifene was less effective at reducing bone resorption, but had a lesser suppressive effect on bone formation than estrogen. Raloxifene was approved for the prevention of osteoporosis in late 1997 and is an option for women who cannot, or will not, take ERT because of concerns about the side-effect profile of estrogen. Recent data have also confirmed a significant decrease in the incidenc of new vertebral fractures. The recommended dose of raloxifene is 60 mg/d. Women who are perimenopausal are not candidates for a SERM due to potential adverse effects on the fetus. The drug is also contra-indicated in women with a past history of thromboembolic disease. Adverse effects include an increased incidence of hot flashes and leg cramps.

Calcitonin

For women who cannot, or will not, take ERT, or a SERM, there are several other antiresorptive options. Synthetic calcitonin, taken as either a subcutaneous injection or nasal spray, is FDA-approved for the treatment of osteoporosis. Calcitonin inhibits osteoclastic bone resorption directly, thus reducing rates of bone loss *(163)*. Randomized clinical trials have shown that both parenteral and nasal spray calcitonin prevent trabecular and cortical bone loss *(164–168)*. Interim analyses of a 5-yr trial of nasal spray calcitonin shows that 200 U/d reduces the risk of new vertebral fractures by 37% relative to placebo [95% confidence interval (0.403 to 0.971, $p = 0.037$] and decreases the risk for new and/or worsening vertebral fractures by 29% *(169)*. Analgesic effects of calcitonin have been found to significantly reduce osteoporotic bone pain in fracture subjects treated with subcutaneous calcitonin when compared with controls *(170)*. This may be associated with an increase in endorphins.

The recommended dose of calcitonin is 200 U intranasally daily (alternating nostrils) or 50–100 U parenterally 3–7 d/wk. The most common side effects of nasal spray calcitonin are rhinorrhea or nasal dryness. The side-effect profile associated with parenteral calcitonin includes dermatologic hypersensitivity, facial flushing, nausea, and anorexia. These side effects are not seen with nasal spray calcitonin. Although calcitonin can be used for any individual who is not a candidate for ERT, its greatest clinical utility is in the management of patients with severe osteoporosis, vertebral fractures, and increased pain *(171)*.

Bisphosphonates

Bisphosphonates are analogs of pyrophosphate in which the oxygen of pyrophosphate has been replaced by a carbon to create a stable therapeutic compound. Bisphosphonates inhibit osteoclastic bone resorption and through their ability to bind to hydroxyapetite, they can also inhibit crystal dissolution and aggregate formation. They appear to shift the balance between resorption and formation to favor small, but significant increases in bone mass.

Bisphosphonates are skeletal-specific and any drug not taken up by the skeleton is renally excreted unchanged. It has a long skeletal retention, but only that drug that is on the cell surface has antiresorptive effects. When given at a high concentration over an extended period of time, the early generation bisphosphonates (e.g., etidronate) interfere with mineralization of newly formed bone *(172)*. To ensure safety, these must thus be administered in cyclical regimens. The new aminobisphosphonates are more potent analogs and can be administered in lower doses that inhibit resorption, but do not inhibit mineralization *(173)*.

Alendronate is the first nonhormonal treatment for osteoporosis approved by the FDA. At doses of 10 mg/d, alendronate increases BMD at the spine and total hip by 7.21 and 5.27%, respectively, over a 2-yr interval with minimal effect on forearm or total-body BMD *(174)*. More than 90% of women receiving alendronate exhibit some increase in BMD. The increase in BMD is clinically significant as it is associated with a reduction in vertebral height loss and a 48% decrease in the incidence of vertebral fractures. In women who have previously experienced a vertebral fracture, alendronate therapy decreased the incidence of hip fractures by 50% *(175)*.

At doses of 5 mg/d, alendronate also prevents bone loss in early postmenopausal women *(176)*. The magnitude of response is only approximately half of that achieved with estrogen. Alendronate has been also approved by the FDA for primary prevention of osteoporosis.

As bisphosphonates are poorly absorbed orally, and absorption is obliterated when taken concurrently with food, it should be taken first thing in the morning, 30–60 min prior to breakfast with 6–8 oz of water. The ideal duration of therapy is not known. Bone loss begins to recur within 1–2 yr after discontinuation of alendronate, but in contrast to HRT, there is no catch-up bone loss *(177)*. Side effects associated with alendronate include abdominal pain, nausea, constipation, diarrhea, and musculoskeletal pain. With approval by the FDA, there have also been reports of esophagitis and severe esophageal ulceration *(178)*. To reduce side effects, individuals should stay upright for at least 30–60 min after dosing.

Bisphosphonate therapy should be withheld in individuals who have evidence of secondary hyperparathyroidism or vitamin D deficiency until treatment of this underlying problem has been initiated. Bisphosphonates decrease serum calcium resulting in a temporary increase in PTH levels *(179)* and may exacerbate secondary hyperparathyroidism. Because bisphosphonates are renally cleared, they are contraindicated in chronic renal failure.

Etidronate, the first-generation drug, has also been utilized for the treatment of osteoporosis, although it is not currently FDA-approved in the United States. Using an intermittent cyclical regimen, etidronate has been shown to increase bone mass at the spine and femur *(180,181)*. The greatest gains occur within the first year, but progressive increases in BMD have been reported through 5 yr of treatment *(182)*. Although its effect on vertebral fracture rate is not definitively established, studies suggest that it may benefit individuals with severe osteoporosis. The recommended dose is 400 mg/d for 2 wk followed by an 11-wk etidronate-free period where 1500 mg/d of calcium is taken. Utilizing this cyclical regimen, there is no acquisition of a mineralization defect and no evidence of frank osteomalacia *(183)*. It remains a therapeutic option for individuals who are candidates for ERT and have been unable to tolerate alendronate because of upper G.I. symptoms.

There has been great interest in the potential use of concurrent HRT and bisphosphonate therapy. In animal models, the combination of alendronate and HRT results in a greater gain in bone mass than seen with either agent alone *(184)*. In women, intermittent cyclical etidronate, plus HRT, resulted in gains of spinal BMD of 11% over 2 yr compared to a 7% increase with either drug given independently *(185)*. Combination studies with alendronate and HRT are in progress.

Fluoride

There are situations where bone formation rates are low and the stimulation of osteoblastic bone formation might be desirable. Unlike estrogen, calcitonin and the bisphosphonates that are all antiresorptive therapies, fluoride stimulates the formation of new bone by enhancing the recruitment and differentiation of osteoblasts. Initial studies using 50–75 mg of sodium fluoride/d showed significant increases in bone mass at the spine (7.8%/yr) and hip (2.5%/yr) with a decline in bone mineral content of the midradius (–1.4%/yr) *(186)*. This reduction in bone density of nonweight-bearing appendicular bones has been confirmed in other studies *(187)*. Despite gains in bone mass, there was no evidence to suggest that there is an associated significant reduction in the rate of new vertebral fractures. In fact, a 4-yr randomized placebo-controlled trial by Riggs et al. showed only a 15% reduction in the number of women with new vertebral fractures with an increase in the number and frequency of nonvertebral fractures *(186)*.

Recent trials have focused on slow-release sodium fluoride and monoflurophosphate. Utilizing cyclical (12 mo on–2 mo off) slow-release sodium fluoride (25 mg b.i.d.) with 800 mg/d of calcium, there is evidence of substantial increases in bone mass at the spine and hip, decreases in loss of height, and a decrease in new vertebral fracture incidence *(188)*. This increase in spine BMD is not maintained after fluoride discontinued. Slow-release sodium fluoride appears to be most beneficial in women who have an initial BMD that is >65% of the average BMD seen in young normal adults. Randomized trials of monoflurophosphate have yielded conflicting results regarding its benefit in reducing fracture. At the present time, neither slow-release sodium fluoride nor monofluro-phosphate are available for clinical use.

Calcitriol

Calcitriol is the synthetic form of 1,25 dihydroxy vitamin D. It increases G.I. calcium and phosphate absorption and increases renal tubular reabsorption of calcium and phosphate resulting in enhanced mineralization of the skeleton. At doses of <0.5 mcg/d, calcitriol is utilized to correct for the 1-alpha hydroxylase defect in elderly subjects, and to prevent the development of secondary hyperparathyroidism. At doses >0.5 mcg/d, some trials have suggested the prevention of cortical and cancellous bone loss *(189)* and a reduction in the incidence of new vertebral fractures *(190)*. The 20% incidence of hypercalciuria and hypercalcemia with this regimen has limited its use.

Experimental Agents

There are many new drugs under development today to address the need for additional therapeutic interventions for the treatment of osteoporosis. Many of these agents are bisphosphonate analogs, but several specific new categories of drugs are worth mentioning.

Trials of growth hormone have shown an increase in height velocity, muscle, and bone mass when given to children with growth hormone deficiency. Therapy with growth hormone also increases muscle and bone mass in growth-hormone-deficient adult patients, although the magnitude of gain is small (<4%/2 yr) Growth hormone given to the elderly has resulted in only minimal benefit and long-term studies have been largely unsuccessful because of high cost and the increased incidence of side effects.

The anabolic effect of PTH on cancellous bone has recently been applied to the treatment of osteoporosis. In humans, intermittent PTH causes activation of lining cells and rapid increases in BMD at the spine despite an increase in remodeling based turnover. Its current use is limited, however, because of the associated increased loss of cortical bone. Combination studies with a bisphosphonate or other agent to preserve cortical bone content are underway.

In summary, although many questions remain, the future for the diagnosis and management for osteoporosis is bright. With improvements in techniques for early detection and the breadth of therapeutic options under development, we may have a significant impact in reducing the disability associated with this common disease.

REFERENCES

1. NIH Consensus Development Conference. Diagnosis, prophylaxis and treatment of osteoporosis. Am J Med 1993;94:646–650.
2. Melton LJ, Chaos EYS, Lane J. Biochemical aspects of fractures. In: BL Riggs, LJ Melton, eds. Osteoporosis: Etiology, Diagnosis and Management. Raven, New York, 1988, p. 111.
3. Kanis JA, Melton LJ, III, Christiansen C, Johnston CC, Khaltaev N. The diagnosis of osteoporosis. J Bone Miner Res 1994;8:1137–1141.
4. Genant HK, Engellae K, Fuerst T, et al. Non-invasive assessment and structure: state-of-art. J Bone Miner Res 1996;11:707–730.
5. Graendak GA, Barrett-Connor E. Outcomes of osteoporosis fractures. In: Marcus R, Freedman D, Kelsey J, eds. Osteoporosis. Academic, Orlando, FL, 1996.
6. Magaziner J, Simonsick EM, Kashne TM, et al. Predictors of functional recovery one year following hospital discharge for hip fracture: a prospective study. J Gerontol 1990;45:M101–M107.
7. Cummings SR, Kelsey JL, Nevitt MC, O'Dowd KJ. Epidemiology of osteoporosis in osteoporotic fractures. Epidemiol Rev 1985;7:178–208.
8. Browner WS, Pressman AR, Nevitt MC, Cummings SC for the Study of Osteoporotic Fractures Research Group. Mortality following fractures in older women: the study of osteoporotic fractures. Arch Intern Med 1996;156:1521–1525.

9. U.S. Congress Office of Technology Assessment. Effectiveness and costs of osteoporosis screening and hormone replacement therapy. Vol 1. Cost effectiveness analysis. OTA-BP-H-160. U.S. Government Printing Office, Washington, DC, 1995.

10. Miller CW. Survival and ambulation following hip fractures. J Bone Joint Surg 1978;60-A:930–934.

11. Melton LJ, III. How many women have osteoporosis now? J Bone Miner Res 1995;10:175–177.

12. Looker AC, Johnston CC, Jr, Wahner HW, et al. Prevalence of low femoral bone density in older US. women from NHANES III. J Bone Miner Res 1995;10:796–802.

13. Melton LJ, III, Chrischilles EA, Cooper C, Lane AW, Riggs BL. Perspective: How many women have osteoporosis? J Bone Miner Res 1992;7:1005–1010.

14. National Osteoporosis Foundation. Osteoporosis: cost effectiveness analysis and review of the evidence for prevention, diagnosis and treatment. Osteoporosis Int 1998;8(suppl 4): S1–S88.

15. Ray NF, Chan JK, Thamer M, Melton LJ, III. Medical expenditures for the treatment of osteoporotic fracture in the United States in 1995: report from the National Osteoporosis Foundation. J Bone Miner Res 1997;12:24–35.

16. Frost H. A new direction for osteoporosis: a review and proposal. Bone 1991;12:429–437.

17. Kanis JA. Estrogens, the menopause and osteoporosis. Bone;1996:19:185S–190S.

18. Baran RE. Anatomy and ultrastructure of bone. In: Fauvus MJ, ed. Primer on the Metabolic Bone Diseases and Disorders of Mineral Metabolism. Lippincott-Raven, Philadelphia, PA, 1996, pp. 3–10.

19. Pacifici R. Estrogen, cytokines and pathogenesis of postmenopausal osteoporosis. J Bone Miner Res 1996;11:1043–1051.

20. Hughes DE, Jilka RL, Manolages S, et al. Sex steroids promote osteoclast apoptosis in vitro and in vivo. J Bone Miner Res 1995;10:S48.

21. Chaudharg LR, Spelsberg TC, Riggs BL. Production of various cytokines by normal human osteoblast-like cells in response to interleukin 1B and tumor necrosis factor a: lack of regulation by 17b estradiol. Endocrinol 1992;130:2528–2534.

22. Pacifici R, Rifas L, McCracken R, et al. Ovarian steroid treatment blocks a postmenopausal increase in blood monocyte IL_1 release. PNAS 1989;86:2398–2402.

23. Ralston SH. Analysis of gene expression in human bone biopsies by polymerase chain reaction. Evidence for enhanced cytokine expression in postmenopausal osteoporosis. J Bone Miner Res 1994;9:883–890.

24. Pacifici R, Vannice JL, Rifas L, Kimble RB. Monocytic secretion of IL_1 receptor antagonist in normal and osteoporotic women. Effects of menopause and estrogen: progesterone therapy. J Clin Endocrinol Metab 1993;77:1135–1141.

25. Sowers M. Pregnancy and lactation as risk factors for subsequent bone loss and osteoporosis. J Bone Miner Res 1996;11:1052–1060.

26. Arlot ME, Sornay-Rendu E, Garnero P, Vey-Marty B, Delmas PD. Apparent pre- and postmenopausal bone loss evaluated by DXA at different skeletal sites in women: the OFELY cohort. J Bone Miner Res 1997;12:683–690.

27. Wasnich RD. Epidemiology of osteoporosis. In: Fauvus, MJ ed. Primer on the Metabolic Bone Diseases and Disorders of Mineral Metabolism. Lippincott-Raven, Philadelphia, PA, 1996, pp. 249–251.

28. Black DM, Cummings SR, Melton LJ, III. Appendicular bone mineral and a woman's lifetime risk of hip fracture. J Bone Miner Res 1992b;7:639–646.

29. Cummings SR, Black DM, Nevitt MC, et al. Appendicular bone density and age predict hip fracture in women The Study of Osteoporotic Fractures Research Group. JAMA 1990;263:665–668.

30. Cummings SR, Black DM, Nevitt MC, et al. for the Study of Osteoporotic Fractures Research Group. Bone density at various sites for prediction of hip fractures. Lancet 1993;341:72–75.

31. Gardsell P, Johnell O, Nilsson BE, Gulberg B. Predicting various fragility fractures in women by forearm bone densitometry: a follow up study. Calcif Tiss Int 1993;52:348–353.

32. Hui SL, Slemenda CW, Johnston CC, Jr. Age and bone mass as predictors of fracture in a prospective study. J Clin Invest 1988;81:1804–1809.

33. Hui SL, Slemenda CW, Johnston CC, Jr. Baseline measurement of bone mass predicts fracture in white women. Ann Int Med 1989;111:355–361.

34. Stevenson JC, Lees B, Davenport M, Cust MD, Ganger KF. Determinants of bone density in normal women: Risk factors for future osteoporosis. B Med J 1989;298:924–928.

35. Slemenda CW, Hui SL, Longcope C, Wellman H, Johnston CC, Jr. Predictors of bone mass in perimenopausal women: a prospective study of clinical data using photon absorptiometry. Ann Intern Med 1990;112:96–101.

36. Bauer DC, Browner WS, Cauley JA, et al. Factors associated with appendicular bone mass in older women. Ann Intern Med 1993;118:657–665.
37. Pocock NA, Eisman JA, Hopper JL, Yeates MG, Sambrook PN, Ebert SE. Genetic determinants of bone mass in adults: a twin study. J Clin Invest 1987;80:706–710.
38. Slemenda CW, Christian JC, William CJ, Norton JA, Johnston CC, Jr. Genetic determinants of bone mass in adult women: a re-evaluation of the model and the potential importance of gene interaction on heritability estimates. J Bone Miner Res 6:561–567.
39. Kelly PJ, Nguyen T, Pocock n, Hopper J, Sambrook PN, Eisman JA. Genetic determination of changes in bone density with age: a twin study. J Bone Miner Res 1993;8:11–17.
40. Lim SK, Park YS, Park JM, Song YD, Lee EJ, Kim KR, Lee HC, Huh KB. Lack of association between vitamin D receptor genotypes and osteoporosis in Koreans. J Clin Endocrinol Metab 1995;80:3677–3681.
41. Kelly PJ, Hopper JL, Macaskill GT, Pocock NA, Sambrook PN, Eisman JA. Genetic factors in bone turnover. J Clin Endocrinol Metab 1991;72:808–814.
42. Morrison NA, Qi JC, Tokita A, Kelly PJ, Croft L, Nguyen TV, Sambrook PN, Eisman JA. Prediction of bone density by vitamin D receptor alleles. Nature 1994;367:284–287.
43. Eisman J Vitamin D receptor gene alleles and osteoporosis: an affirmative view. J Bone miner Res 1995;10:1289–1293.
44. Ferrari S, Rizzoli R, Chevalley T, Slosman D, Eisman JA, Bonjour J-P. Vitamin D receptor gene polymorphisms and the rate of change of lumbar spine bone mineral density in elderly men and women. Lancet 345:423–424.
45. Fleet JC, Harris SS, Wood RJ, Dawson-Hughes B. The BsmI vitamin D receptor restriction length polymorphism (BB) predicts low bone density in premenopausal black and white women. J Bone Miner Res 10:985–990.
46. Garnero P, Borel O, Sornay-Rendu E, Delmas PD. Vitamin D receptor polymorphisms do not predict bone turnover and bone mass in healthy premenopausal women. J Bone Miner Res 10:1283–1288.
47. Krall EA, Parry P, Lichter JB, Dawson-Hughes B. Vitamin D receptor alleles and rate of bone loss: influences of years since menopause and calcium intake. J Bone Miner Res 1995;10:978–984.
48. Matsuyama T, Ishii S, Tokita A, Yabuta K, Yamamori S, Morrison NA, Eisman JA. VDR gene polymorphisms and vitamin D analog treatment in Japanese. Lancet 1995;345:1238–1239.
49. Morrison NA, Yeoman R, Kelly PJ, Eisman JA. Contribution of transacting factor alleles to normal physiological variability: vitamin D receptor gene polymorphisms and circulating osteocalcin. Proc Natl Acad Sci USA 1992;89:6665–6669.
50. Nguyen TV, Kelly PJ, Morrison NA, Sambrook PN, Eisman JA. Vitamin D receptors genotypes in osteoporosis. Lancet 1994;344:1580,1581
51. Riggs BL, Nguyen TV, Melton LJ, III, Morrison NA, O'Fallon WM, Kelly PJ, Logan KS, Sambrook PN, Muhs JM, Eisman JA. Contribution of vitamin D receptor gene alleles to the determination of bone mineral density in normal and osteoporotic women. J Bone Miner Res 1995;10:991–996.
52. Spector TD, Keen RW, Arden NK, Major PJ, Baker JR, Morrison NA, Nguyen TV, Kelly PJ, Sambrook PN, Lanchbury JS, Eisman JA. Vitamin D receptor gene (VDR) alleles and bone density in postmenopausal women: a UK study. Br Med J 1995;310:1357–1360.
53. Cooper GS, Umbach DM. Are vitamin D receptor polymorphisms associated with bone mineral density? A meta-analysis. J Bone Miner Res 1996;11:1841–1849.
54. Sano M, Inoue S, Hosoi T, Ouchi Y, Emi M, Shiraki M, Orimo H. Association of estrogen receptor dinucleotide repeat polymorphism with osteoporosis. Biochem Biophys Res Comm 1995;217:378–383.
55. Kobayashi S, Inoeie S, Hosoi T, Auchi Y, Shiroki M, Orlmo H. Association of bone mineral density with polymorphism of the estrogen receptor gene. J Bone Miner Res 1996;11:306–311.
56. Shiroki M, Shiroki Y, Aoki C, et al. Association of bone mineral density with apolipoprotein E phenotype. J Bone Miner Res 1996;11:S436.
57. Grant SF, Reid DM, Blake G, Herd R, Fogelman I, Ralston SH. Reduced bone density and osteoporosis associated with a polymorphic Sp1 binding site in the collagen type 1 alpha 1 gene. Nature 1994;367:284–287.
58. Franceschi S, Schinella D, Bidoli E, et al. The influence of body size, smoking and diet on bone density in pre- and post-menopausal women. Epidemiology 1996;7:411–414.
59. Orwoll ES, Bauer DC, Vogt TM, et al. Axial bone mass in older women. Ann Intern Med 1996;124:187–196.
60. Kritz-Silverstein D, Barrett-Connor E. Early menopause, number of reproductive years, and bone mineral density in post-menopausal women. Am J Public Health 1993;83:983–988.
61. Stevenson JC, lees B, Davenport M, Cust MP, Ganger KF. Determinants of bone density in normal women: risk factors for future osteoporosis? BMJ 1989;298:924–928.

62. Kiel DP, Zhang Y, Hannon MT, et al. The effect of smoking at different life stages on bone mineral density on elderly men and women. Osteoporosis Int 1996;6:240–248.

63. Egger P, Suggleby S, Hobbs R, Fall C, Cooper C. Cigarette smoking and bone mineral density in the elderly. Epidemiol Community Health 1996;50:47–50.

64. Felson DT, Zhang Y, Hannan MT, Kannel WB, Kiel DP. Alcohol intake and bone mineral density in elderly men and women: the Framingham Study. Am J Epidemiol 1995;142:485–492.

65. Vuori I. Peak bone mass and physical activity: a short review. Nutr Rev 1996;54:511–514.

66. Paginini-Hill A, Chao A, Ross RK, Henderson BE. Exercise and other factors in the prevention of hip fractures. The Leisure World study. Epidemiology 1991;2:16–25.

67. Heany RP. Nutrition and risk for osteoporosis. In: Marcus R, Feldman D, Kelsey J, eds. Osteoporosis. Academic Press, San Diego, 1996, pp. 483–505.

68. Chan GM, Hess M, Hollis J, Book LS. Bone mineral status and childhood accidental fractures. Am J Dis Child 1984;138:569–70.

69. Matkovic V, Koshal K, Simonovic I, et al. Bone status and fracture risks in two regions of Yugoslavia. Am J Clin Nutr 1979;32:540–549.

70. Faulkner KG, Cummings SR, Black D, et al. Simple measurement of femoral geometry predicts hip fracture: the study of osteoporotic fractures. J Bone Miner Res 1993;8:1211–1217.

71. Heany RP. Pathogenesis of osteoporosis. In: Fauvus, MJ, ed. Primer on the Metabolic Bone Diseases and Disorders of Calcium Metabolism. Lippincott-Raven, Philadelphia, PA, 1996, pp. 252–258.

72. Cummings SR, Nevitt MC, Browner WS for the Study of Osteoporotic Fractures Research Group. Risk factors for hip fractures in white women. N Engl J Med 1995;332:767–773.

73. Dargent-Molina P, Favier F, Granjean H et al for the EPIDOS Study Group. Fall- related factors and risk of hip fracture. The EPIDOS prospective study. Lancet 1996;348:145–149.

74. Johnell O, Gullberg B, Kanis JA, et al. Risk factors for hip fracture in European women-The MEDOS study. J Bone Miner Res 1995;10:1802–1815.

75. Nelson HD, Nevitt MC, Scott JC, Stone K, Cummings SR. Effects of smoking and alcohol on neuro-muscular function in older women. JAMA 1994;272:1825–1831.

76. Earnshaw SA, Hosking DJ. Clinical usefulness of risk factors for osteoporosis. Am Rheum Dis 1996;55:338–339.

77. Kroger H, Tupparainen M, Hunkanen R, Alhava E, Saarokoski S. Bone mineral density and risk factors for osteoporosis-a population-based study of 1600 perimenopausal women. Calcif Tiss Int 1994;55:1–7.

78. Ribot C, Pouilles JM, Bonneu M, Tremolliere F. Assessment of the risk of post-menopausal osteoporosis using clinical factors. Clin Endocrinol 1992;36:225–228.

79. Kleerekoper M, Peterson E, Nelson D, et al. Identification of women at risk for developing post-menopausal osteoporosis with vertebral fractures: role of history and single photon absorptiometry. Bone Miner 1989;7:171–186.

80. Cummings SR. Treatable and untreatable risk factors for hip fracture. Bone 1996;18:165S–167S.

81. Ross PD, Davis JW, Epstein RS, Wasnich RD. Pre-existing fractures and bone mass predict vertebral fracture incidence in women. Ann Int Med 1991;114:919–923.

82. Wasnich RD, Davis JW, Ross PD. Spine fracture risk is predicted by non-spine fractures. Osteoporosis Int 1994;4:1–5.

83. Farmer ME, Harris T, Madans JH, et al. Anthropometric indicators and hip fracture: The NHANES I Epidemiologic Follow-up Study. J Am Geriatr Soc 1989;37:9–16.

84. Grisso JA, Kelsey JL, Strom BL, et al. Risk factors for falls as a cause of hip fracture in women. N Engl J Med 1991;324:1326–1331.

85. Langlois JA, Harris T, Looker AC, Madans JH. Weight change between the age of 50 years and old age is associated with risk of hip fracture in white women aged 67 years and older. Arch Int Med 1996;156:989–994.

86. Cooper C, Barker DJP, Wickham C. Physical activity, muscle strength and calcium intake in fracture of the proximal femur in Britain. BMJ 1988;297:1443–1446.

87. Krall EA, Dawson-Hughes B. Smoking and bone loss among post-menopausal women. J Bone Miner Res 1991;6:331–338.

88. Hoppe JL, Seeman E. The bone density of female twins discordant for tobacco use. N Engl J Med 1994;330:387–392.

89. Williamson MR, Boyd CM, Williamson SL. Osteoporosis: Diagnosis by plain chest film versus dual photon bone densitometry. Skeletal Radiol 1990;19:27–30.

90. Virtama P. Uneven distribution of bone mineral and covering effect of non-mineralized tissue as reasons for impaired detectability of bone density from roentgenograms. Ann Med Int Fenn 1960;49:57–60.

91. Finsen V, Anda S. Accuracy of visually estimated bone mineralization in routine radiographs of the lower extremity. Skeletal Radiol 1988;17:270–275.

92. Melton LJ, III, Atkinson EJ, O'Fallon WM, Wahner HW, Riggs BL. Long-term fracture prediction by bone mineral assessed at different skeletal sites. J Bone Miner Res 1993;8:1227–1233.

93. Smith DM, Khairi MRA, Johnston CC, Jr. The loss of bone mineral with aging and its relationship to risk of fracture. J Clin Invest 1975;56:311–318.

94. Wasnich RD, Ross PD, Heilbrun LK, Vogel JM. Prediction of postmenopausal fracture risk with use of bone mineral measurements. Am J Obstet Gynecol 1985;153:745– 751.

95. Nevitt MC, Johnell O, Black DM, et al. Bone mineral density predicts non-spine fractures in very elderly women. Study of Osteoporotic Fractures Research Group. Osteoporos Int 1994;4:325–331.

96. Cosman F, Harrington B, Himmelstein S, Lindsay R. Radiographic absorptiometry: a simple method for determination of bone mass. Osteoporos Int 1991;2:34–38.

97. Grampp S, Genant HK, Mathur A, et al. Comparisons of non-invasive bone mineral measurements in assessing age-related loss, fracture discrimination and diagnostic classification. J Bone Miner Res 1997;12:697–711.

98. Kelly TL, Crane G, Baran DT. Single x-ray absorptiometry of the forearm: precision, correlation and reference data. Calcif Tiss Int 1994;54:212–218.

99. Mazess R, Chesnut III CH, McClung M, Genant HK. Enhanced precision with dual- energy x-ray absorptiometry. Calcif Tiss Int 1992;51:14–17.

100. Cann CE, Genant HK, Kolb FQ, Ettinger BE. Quantitative computed tomography for prediction of vertebral fracture risk. Bone 1988;6:1–7.

101. Steiger P, Cummings SR, Black DM, Spencer NE, Genant HK. Age-related decrements in bone mineral density in women over 65. J Bone Miner Res 1992;7:625–632.

102. Silverman SL, Greenwald M, Klein RA, Drinkwater BL. Effect of bone density information on decisions about hormone replacement therapy: a randomized trial. Obstet Gynecol 1997;89:321–325.

103. Phillipov G, Mos E, Scinto S, Phillips PJ. Initiation of hormone replacement therapy after diagnosis of osteoporosis by bone densitometry. Osteoporos Int 1997;7:162– 164.

104. Garnero P, Delmas PD. New developments in biochemical markers for osteoporosis. Calcif Tiss Int 1996;59: S2–S9.

105. Calvo MS, Eyre DR, Gundberg CM. Molecular basis and clinical application of biological markers of bone turnover. Endocrine Rev 1996;17:333–368.

106. Panteghini M, Pagini. Biologic variation in urinary excretion of pyridinium cross-links: recommendation for the optimum specimen. Ann Clin Biochem 1996;33:36–42.

107. Popp-Snijders C, Lips P, Netelenbos JC. Intra-individual variation in bone resorption markers in the urine. Ann Clin Biochem 1996;33:347–348.

108. Garnero P, Hauseherr E, Chaupy MC, et al. Markers of bone resorption predict hip fracture in elderly women. The EPIDOS prospective study. J Bone Miner Res 1996;11:1531–1538.

109. Riis BJ, Hansen MA, Jensen AM, Overgaard K, Christiansen C. Low bone mass and fast rate of bone loss at menopause are equal risks for future fracture: a fifteen year follow up study. Bone 1996;19:9–12.

110. Lloyd T, Rollins N, Ander MB, et al. Enhance bone gain in early adolescence due to calcium supplementation does not persist in late adolescence. J Bone Miner Res 1996;11:S154.

111. Lee WTK, Leung SSF, Leung DMY, Chang JC. A follow-up study on the effects of calcium supplement withdrawal and puberty on bone acquisition of children. Am J Clin Nutr 1996;64:71–77.

112. Dawson-Hughes B, Dallal GE, Krall EA, et al. A controlled trial of the effect of calcium supplementation on bone density in post-menopausal women. N Engl J Med 1990;323:878–883.

113. Kinyomu HK, Gallagher JC, Balhorn KE, et al. Serum vitamin D metabolites and calcium in normal young and elderly free-living women and in women living in nursing homes. Am J Clin Nutr 1997;65:71–77.

114. Dawson-Hughes B, Harris SS, Dallal GE. Plasma calcidiol, season, and serum parathyroid hormone concentrations in healthy elderly men and women. Am J Clin Nutr 1997;65:67–71.

115. Lips P. Vitamin D deficiency and osteoporosis. The role of vitamin D deficiency and treatment with vitamin D and analogues in the prevention of osteoporosis-related fractures. Eur J Clin Invest 1996;26:436–442.

116. Prince R, Devine A, Dick I, et al. The effects of calcium supplementation (milk powder or tablets) and exercise on bone density in post-menopausal women J Bone Miner Res 1995;10:1068–1075.

117. Reid IR, Ames RW, Evans MC, et al. Long-term effects of calcium supplementation on bone loss and fractures in post-menopausal women: a randomized controlled trial. Am J Med 1995;98:331–335.

118. Riis B, Thomsen K, Christiansen C. Does calcium supplementation prevent post-menopausal bone loss. A double-blind controlled clinical trial. N Engl J Med 1987;316:173–177.
119. Chapuy MC, Arlot ME, Dobouf F, et al. Vitamin D_3 and calcium to prevent hip fractures in elderly women. N Engl J Med 1992;327:1637–1642.
120. Chapuy MC, Arlot ME, Delmas PD, et al. Effect of calcium and cholecalciferol treatment for three years on hip fractures in elderly women. BMJ 1994;308:1081–1082.
121. Dawson-Hughes B, Harris SS, Krall EA, Dallal GE. Effect of calcium and vitamin D supplementation on bone density in men and women 65 years of age and older. N Engl J Med 1997;337:670–676.
122. NIH Consensus Conference. Optimal calcium intake. JAMA 1994;272:1942–1948.
123. Saunders D, Sillery J, Chapman R. Effect of calcium carbonate and aluminum hydroxide on human intestinal function. Dog Dis Sci 1988;33:409–413.
124. Nordstrom P, Thorsenk K, Bergstrom E, Lorentzon R. High bone mass and altered relationships between bone mass, muscle strengthh and body constitution in adolescent boys on a high level of physical activity. Bone 1996;19:189–195.
125. Boot AM, deRidder MAJ, Pols HAP, et al. Bone mineral density in children and adolescents: relation to puberty, calcium intake and physical activity. J Clin Endocrinol Metab 1997;82:57–62.
126. Hapasalo H, Sievanan H, Kannus P, et al. Dimensions and estimated mechanical characteristics of the humerus after long-term tennis loading. J Bone Miner Res 1996;11:864–872.
127. Etherington J, Harris PA, Nandra D, et al. The effect of weight-bearing exercise on bone density: a study of female ex-athletes and the general population. J Bone Miner Res 1996;11:1333–1338.
128. Karlsson MK, Hasserius R, Obrant KJ. Bone mineral density in athletes during and after career: a comparison between loaded and unloaded skeletal regions. Calcif Tiss Int 1996;59:245–248.
129. Huddleston AL, Rockwell D, Kuland DN, et al. Bone mass in lifetime tennis players. JAMA 1980;244:1107–1109.
130. Friedlander AL, Genant HK, Sadowsky S, Byl NN, Gluer CC. A two year program of aerobics and weight training enhances bone mineral density of young women. J Bone Miner Res 1995;10:574–585.
131. Lohman T, Going S, Pamonter S, et al. Effects of resistance raining on regional and total bone mineral density in premenopausal women: a randomized prospective study. J Bone Miner Res 1995;10:1015–1024.
132. Pruitt LA, Jackson RD, Bartels RL, Lehnard HJ. Weight training effects on bone. mineral density in early postmenopausal women. J Bone Miner Res 1992;7:179–185.
133. Dalsky G, Stocke KS, Eshani AA, et al. Weight bearing exercise training and lumbar bone mineral content in post-menopausal women. Ann Int Med 1988;108:824–828.
134. Menkes A, Mazel S, Richmond RA, et al. Strength training increases regional bone mineral density and bone remodeling in middle-aged and older men. J Appl Physiol 1993;74:2478–2484.
135. Cavanaugh DJ, Cann CE. Brisk walking does not stop bone loss in post-menopausal women. Bone 1988;9:201–204.
136. Notelovitz M, Martin D, Tesar R, et al. Estrogen therapy and variable resistance weight training increase bone mineral in surgically menopausal women. J Bone Miner Res 1991;6:583–590.
137. Province MA, Hadley EC, Hornbrook MC, et al. The effects of exercise on falls in elderly patients. JAMA 1995;273:1341–1347.
138. Sinaki M, Mikkelsen BA. Postmenopausal spinal osteoporosis: flexion versus extension exercises. Arch Phys Med Rehabil 1984;65:593–596.
139. Lindsay R, Bush TL, Grady D, Speroff L, Lobo RA. Therapeutic controversy. Estrogen replacement in menopause. J Clin Endocrinol Metab 1996;81:3829–3838.
140. Vedi S, Compston JE. The effects of long-term hormone replacement therapy on bone remodeling in post-menopausal women. Bone 1996;19:535–539.
141. Steiniche T, Hasling C, Charles P, et al. A randomized study on the effects of estrogen gestagen or high dose oral calcium on trabecular bone remodeling in postmenopausal osteoporosis. Bone 1989;10:313–320.
142. Ericksen EF, Langdahl B, Glerup A, et al. Hormone replacement therapy (HRT) preserves bone balance by preventing osteoclastic hyperactivity in post-menopausal women: a randomized prospective histomorphometric study. J Bone Miner Res 1996;11: s1.
143. Hughes DE, Dai A, Tiffae JC, et al. Estrogen promotes apoptosis of murine osteoclasts mediated by TGF-B. Nat Med 1996;2:1132–1136.
144. Brockstedt H, Kassom M, Eriksen EF. Estrogen prevents cortical bone loss in early post-menopausal women: a histomorphometric study. Bone 1996;19: S133.
145. Civitelli R, Agnus Dei D, Nardi P, et al. Effect of one year treatment with estrogens on bone mass, intestinal calcium absorption and 25 hydroxy vitamin D 1 alpha hydroxylase reserve in post-menopausal osteoporosis. Calcif Tiss Int 1988;42:77–86.

146. Christiansen C, Christiansen Ms, Transbol I. Bone mass in postmenopausal women after withdrawal of oestrogen/gestagen replacement therapy. Lancet 1981;1:459–461.

147. Ettinger B, Genant HK, Cann CE. Long-term estrogen replacement therapy prevents bone loss and fractures. Ann Int Med 1985;102:319–324.

148. Ettinger B, Genant HK, Cann CE. Postmenopausal bone loss is prevented by treatment with low-dose estrogen and calcium. Ann Intern Med 1987;106:40–43.

149. Lindsay R, Tohme JF. Estrogen treatment of patients with established postmenopausal osteoporosis. Obstet Gynecol 1990;76:290–295.

150. Prince RL, Smith M, Dick IM, et al. Prevention of postmenopausal osteoporosis. A comparative study of exercise, calcium supplementation and hormone-replacement therapy. N Engl J Med 1991;325:1189–1195.

151. Hutchinson TA, Polansy SM, Feinstein AR. Postmenopausal estrogens protect against fractures of the hip and distal radius. Lancet 1979;2:705–707.

152. Johnson RE, Specht EE. The risk of hip fracture in postmenopausal females with and without estrogen exposure. Am J Publ Health 1981;71:139–144.

153. Paganini-Hill A, Ross PD, Gerkins VR, et al. Menopausal estrogen therapy and hip fractures. Ann Int Med 1981;95:28–31.

154. Cauley JA, Seely DG, Ensrud K, et al. Estrogen replacement therapy and fractures in older women. Ann Int Med 1995;122:9–16.

155. Schneider Dl, Barrett-Connor EL, Martin DJ. Timing for postmenopausal estrogen for optimal bone mineral density-The Rancho Bernardo Study. JAMA 1997;277:543–547.

156. Marx CW, Dailey GE III, Cheney C, et al. Do estrogens improve bone mineral density in osteoporotic women over age 65? J Bone Miner Res 1992;7:1275–1279.

157. Quigley MET, Martin PL, Burnier AM, et al. Estrogen therapy arrests bone loss in elderly women. Am J Obstet Gynecol 1987;156:1516–1523.

158. Grady D, Rubin SM, Petitti DB, et al. Hormone replacement therapy to prevent disease and prolong life in post-menopausal women. Ann Int Med 1992;117:1016– 1037.

159. Goldstein F, Stamfer MJ, Manson JE, et al. Postmenopausal estrogen and progestin use and the risk of cardiovascular disease. N Engl J Med 1996;335:453–461.

160. The Writing Group for the PEPI Trial. Effects of hormone therapy on bone mineral density: Results from the Postmenopausal Estrogen/Progestin Interventions Trial. JAMA 1996;276:1389–1396.

161. Lindsay R, Hart DM, MacLean A, et al. Bone response to termination of estrogen treatment. Lancet 1978;1:1325–1327.

162. Eiken P, Kolyhoff N, Nielson SP. Effect of 10 years hormone replacement therapy on bone mineral content in post-menopausal women. Bone 1996;19: S191–S193.

163. Reginster JY. Effect of calcitonin on bone mass and fracture rates. Am J Med 1991;92:19S–22S.

164. Gennari C, Cheichetti SM, Bigazzi S, et al. Comparative effects on bone mineral content of calcium or calcium plus salmon calcitonin given in two different regimens in post-menopausal osteoporosis. Curr Ther Res 1985;38:455–464.

165. Gennari C, Agnusdei D, Montagnani M, Gonnelli S, Civitelli R. An effective regimen of intranasal salmon calcitonin in early post-menopausal bone loss. Calcif Tiss Int 1992;50:381–383.

166. MacIntyre I, Stevenson JC, Whitehead MI, et al. Calcitonin for the prevention of postmenopausal bone loss. Lancet 1988;1:900–902.

167. Overgaard K, Hansen MA, Jensen SB, Christiansen C. Effect of salcatonin given intra nasally on bone mass and fracture rates in established osteoporosis: a dose-response study. BMJ 1992;305:556–561.

168. Reginster JY, Deroisy R, Lecart MP, et al. A double-blind placebo controlled dose-finding trial of intermittent nasal calcitonin for the prevention of postmenopausal lumbar spine loss. Am J Med 1995;98:4452–4458.

169. Stock JL, Avioli LV, Baylink DJ, et al for the PROOF Study Group. Calcitonin-salmon nasal spray reduces the incidence of new vertebral fractures in postmenopausal women: Three year interim results of the PROOF study. J Bone Miner Res 1997;12:s149.

170. Pun KK, Chan LWL. Analgesic effect of intranasal salmon calcitonin in the treatment of osteoporotic compression fractures. Clinical Ther 1989;11:205–209.

171. Healey JH. Orthopedic management of osteoporosis. Curr Opin Orthop 1996;7:1–4.

172. Boyce BF, Fogelman I, Ralston S, et al. Focal osteomalacia due to low-dose diphosphonate therapy in Paget's disease. Lancet 1984;1:821–824.

173. Seedor JG, Balena R, Masarachia P, et al. Comparison of the therapeutic potencies of two bisphosphonates. Bone 1992:13:S116.

174. Liberman UA, Weiss SR, Broll J, et al. for the Alendronate Phase III Osteoporosis Treatment Study Group. Effect of oral alendronate on bone mineral density and the Incidence of fractures in postmenopausal osteoporosis. N Engl J Med 1995;333:1437–1443.

175. Black DM, Cummings SR, Karpf DB, et al. Randomized trial of the effect of alendronate on risk of fracture in women with existing vertebral fractures. Lancet 1996;1:1535–1541.

176. Eisman JA, Christiansen C, McClung M, et al. Alendronate prevents bone loss at the spine and hip in recently postmenopausal women. J Bone Miner Res 1995;10:s.

177. Stock J, Bell N, Chesnut C, et al. Resolution of alendronate effects on bone turnover and BMD after multi year treatment of osteoporotic women. J Bone Min Res 1995;10: s.

178. DeGroen PC, Lubbe DF, Hirsch LJ, et al. Esophagitis associated with the use of alendronate. N Engl J Med 1996;335:1016–1021.

179. Tucci JR, Tonino RP, Emkey RD, et al. Effect of three years of oral alendronate treatment in postmenopausal women with osteoporosis. Am J Med 1996;101:488– 501.

180. Watts NB, Harris ST, Genant HK, et al. Intermittent cyclical etidronate treatment of postmenopausal osteoporosis. N Engl J Med 1990;323:73–79.

181. Storm T, Thamsborg G, Steiniche T, Genant HK, Sorensen OH. Effect of intermittent cyclical etidronate therapy on bone mass and fracture rate in women with postmenopausal osteoporosis. N Engl J Med 1990;32:1265–1271.

182. Harris ST, Watts NB, Jackson, RD, et al. Four year study of intermittent cyclical etidronate treatment of postmenopausal osteoporosis: Three years of blinded treatment followed by one year of open therapy. Am J Med 1993;95:557–567.

183. Storm T, Sorensen HA, Thamsborg G, et al. Bone histomorphometric changes after up to seven years of cyclical etidronate treatment. J Bone Miner Res 1995;10:s198.

5

Lower Urinary Tract Changes of Aging Women

Renee M. Caputo, MD

CONTENTS

INTRODUCTION

The percentage of elderly persons is increasing in the United States. Nearly two-thirds of the elderly are women, and the proportion of women increases with increasing age. In the industrialized West, 95% of women are expected to reach the menopause and 60% will live past age 75 *(1)*. According to United States Census projections, within just six years, the average life expectancy for women will be 80 yr *(2)*.

Lower urogenital dysfunction is more prevalent in the elderly, but should never be accepted as normal in this population. This misconception has unfortunately led patients with urogenital dysfunction and their healthcare providers to either tolerate or ignore symptoms, which can have devastating consequences. Because lower urinary tract dysfunction increases with age, it is often assumed that there is a causal relationship between it and hormonal deficiency. This chapter will explore the effects of menopause on the female lower urinary tract function with an emphasis placed on sex hormonal influences. Common clinical presentations by menopausal women regarding the lower urinary tract and the effects of hormonal therapy on these symptoms will be discussed.

LOWER URINARY TRACT ANATOMY AND PHYSIOLOGY

The lower urinary tract serves two purposes, the storage and evacuation of urine. Although seemingly simple functions, the mechanisms behind them are quite complex and poorly understood.

From: *Contemporary Endocrinology: Menopause: Endocrinology and Management*
Edited by: D. B. Seifer and E. A. Kennard © Humana Press Inc., Totowa, NJ

The urinary and genital tracts share a common embryologic origin explaining why congenital abnormalities in one system often co-exist with abnormalities in the other. Estrogen and progesterone receptors have been found in the urethra and bladder trigone (3). Therefore, a reasonable assumption would be that the lower urinary tract and genital system are both sex-hormone sensitive.

The bladder and proximal urethra are lined by transitional epithelium. The distal urethral is lined by squamous epithelium that may migrate proximally throughout a woman's reproductive years to include the trigone (4). Changes in urethral smears and urinary cytology have been shown to correlate with the different phases of reproductive life such as the menstrual cycle, pregnancy, and the menopause (5). In the premenopause, the urethral mucosa is supple and arranged in multiple folds, which allow for a water-tight seal (6). This phenomenon may be estrogen dependent as the mucosal folds are not as prominent in the menopause (7).

Below the urethral mucosa is a vascular plexus that compresses the urethral mucosa circumferentially (8). The submucosal vascular plexus is felt to be estrogen sensitive because vascular pulses corresponding to heart rate recorded during urethral-pressure measurements decrease in size in menopausal women. This decrease is reversed with estrogen therapy (9,10). Together, the urethral mucosa and submucosal vascular plexus contribute approximately one-third of the resting urethral-closing pressure (11,12).

The urethral muscle is comprised of smooth and skeletal components. The urethral smooth muscle is organized into two distinct layers, a circular outer layer, and a more prominent inner-longitudinal layer. Although contiguous with the smooth muscle of the bladder, the urethral smooth muscle functions separately—contributing another one-third of the resting-urethral pressure (12). The urethral smooth muscle is sympathetically innervated via alpha adrenergic receptors. Semmelink et al., using histomorphometric parameters, observed an abrupt, age-independent decrease of smooth muscle tissue in the proximal and distal portions of the female urethra at the age of about 51 yr (13). Estrogen has been shown to potentiate alpha-adrenergic stimulation of the urethral smooth muscle (14–16). In a rabbit animal model, castration decreased alpha-adrenergic sensitivity that was subsequently reversed by the administration of estrogen therapy (17).

The skeletal muscle of the urethral sphincter is comprised of three portions that function as a single unit: a proximal circularly oriented sphincteric portion and two more distal muscle bands that arch over the ventral surface of the urethra. Overall, the skeletal muscle surrounds the urethral lumen over 20–80% of urethral length (18). The skeletal muscle sphincter contributes one-third of the resting urethral pressure (12). It is the only portion of the urethral sphincter that can reflexively and voluntarily contract in response to increases in intra-abdominal pressure. This can be demonstrated by increases in elec-tromyographic muscle fiber recruitment and urethral-pressure measurements during these times (19). Portions of the urethral skeletal muscle decrease in thickness and disappear with advancing age (20).

Extrinsic supports include skeletal muscle and fibromuscular attachments of the pe-riurethral tissue and lateral vagina to the levator ani and obturator internus fascia, respec-tively. This arrangement converts the anterior vaginal wall into a "backstop" against which the urethra is compressed during reflex contraction of the levator ani in response to increases in intra-abdominal pressure (21). Although there is no understood mecha-nism through which estrogen may act on the skeletal muscle sphincter and supports, recent data suggest that estrogen therapy has a measurable positive effect on contractility and tone of the pelvic floor musculature (22). Significant levels of estrogen-receptor expression have been found in pubococcygeal muscles of adult females (23). Bump and Friedman reported that estrogen replacement enhances the urethral sphincter mechanism in the castrate female baboon by effects that were unrelated to the skeletal muscle component (24). These data suggest that the effects might be related not just to changes in urethral smooth muscle, but may also be because of changes in the urethral mucosa, submucosal vascular plexus, and connective tissue components of the urethral sphincter.

Collagen is found intrinsic to the urethra, as well as extrinsically in the urethra's supporting structures. In the skin, collagen content declines after the menopause, but this is reversed by estrogen replacement therapy (25,26). The mechanism by which estrogen exerts this effect is felt to be because of a reduction in collagen breakdown via the negative regulation of the synthesis of procollagenase (27,28). Clinically, urethral pressure parameters positively correlate with skin collagen content in postmenopausal women (29). In addition, several studies have shown a decrease in tissue collagen content in women with urinary incontinence compared to controls (30–32) It is reasonable to assume then that estrogen has a positive effect on the collagen content of the urethral sphincter and supports.

The bladder is a hollow organ whose walls are made of smooth muscle and are lined by transitional epithelium and a loose submucosa. It is comprised of the body and base also referred to as the detrusor and trigone, respectively. The body portion of the bladder lies superior to and the base inferior to the level of entrance of the ureters into the dorsal wall of the bladder. The smooth muscle of the bladder is arranged in an interlacing fashion without any specific pattern or layering that continues into the bladder neck. The normal bladder body is able to maintain low intravesical pressures with increasing volume. The pressure ratio of change in intravesical volume to intravesical pressure is called compliance. Normal compliance is a function of the elastic and vesicoelastic properties of the bladder wall. In contrast, the bladder base is relatively thick and nondistensible.

Normal contractility of the detrusor muscle is essential for efficient, complete emptying of the bladder. To achieve complete emptying, a detrusor contraction must be strong, fast, summated throughout the detrusor, and sustained. Unlike skeletal muscle, actin and myosin filament in smooth muscle lack periodic spatial arrangement. Smooth muscle-filaments contain one-twelfth to one-fifteenth the number of actin filaments as skeletal muscle, but it is felt that sufficient cross bridges exist to interact with the actin filaments. Overall, the contractile process is similar, but develops much slower in smooth muscle. There is, however, some uncertainty as to the mechanism of spread of the contractile impulse within bladder smooth muscle. The bladder seems to share characteristics of multiunit smooth muscle, having a 1:1 ratio between nerve endings and muscle fibers, and unitary smooth muscle, which receives much less innervation and relies on cell-to-cell contact and "gap junctions" through which ions can flow (33). Detrusor biopsies from elderly women with normal bladder function examined by electron microscopy have identified a structural pattern known as the dense band pattern. This pattern is characterized by normal configuration of muscle cells, cell junctions, and muscle cell membranes (sarcolemma) dominated by dense bands with depleted caveolae, widening of spaces between muscle cells and little collagen content. Caveolae are felt to be involved in the contractile mechanism of smooth muscle. The author proposed that the dense band pattern represents the structural norm of the aging detrusor (34). Because there is evidence for estrogen influence of detrusor function, the author also proposed the role of a hormonal factor in the depletion of caveolae that was observed.

Estrogen and progesterone receptors have been demonstrated in the bladder *(3,23,35,36)*. Hormone-receptor content tends to decrease from the distal to the proximal part of the lower urinary tract, which may reflect its embryologic origin *(3)*. Because progesterone effects relaxation of uterine smooth muscle, one would expect it to have the same effect on the lower urinary tract. Bladder strips from gravid rabbits exhibited less tension compared to controls when exposed to a cholinergic agonist leading the author to conclude that progesterone has a relaxation effect on bladder smooth muscle *(14)*. Bladder capacity in women increases during pregnancy further supporting a progesterone relaxation effect on the bladder *(37)*. In contrast, a study of more than 200 women with premature ovarian failure receiving cyclic hormone replacement therapy (HRT) revealed an increase in the symptom of urinary urgency during the progesterone part of the therapy *(38)*. Estrogen, on the other hand, may increase bladder smooth muscle tone. Data from ovariectomized rats have shown significant decreases in contractile responsiveness of bladder muscle strips that were prevented by estradiol *(39,40)*.

The lower urinary tract is innervated by the autonomic and somatic nervous systems. Autonomic innervation of the bladder and urethra emanates from ganglia that generally lie close to or within these structures. All peripheral ganglia are composed of cholinergic, adrenergic and SIF (small intensely fluorescent) cells where modulation of one neural component by another can occur.

The sympathetic component of the autonomic nervous system originates in the intermediolateral nuclei of spinal cord segments T11 to L2, transverses lumbar sympathetic ganglia, and joins the superior hypogastric plexus. It then divides into the right and left hypogastric nerves. The sympathetic component is responsible for bladder storage via alpha and beta adrenergic receptors. There are proportionally more beta receptors in the bladder body than the urethra and more alpha receptors in the urethral smooth muscle *(41)*. Thus, the overall effect of sympathetic stimulation is increased urethral tone and bladder relaxation, which promotes continence. The parasympathetic component originates from the intermediolateral region of the gray matter of sacral spinal cord segments S2–4 emerging in the ventral nerve roots. This preganglionic supply is conveyed by the pelvic nerve that meets the hypogastric to form the pelvic plexus. The parasympathetic component controls bladder emptying via stimulation of cholinergic receptors.

The skeletal muscle sphincter is somatically innervated by the pudendal nerve, S2–4. There is evidence, however, to suggest that its innervation is more complex, possibly involving the autonomic system as well *(42)*.

Sensory information from the bladder is conveyed by both hypogastric and pelvic nerves. Afferent fibers responsible for the sensation of bladder distention originate in tension receptors in the bladder wall and travel in the pelvic nerves. Afferent fibers responsible for sensations of pain, temperature, conscious touch, and distention originate in the trigone and anterior bladder neck region and travel in the hypogastric nerve. Afferent pathways from the striated sphincter and urethral, which transmit sensations of temperature, pain, urethral wall distention, and urine passage, travel in the pudendal nerve.

The ultimate control of bladder storage and emptying resides at higher neurologic levels that facilitate and inhibit bladder and urethral activities via the peripheral nervous system. Barrington's center, located in the pontine-mesencephalic gray matter of the brain stem, is considered to be the origin of facilitory impulses to the bladder *(43)*. Input to this area is derived from the spinal cord, cerebellum, basal ganglia, thalamus and hypothalamus, and cerebral cortex. This network is quite complex, which unfortunately makes it vulnerable to injury and the alterations in central neurotransmitters and neuroreceptors that are known to occur with aging *(44)*.

PATHOPHYSIOLOGY OF THE AGING BLADDER

Effects of aging on the intrinsic factors responsible for normal function of the lower urinary tract can lead to varying degrees of impairment. Urogenital atrophy occurs, which leads to thinning of the trigonal urothelium and possibly an increase in irritative symptoms or urinary tract infections *(45,46)*. Urethral mucosa thinning also occurs, which decreases coaptation and predisposes a woman to stress urinary incontinence. Leakiness of the endothelium increases with advancing age, but the clinical significance of this is unknown *(47)*. A decline in the volume of blood flow through the submucosal vascular plexus probably also contributes to the loss of urethral mucosal coaptation. Connective tissue changes occur including decreased elasticity, reduced total amounts of collagen, and increased crosslinking of collagen. These changes in conjunction with atrophy of skeletal muscle may lead to deficiencies in the urethral supports. Neurologic changes associated with aging can reduce the number of adrenergic receptors effecting the responsiveness of urethral smooth muscle and slowing nerve conduction times. These changes result in varying degrees of sensory and motor impairment.

In addition to changes in factors intrinsic to the lower urinary tract, changes in other organ systems that occur with aging can also have a profound impact on lower urinary tract function in the elderly female. Neurologic diseases such as stroke, Alzheimer's disease, Parkinson's disease, or lumbosacral disc disease have the potential of interfering with the complex neuronal network responsible for bladder storage and emptying *(48,49)*. Neurologic diseases that affect cognitive functioning can interfere with the awareness of bladder fullness or inhibition of detrusor contractions. Peripheral neuropathy associated with diabetes, hypothyroidism, uremia, peripheral vascular disease, and vitamin B12 deficiency can interrupt the autonomic component of lower urinary tract innervation or affect mobility. Changes in lower urinary tract functioning can also occur after radical pelvic surgery or radiation for pelvic malignancies *(50)*. Third-spacing of fluid, which often occurs with cardiovascular disease, may cause mobilization of retained fluid when the patient becomes supine and result in nocturia or nocturnal enuresis. Age-related changes in glomerular filtration rate, renal blood flow, and renal tubular function with loss of concentrating ability can account for increased volume and diurnal increased frequency. Nocturnal diuresis, a common phenomenon also associated with the aging process, will also contribute to increasing nocturia or nocturnal enuresis *(51)*. Diabetes can increase urine output. Pulmonary diseases that increase coughing frequency and intensity can have a negative affect on pelvic floor support mechanisms. Mobility and dexterity are often lost with aging because of multiple factors that may make it more difficult to get to the bathroom and remove clothing in a timely fashion. Many medications used for various medical conditions can secondarily affect lower urinary tract function.

Changes in the intrinsic factors associated with aging are usually attributed to the loss of estrogen that follows the menopause. Although the loss of estrogen is not responsible for most of the age-related changes observed in other organ systems, it can increase the impact of some of these changes on the lower urinary tract. Estrogen deficiency at menopause is primarily associated with the accelerated phase of cancellous-bone loss in women due to a dramatic increase in bone resorption. With aging, the risk for osteoporosis and osteoporotic bone fracture rates increase, especially for hip, pelvis, spine, and ribs (52–54). An osteoporotic fracture can impinge upon neurologic pathways and restrict mobility. Women are more than three times more likely to develop dementia than men (2). Increasing evidence indicates that 17 beta-estradiol enhances memory functions in women throughout their adult life and that loss of estrogen, either through medically induced or natural menopause, results in a decline in memory and cognitive function (55–58). Dementia is a commonly identifiable cause of urinary incontinence. Cardiovascular disease is by far the leading cause of death among postmenopausal women. Recent data have suggested an overall 50% reduction in cardiovascular mortality in women taking estrogen replacement therapy (ERT) and the number of studies supporting this is growing (59). Cardiovascular disease can impact on urinary control and changes in voiding patterns due to third-spacing of fluid with mobilization of excess fluid at night. Diuretics, alpha and beta adrenergic antagonists, and medications commonly used in patients with these disorders, can have dramatic effects on the lower urinary tract.

CLINICAL PRESENTATIONS

Irritative Symptoms

Irritative symptoms of the lower urinary tract include frequency (more than seven voids per d given normal fluid intake of 1500–2000 cc/d), nocturia (the need to urinate more than once per night), dysuria, urgency, or bladder pain. Although irritative symptoms are most commonly caused by urinary tract infections, they are often experienced by postmenopausal women in the absence of an infection. Some have suggested these symptoms are caused by the loss of estrogen and a so called "senile atrophic urethritis" (45). Irritative symptoms have been correlated with changes in urethral cytology in postmenopausal women and both have responded to estrogen therapy (60).

The symptoms of frequency and urgency increase and peak between 45 and 50 yr, declining thereafter (61). This is evidence against hypoestrogenism being the absolute cause of these symptoms. It has been postulated that because frequency and urgency occur with greatest frequency during the climacteric, fluctuations in estrogen levels may be more responsible for these symptoms (62).

Voiding frequency and nocturia, however, seem to increase with age. About 30% of menopausal patients are noted to have urinary frequency. This rate increases two years after the menopause, as does nocturia (62,63). Nocturia is the most common urinary symptom in the elderly and it increases in severity with age. It is present in 31% of women age 45–64, and in 61% of elderly women (64). There is an increase in nighttime diuresis, despite an overall reduction in fluid intake in elderly women. This phenomenon is attributed to a decrease in kidney filtration with age, which tends to compensate during the night. The nocturnal diuresis may be exacerbated by conditions that increase third spacing of fluid or the decrease in bladder capacity often observed in this population (65).

Irritative symptoms can be explained by specific urodynamic findings in elderly women. Resnik concluded that bladder capacity, the ability to postpone voiding, and bladder compliance decline with age (49). Brocklehurst found that the majority of elderly nonincontinent women have uninhibited bladder contractions and decreased bladder capacities on cystometrogram (66).

Versi, however, using strict urodynamic criteria, did not demonstrate early first sensation and reduced bladder capacity in a group of patients who had recently undergone menopause. One reason cited for this discrepancy is that irritative symptoms and the associated urodynamic changes may be more commonly seen only after atrophic changes have been present for a longer time *(62)*.

URINARY TRACT INFECTIONS

The prevalence of urinary tract infections increases with age, rising in a linear fashion even many years after the menopause *(67)*. The incidence of bacteriuria has been shown to be greater in women over age 65. Risk factors for urinary tract infections identified in this age group include a voiding dysfunction (elevated postvoid residual) and urogenital atrophy *(68)*. Atrophy of the vaginal epithelium results in a decrease in the secretion of glycogen. This reduces the colonization of lactobacilli, which then elevates vaginal pH. Decreased vaginal acidity may encourage the overgrowth of gram negative organisms making the vagina a reservoir of uropathogens *(69)*. Significant correlations have been identified between a vaginal pH greater than 4.4 and culture positivity *(70)*. Estrogen replacement has been shown to increase lactobacilli concentration and decrease vaginal pH *(71)*. Randomized controlled studies have shown that oral and vaginal estrogen significantly decreases the number of urinary tract infections and restores vaginal flora and pH to a premenopausal state in elderly women treated versus placebo *(72)*. Other studies have confirmed these findings following administration of exogenous estrogen *(73–76)*.

VOIDING DYSFUNCTION SYMPTOMS

A voiding dysfunction is defined as incomplete bladder emptying. Voiding dysfunctions occur because of either increased urethral resistance or an inability of the detrusor muscle to initiate and sustain a contraction of sufficient amplitude. Depending on the cause, women with a voiding dysfunction may be asymptomatic or complain of urinary hesitancy, frequency, urgency, painful voiding, a slow or interrupted urine stream, and feelings of incomplete bladder emptying.

The process of normal voiding is complex, whereby initiation is voluntary, but the maintenance and completion are autonomically mediated. The first event that must occur is awareness of bladder fullness. Voluntary relaxation of the pelvic floor skeletal musculature and subsequent relaxation of the urethral sphincter then follow. This initiates the detrusor reflex, which results in a sustained, coordinated contraction of bladder smooth muscle. Coordination of urethral relaxation with the detrusor contraction must also occur. All of these events are neurologically mediated through peripheral and central pathways.

Causes of voiding dysfunction are many and are usually classified according to whether urethral or bladder function is disrupted. In the healthy postmenopausal female, maximum and mean urine flow rates are decreased when compared to healthy premenopausal women *(77)*. Postvoid residual urine usually increases up to 100 cc in the elderly. In one study of geriatric outpatients, 28% of the incontinent and 39% of the continent women had residual volumes greater than 100 mL *(78)*. It has not been determined whether these findings are secondary to decreased bladder contractility or increased urethral resistance. Some authors have suggested that estrogen deficiency may contribute to distal urethral stenosis, but true urethral stenosis is relatively rare in the female population *(79)*. If one considers the combination of changes that occurs in the intrinsic and extrinsic factors responsible for normal lower urinary tract function, voiding dysfunction in the aging female is more commonly the result of decreased bladder contractility. Urethral closing pressure typically decreases with age. Karram et al. assessed the effects of aging, childbirth, menopausal status, and anterior vaginal wall relaxation on detrusor contraction strength during voiding. Menopausal status was the only factor identified that significantly affected maximum detrusor pressure during voiding *(80)*. Hilton and Stanton showed a significant subjective improvement in voiding dysfunction symptoms following vaginal estrogen cream *(81)*. There are no clinical trials available that evaluate an objectively measurable effect of HRT on voiding efficiency in postmenopausal women.

URINARY INCONTINENCE

Urinary incontinence is the involuntary loss of urine that is a social or hygienic problem for the patient. Women are two times more likely to experience urinary incontinence than men. In a recent study, the prevalence of reported urinary incontinence in community-dwelling women over 69 yr of age was 41% with 14% reporting daily incontinence *(82)*. In this study, age, hysterectomy, obesity, poor overall health, presence of certain medical conditions (stroke, chronic obstructive pulmonary disease, and diabetes), and gait speed were identified as important independent factors associated with daily urinary incontinence. Obesity and hysterectomy accounted for the largest attributable risk proportion. It is well known that the prevalence of incontinence increases with age *(83,84)*. This increase in prevalence with aging however, does not seem to correspond with the onset of menopause.

Incontinence can be transient in up to one-third of community dwelling elderly and up to 50% of inpatients *(85)*. Transient incontinence most likely occurs in individuals who have underlying lower urinary tract dysfunction and whose continence status is tenuous. These individuals are then exposed to a condition or agent that further compromises their continence status and incontinence ensues. Causes of transient incontinence include confusion, infection, atrophic urogenital mucosa, medications that interfere with lower urinary tract function, excessive urine output such as with diuretics or metabolic disorders, restricted mobility, or fecal impaction.

There are four types of urinary incontinence, stress, urge, mixed (stress and urge), and overflow. The prevalence of the different types of urinary incontinence depends on the age of the population. In the elderly population, urge incontinence is the most common type of incontinence and is associated with two-thirds of established incontinence in older individuals *(86,87)*. Urge incontinence is defined by an involuntary detrusor contraction that occurs either spontaneously or with provocation while the patient is trying to inhibit micturition. In support of this, the most common urodynamic finding in the incontinent elderly is the uninhibited increase in detrusor pressure during a retrograde cystometrogram occurring in up to 75% of patients studied *(48)*. The prevalence of urge incontinence increases with age, but there is no proven association with timing of the menopause *(88,62)*.

Patients with urge incontinence often complain of a sudden urge to urinate and the involuntary leakage of urine shortly thereafter. The amount of leakage is usually large and the frequency of occurrence is unpredictable, making urge incontinence the most distressing of the different types of urinary incontinence. Other symptoms often associated with urge incontinence include frequency of urination, urgency, nocturia, and nocturnal enuresis (bedwetting).

When urge incontinence is associated with a neurologic disease, it is referred to as detrusor hyperreflexia. If there is no identifiable neurologic disease present, this condition is called detrusor instability. This distinction can be blurred given frequent neurologic compromise in the elderly patient. A third subset of urge incontinence is detrusor hyperactivity with impaired contractions or DHIC. Patients with this disorder have urge incontinence, but also empty their bladders incompletely. DHIC is the second most-common type of incontinence in institutionalized patients (87). This diagnosis carries important implications with regard to therapy because anticholinergic agents, often used to control uninhibited detrusor contractions, may worsen the voiding dysfunction or cause urinary retention.

The spontaneous detrusor activity that defines urge incontinence is because of specific changes at the smooth muscle–cell junctions. Whether these changes are neurologically mediated or are inherent to the smooth muscle or neuroreceptor affinity cannot be determined with certainty in any one individual. Electron microscopic examination of aging detrusor smooth muscle in patients with overactive, unobstructed bladders has shown distinctive cell-to-cell contact areas called protrusion junctions and ultraclose abutments which are not found in the normal detrusor (89). Elbadawi proposed that these junctions are mediators of uninhibited bladder contractions via electrical cell coupling. The linkage of smooth muscle cells by these junctions creates a syncytium around a loci of muscle cells that are sensitive to various stimuli (stretch, neural stimuli, etc.). Contractions originating in one foci could then be propagated electrically to other parts of the detrusor. Measurable involuntary contractions would result if this propagation involved a large area of the detrusor. It is not known whether aging *per se* or hormone depletion are the cause of smooth muscle–cell junction changes in elderly women, but Elbadawi observed no gender differences in the structural features of the dysjunction pattern. A study of humans of varying ages concluded that there was a reduction in the number of axons in the bladder with aging (90). Conflicting findings regarding changes in cholinergic and adrenergic receptor responsiveness in the bladder with age have been reported in rats (78,91–93). However, estrogen caused a significant increase in the response of the bladder body of immature rabbits to alpha-adrenergic and muscarinic cholinergic agonists (94). No changes were observed in the beta-adrenergic receptors.

Stress incontinence is caused by a weakness in the urethral sphincteric mechanism such that an increase in intra-abdominal pressure causes bladder pressure to exceed urethral pressure in the absence of a bladder contraction. It is the second most common cause of urinary incontinence in elderly women (95). Women with stress incontinence will complain of leakage of urine with physical activity such as a cough, sneeze, lifting, or a change in position. Stress incontinence episodes tend to be small and can be controlled somewhat by the level and intensity of activity performed. The severity of stress incontinence depends on the degree of urethral sphincteric dysfunction. How this is quantified is a matter of controversy, but usually consists of a combination of urethral-pressure studies and bladder-neck imaging.

Most of the components of the urethral sphincter are sensitive to estrogen stimulation, however, it is not clear clinically whether urethral function is estrogen-dependent. Maximum urethral-closing pressure (the difference between resting-urethral pressure and total bladder pressure) in normal women reaches a peak between age 20 and 25 and then decreases with age (19,96). This suggests that menopause does not play a role in the decline of urethral-pressure parameters. However, Versi has shown that urethral function at rest does deteriorate following ovarian failure. This difference could not be accounted for by age differences alone and was statistically significant (97). Findings in other studies evaluating the effects of estrogen on resting urethral pressures have been inconsistent with some showing significant increases in urethral pressures at rest and others showing no changes in urethral resting pressures *(81,98–101)*.

Although resting-urethral pressure is an important factor for maintaining continence, urethral function is defined by the status of the urethral pressure relative to the total bladder pressure during times of increased intra-abdominal pressure. This dynamic role is fulfilled by the skeletal muscle components of the urethral sphincter and supports *(102)*. The ability of the urethral sphincteric unit to reflexively increase its pressure in response to increases in intra-abdominal pressure is measured urodynamically by the pressure transmission ratio. Higher pressure transmission ratios reflect larger increases in the urethral pressure above resting pressure. Although estrogen may have a positive effect on skeletal muscle tone, studies evaluating the effect of estrogen on pressure transmission ratios have yielded inconsistent results *(81,100,101,103–105)*.

HORMONAL THERAPY FOR URINARY INCONTINENCE

Although there is evidence of specific hormonal effects on various components of the lower urinary tract, very little has been done to prove a significant clinical benefit from hormonal therapy in women with urinary incontinence. The effect of progesterone on the lower urinary tract in general is poorly understood and therefore will not be discussed here. Most of the early studies evaluating the efficacy of estrogen therapy in postmenopausal women were uncontrolled and used subjective outcome measures making it impossible to account for a placebo effect. In the first report published in 1941, Salmon et al. treated 16 women with dysuria and incontinence with intramuscular estradiol *(106)*. After several weeks, 12 of the women reported symptomatic improvement, only to have their symptoms worsen when the drug was stopped and again improve when estrogen therapy was subsequently repeated. Cellular maturation was observed in vaginal smears. Bhatia used conjugated estrogen vaginal cream daily in 11 postmenopausal women with genuine stress urinary incontinence (urodynamically proven) for 6 wk *(107)*. Six were either cured or significantly improved and this improvement correlated with an increase in resting urethral pressures and transmission ratios, as well as changes in urethral cytology.

The first randomized, placebo-controlled, double-blind trial published showed a significant reduction in the frequency of incontinence in hospitalized elderly women after 5 wk of treatment with quinestradol, a synthetic estrogen *(108)*. No significant placebo effect was found. Another randomized study by Walter et al. evaluated the effect of oral estradiol and estriol versus placebo in 29 postmenopausal women with urinary incontinence *(101)*. Patients were treated for a total of four months. There was a statistically significant increase in the serum estradiol level in the treated group compared to the placebo group. In addition, there was an obvious maturation of vaginal and bladder biopsies in the estrogen-treated group not observed in the placebo group. With regard to urge incontinence and bladder irritative symptoms, there was a significant subjective improvement in the treated group versus the placebo group. However, stress incontinence symptoms and changes in urethral function studies were not significantly different between groups after treatment. In a study of 34 incontinent elderly women, Samsioe et al. evaluated placebo versus oral estriol in a double-blind crossover fashion *(109)*. There was no significant difference in response between estriol and placebo in the stress-incontinent patients, but estrogen therapy did improve symptoms in patients with urge and mixed incontinence compared to placebo. Wilson et al. reported subjective improvement in incontinence symptoms among women receiving oral estrogen replacement versus placebo, but no statistically significant differences were found between groups with respect to urethral studies or amount of urine loss *(110)*.

In his first published study regarding estrogen therapy and urinary incontinence, Fantl compared clinical and urodynamic variables of 49 nonestrogen-supplemented and 23 estrogen-supplemented postmenopausal women with urinary incontinence *(111)*. In patients with detrusor instability, the difference between the bladder volume at maximum cystometric capacity and first desire to void was larger in the estrogen-supplemented group and this approached statistical significance. There was also a significantly lower frequency of nocturia, a significantly higher prevalence of a positive bulbocavernosus reflex, and a lower prevalence of the symptoms of urge incontinence in the estrogen-supplemented subjects supporting a sensory modulating effect of estrogen therapy. None of the urethral sphincteric function studies were independently affected by estrogen therapy. Fantl et al. subsequently applied a meta-analysis to available data to evaluate the efficacy of estrogen therapy in the management of postmenopausal urinary incontinence *(112)*. From 23 eligible articles reviewed, a significant effect of estrogen therapy on subjective improvement was found for all subjects. There was no significant effect on the amount of urine loss. Although a significant effect on maximum urethral closure pressure was demonstrated, the author points out that this result was influenced by only one study showing a large effect. In a prospective, randomized, double-blind, placebo-controlled trial, Fantl et al. assessed the efficacy of three months of cyclic postmenopausal hormone replacement in treating urinary incontinence in hypoestrogenic women *(113)*. No significant differences in the number of incontinent episodes or the amount of urine lost after treatment was observed in the treatment and control groups. There were no significant differences for either day or nighttime frequency, quality-of-life measures, or patient's subjective improvement. Significant changes in plasma estradiol levels and cytologic maturational index of vaginal smears were observed in the estrogen-treated group.

Theoretically, estrogen therapy through several mechanisms should enhance urethral sphincteric function and improve outlet resistance. Unfortunately, clinical studies of the effect of estrogen therapy on urethral function have not shown consistent improvement in urethral-pressure measurements or symptoms of stress incontinence. One of the proposed mechanisms through which estrogen exerts a positive effect on urethral pressure, which has been previously described, is the increased sensitivity of alpha-adrenergic receptors in the smooth muscle sphincter. Clinical experience supports an additive effect when estrogen and alpha-adrenergic agonist are given simultaneously. Ek et al. found significant symptomatic improvement in women with stress urinary incontinence following treatment with estradiol and norephedrine but not estradiol alone *(114)*. Urethral closure pressure increased in the combination group and in the norephedrine alone group but not the estradiol group. A study by Kinn revealed a significant improvement in incontinence symptoms and patient satisfaction with both estriol and phenylpropanolamine compared to either drug alone *(115)*. Urethral pressure increased and urine loss decreased in patients receiving combination therapy and phenylpropanolamine. Ahlstrom et al. showed a better response in postmenopausal women with stress urinary incontinence receiving combined estriol and phenylpropanolamine than those receiving estriol alone *(116)*. Also, a significant increase in the maximum urethral closure pressure was identified in the group receiving combined therapy. Maturation indices in this study revealed a positive effect. Thus, the clinical effect of estrogen and alpha-adrenergic combination therapy on symptoms of stress urinary incontinence seems to be consistent.

SUMMARY

Although lower urinary tract dysfunction is not normal at any age, its prevalence increases with aging. Women are more commonly affected by these conditions than men. Thus, a likely assumption has been that a decline in hormonal support with menopause plays a role in the development of urinary storage and evacuation disorders in women. Hormonal receptors have been identified in the lower urinary tract and there is an abundance of literature which demonstrates effects of hormonal therapy, particularly estrogen, on the bladder and urethra. Clinical studies, however, have inconsistently revealed improvement in postmenopausal women with lower urinary tract dysfunction symptoms receiving estrogen replacement, particularly with regard to objective outcome measures. Because certain subsets of postmenopausal women with urinary symptoms have been shown to benefit from estrogen replacement, the recommendation is that estrogen be included among the options given to these women presenting for treatment.

REFERENCES

1. Studd JWW, Chakravarti S, Oram D. The climacteric. Clin Obstet Gynaecol 1977;4:3–29.
2. US. Bureau of the Census, Statistical Abstract of the United States, 113th ed. Washington, DC. 1993.
3. Wolf H, Wandt H, Jonat W. Immunohistochemical evidence of estrogen and progesterone receptors in the female lower urinary tract and comparison with the vagina. Gynecol Obstet Invest 1991;32:227–231.
4. Packham DA. The epithelial lining of the female trigone and urethra. Br J Urol 1971;43:201–205.
5. McCallin PE, Stewart-Taylor E, Whitehead RW. A study of the changes in the cytology of urinary sediment during the menstrual cycle and pregnancy. Am J Obstet Gynecol 1950;60:64–74.
6. Zinner NN, Sterling AM, Ritter RC. Evaluation of inner urethral softness. Urology 1983;22:446–448.
7. Versi E. Incontinence in the climacteric. Clin Obstet Gynecol 1990;33:392–398.
8. Huisman AB. Morfologie van de vrouwelijke urethra. Thesis. Groningen, The Netherlands, 1979.
9. Versi E, Cardozo LD. Urethral vascular pulsations. Proc Int Cont Soc 1985;15:503–504.
10. Batra S, Bjellin L, Iosif S, et al. Effects of oestrogen and progesterone on the blood flow in the lower urinary tract of the rabbit. Acta Physiol Scand 1985;123:191–194.
11. Raz S, Caine M, Zeigler M. The vascular component in the production of intraurethral pressure. J Urol 1972;108:93–98.
12. Rud T, Andersson KE, Asmussen M, et al. Factors maintaining the urethral pressure in women. Invest Urol 1980;17:343–347.
13. Semmilink HJF, deWilde PCM, van Houwelingen JC, et al. Histomorphometric study of the lower urogenital tract in pre and postmenopausal women. Cytometry 1990;11:700–707.
14. Levin RM, Tong VC, Wein AJ. Effect of pregnancy on the autonomic response of the rabbit urinary bladder. Neurourol Urodynam 1991;10:313–316.
15. Ekstrom J, Iosif CS, Malmburg L. Effects on long-term treatment with estrogen and progesterone on in vitro muscle responses of the female rabbit urinary bladder and urethra to autonomic drugs and nerve stimulation. J Urol 1993;150:1284.
16. Schreiter F, Fuchs P, Stockamp K. Estrogenic sensitivity of the alpha receptors in the urethral musculature. Urol Int 1976;31:13.
17. Hodgsen BJ, Dumas S, Bolling DV, et al. Effect of estrogen on sensitivity of rabbit bladder and urethra to phenylephrine. Invest Uro 1978;16:67.
18. DeLancey JOL. Correlative study of paraurethral anatomy. Obstet Gynecol 1986;68:91–97.
19. Constantinou CE. Resting and stress urethral pressures as a guide to the mechanism of continence in the female patient. Urol Clin North Am 1985;12:247–258.
20. Petrucchini D, DeLancey JOL, Ashton-Miller JA. Regional striated muscel loss in the urethra: Where is striated muscle vulnerable? Int Urogynecol J 1997;8:242.
21. DeLancey JOL. Structural aspects of the extrinsic continence mechanism. Obstet Gynecol 1988;72:296–301.

22. Bacho C, Winandy A. Preliminary study of the hormonal effect on various parameters on the pelvic floor in genitally active women without hormone therapy and in menopausal women. Acta Urol Belg 1992;60:45–60.
23. Ingelman-Sundberg A, Rosen K. Gustafsson SA, et al. Cytosol estrogen receptors in the urogenital tissues in stress incontinent women. Acta Obstet Gynecol Scand 1981;60:585.
24. Bump RC, Freidman CI. Intraluminal urethral pressure measurement in the female baboon: effects of hormonal manipulation. J Urol 1986;136:508.
25. Brincat M, Moniz CJ, Studd JWW, et al. The long-term effects of the menopause and sex hormones on skin thickness. Br J Obstet Gynecol 1985;92:256–259.
26. Holland EF, Studd JW, Mansell JP, et al. Changes in collagen composition and cross-links in bone and skin of osteoporotic postmenopausal women treated with percutaneous estradiol implants. Obstet Gynecol 1994;83:180–183.
27. Katz FH, Kappas A. Influence of oestradiol and oestriol on urinary excretion of hydroxyproline in man. J Lab Clin Med 1968;71:65–71.
28. Sato T, Ito A, Mori V, et al. Hormonal regulation of collagenolysis in uterine cervical fibroblasts: modulation of synthesis of procollagenase, prostromelysin and tissue inhibitor of metalloproteinases (TIMP) by progesterone nad oestradiol-17beta. Biochem J 1991;275:645.
29. Versi E, Cardozo L, Brincat M, et al. Correlation of urethral physiology and skin collagen in postmenopausal women. Br J Obstet Gynaecol 1988;95:505–506.
30. Ulmsten U, Ekman G, Giertz G, et al. Different biochemical composition of connective tissue in continent and stress incontinent women. Acta Obstet Gynecol Scand 1987;66:455.
31. Rechberger T, Donica H, Baranowski W, et al. Female urinary stress incontinence in terms of connective tissue biochemistry. Eur J Obstet Gynecol Reprod Biol 1993;49:187.
32. Bergman A, Elia G, Cheung D, et al. Biochemical composition of collagen in continent and stress incontinent women. Gynecol Obset Invest 1994;37:48.
33. Vanarsdalen K, Wein AJ. Physiology of micturition and continence. In: Krane RJ, Siroky MB, eds. Clinical Neuro-urology. Little, Brown and Co., Boston, MA, 1991, pp. 25–82.
34. Elbadawi A, Yalla SV, Resnik NM. Structural basis of geriatric voiding dysfunction II: aging detrusor: normal vs impaired contractility. J Urol 1993;150:1657–1667.
35. Batra SC, Iosif LS. Progesterone receptors in the female lower urinary tract. J Urol 1987;138:1301–1304.
36. Iosif CS, Batra S, Ek A, et al. Estrogen receptors in human female lower urinary tract. Am J Obstet Gynecol 1981;141:817.
37. Youssef AF. Cystometric studies in gynecology and obstetrics. Obstet Gynecol 1956;8:181–188.
38. Burton G, Cardozo LD, Abdalla H, et al. The hormonal effects on the lower urinary tract in 282 women with premature ovarian failure. Neurourol Urodynam 1992;10:318–319.
39. Eika B, Salling LN, Christensen LL, et al. Long-term observation of the detrusor smooth muscle in rats-its relationship to ovariectomy and estrogen treatment. Urol Res 1990;18:439–442.
40. Longhurst PA, Kauer J, Legee HRE, et al. The influences of ovariectomy and estradiol replacement on urinary bladder function in rats. J Urol 1992;148:915.
41. Elbadawi A, Schenk E. Dual innervation of the mammalian urinary bladder. A histochemical study of the distribution of cholinergic and adrenergic nerves. Am J Anat 1966;119:405–427.
42. Elbadawi A, Schenk E. A new theory of the innervation of bladder musculature: III Innervaton of the vesicourethal junction and external urethral sphincter. J Urol 1974;111:613.
43. Barrington FJF. The relation of the hindbrain to micturition. Brain 1921;44:23.
44. Roth GS. Effects of aging on mechanisms of hormone and neurotransmitter action during aging: current status of the role of receptor and post-receptor alterations. A review. Mech Aging Dev 1982;20:175–194.
45. Everett HS. Urology in the female. Am J Surg 1941;52:521–530.
46. Smith P. Age changes in the female urethra. Br J Urol 1972;44:667–676.
47. Brocklehurst JC. The aging bladder. Br J Hosp Med 1986;35:8–10.
48. Brocklehurst JC, Dillane JB. Studies of the female bladder in old age II. Cystometrograms in 100 incontinent women. Geront Clin 1966;8:306–319.
49. Resnik NM, Yalla SV. Aging and its effects on the bladder. Sem Urol 1987;5:82–86.
50. Minini GF, Simeone C, Zambolin T, et al. Long-term functional sequelae of the urinary tract following radical surgical treatment of carcinoma of the cervix with and without extended radiation therapy. Int Urogynecol J 1992;3:8–11.
51. Staskin DR. Age-related physiologic and pathologic changes affecting lower urinary tract function. Clin Geriat Med 1986;2:701–710.

52. Nachtigall CE, Nachtigall RH, Nachtigall RD, et al. Estrogen replacement therapy I: A 10–year prospective study in the relationship to osteoporosis. Obstet Gynecol 1979;53:277–281.

53. Ettinger B, Genant HK, Cann CE. Long term estrogen replacement therapy prevents bone loss and fractures. Ann Intern Med 1985;102:319–324. .

54. Lindsay R. Sex steroids in the pathogenesis and prevention of osteoporosis. In: Riggs BL, Melton LJ, III, eds. Osteoporosis: Etiology, Diagnosis, and Management. Raven, New York, 1988, pp. 333–358.

55. Birge S. Is there a role for estrogen replacement therapy in the prevention and treatment of dementia? J Am Geriat Soc 1996;44:865–870.

56. Sherwin BB, Phillips S. Estrogen and cognitive function in surgically menopausal women. Ann NY Acad Sci 1990;592:474–475.

57. Tang MX, Jacobs D, Stern Y, et al. Effect of oestrogen during menopause on risk and age at onset of Alzheimer's disease. Lancet 1996;348:429–432.

58. Henderson VW, Paganini-Hill A, Emanuel CK, et al. Estrogen replacement therapy in older women. Arch Neurology 1994;51:896–900.

59. Grodstein F, Stampfer MJ. The epidemiology of coronary heart disease and estrogen replacement in postmenopausal women. Prog Cardiovasc Dis 1995;18:199.

60. Smith PJB. The effects of oestrogen on bladder function in the female. In: Campbell S, ed. The Management of the Menopause and Postmenopausal Years. MTP Press, London, UK, 1976, pp. 291–298.

61. Bungay GT, Vessey MP, McPherson CK. A study of symptoms in middle life with special reference to the menopause. Br Med J 1980;281:181–183.

62. Versi E. The bladder in menopause: lower urinary tract dysfunction during the climacteric. Curr Probl Obstet Gynecol Fertil 1994;17:193–232.

63. Glenning PP. Urinary voiding patterns of apparently normal women. Aust N Z J Obstet Gynaecol 1985;25:62–65.

64. Finkbeiner AE. The aging bladder. Int J Urogynecol 1993;4:168–174.

65. DeLancey JOL, Norton P, Wall L. Special considerations in the elderly. In: DeLancey JOL, Norton P, Wall L, eds. Practical Urogynecology. Williams and Wilkins, Baltimore, MD, 1993, pp. 316–331.

66. Brocklehurst JC, Dillane JB. Studies of the female bladder in old age, I. Cystometrograms in non-incontinent women. Geront Clin 1966;8:285–305.

67. Molander U, Milsom I, Ekelund P, et al. An epidemiological study of urinary incontinence and relaxed urogenital symptoms in elderly women. Maturitas 1990:12:51–60.

68. Brocklehurst JC, Dillane JB, Griffiths L, et al. The prevalence of symptomatology of urinary infection in an aged population. Gerontol Clin 1968;10:242–253.

69. Fair WR, Timothy MM, Millar MA, et al. Bacteriologic and hormonal observations of the urethra and vaginal vestibule in normal premenopausal women. J Urol 1970;104:426.

70. Stamey TA, Timoth MM. Studies of introital colonization in women with recurrent urinary infections I. The role of vaginal pH. J Urol 1975;114:261.

71. Molander U, Milsom I, Ekelund P, et al. A health care program for the investigation and treatment of elderly women with urinary incontinence and related urogenital symptoms. Acta Obstet Gynecol Scand 1991;70:137.

72. Raz R, Stann WE. A controlled trial of intravaginal estriol in postmenopausal women with recurrent urinary tract infections. N Engl J Med 1993;329:73–75.

73. Marshal S, Linfoot J Influence of hormones on urinary tract infection. Urology 1977;9:675.

74. Parsons CL, Schmidt JD. Control of recurrent lower urinary tract infection in the postmenopausal woman. J Urol 1982;128:1224.

75. Privette M, Cade R, Peterson J, et al. Prevention of recurrent urinary tract infections in postmenopausal women. Nephron 1988;50:24. .

76. Kirkengen AL, Andersen P, Gjersoe E, et al. Oestriol in the prophylactic treatment of recurrent urinary tract infections in postmenopausal women. Scan J Prim Health Care 1992;10:139–142.

77. Sorensen S, Jonler M, Knudsen LLB, et al. The influence of a urethral catheter and age on recorded urinary flow rates in healthy women. Scand J Urol Nephrol 1989;23:261–266.

78. Ouslander JG, Hepps K, Raz S, et al. Genitourinary dysfunction in a geriatric outpatient population. J Am Geriatr Soc 1986;34:507–514.

79. Roberts M, Smith PJB. Non-malignant obstruction of the female urethra. Br J Urol 1968;40:694–702.

80. Karram MM, Partoll L, Bilotta V, et al. Factors affecting detrusor contraction strength during voiding in women. Obstet Gynecol 1997;90:723–726.

81. Hilton P, Stanton SL. The use of intravaginal oestrogen cream in genuine stress incontinence. Br J Obstet Gynaecol 1983;90:940–944.

82. Brown JS, Seeley DG, Fong J, et al. Urinary incontinence in older women. Who is at risk? Obstet Gynecol 1996;87:715–721.

83. Thomas TM, Plymat KR, Blannin J, et al. Prevalence of urinary incontinence. Br Med J 1980;281:1243–1245.

84. Milsom I, Ekelund P, Molander U, et al. The influence of age, parity, oral contraception, hysterectomy and menopause on the prevalence of urinary incontinence in women. J Urol 1993;149:1459–1462.

85. Resnik NM. Urinary incontinence. Lancet 1995;346:94–98.

86. Brown ADG. Postmenopausal urinary problems. Clin Obstet Gynaecol 1977;4:181–207.

87. Resnik NM, Yalla SV. Detrusor hyperactivity with impaired contractile function. JAMA 1987;257:3076–3081.

88. Kondo A, Saito M, Yamada Y, et al. Prevalence of handwashing urinary incontinence in healthy subjects in relation to stress and urge incontinence. Neurourol Urodynam 1992;11:519–523.

89. Elbadawi A, Yalla SV, Resnik NM. Structural basis of geriatric voiding dysfunction. III Detrusor overactivity. J Urol 1993;150:1668–1680.

90. Gilpin SA, Gilpin CJ, Dixon JS, et al. The effect of age on autonomic innervation of the urinary bladder. Br J Urol 1986;58:378–381.

91. Kolta MG, Wallace LJ, Gerald MC. Age-related changes in sensitivity of rat urinary bladder to autonomic agents. Mech Aging Dev 1984;27:183–188.

92. Wallace LJ, Kolta MG, Gerald MC, et al. Dietary choline affects response to acetylcholine by isolated urinary bladder. Life Sci 1985;36:1377–1380.

93. Johnson JM, Skau KA, Gerald MC, et al. Regional noradrenergic and cholinergic neurochemistry in the rat urinary bladder: effects of age. J Urol 1988;139:611–615.

94. Levin RM, Shofer FS, Wein AJ. Estrogen induced alterations in the autonomic responses of the rabbit urinary bladder. J Pharmacol Exp Ther 1980;215:614–618.

95. Resnik NM. Voiding dysfunction in the elderly. In: Yalla SV, McGuire EJ, Elbadawi A, Blaivas JG, eds. Neurology and Urodynamics: Principles and Practice. Macmillan, New York, 1988, pp. 303–330.

96. Rud T. Urethral pressure profile in continent women from childhood to old age. Acta Obstet Gynecol Scand 1980;59:331–335.

97. Versi E. The bladder in the menopausal woman. In: Greenblatt RB, Heithhecker R, eds. Modern Approach to the Perimenopausal Years. New Developments in Biosciences 2. W de Gruyter, Berlin, 1986, pp. 88–102.

98. Faber P, Heidenreich J Treatment of stress incontinence with estrogen in postmenopausal women. Urol Int 1977;32:221–223.

99. Beisland HO, Fossberg E, Moera, et al. Urethral sphincteric insufficiency in postmenopausal females: treatment with phenylpropanolamine and oestriol separately and in combination. Urol Int 1984;39:211–216.

100. Rud T. The effect of oestrogen and gestagens on the urethral pressure profile in urinary continent and stress incontinent women. Acta Obstet Gynecol Scand 1980;59:265–270.

101. Walter S, Wolf H, Barlebo H, et al. Urinary incontinence in postmenopausal women treated with estrogens: a double-blind clinical trial. Urol Int 1978;33:135–143.

102. Bump RC, Huang KC, McClish DK, et al. Effect of narcotic anesthesia and skeletal muscle paralysis on passive and dynamic urethral function of stress continent and incontinent women. Neurourol Urodyn 1991;10:523–532.

103. Iosif CS. Effects of protracted administration of estriol on the lower genitourinary tract in postmenopausal women. Arch Gynecol Obstet 1992;251:115–120.

104. Yeko TR, Sauer MV, Bhatia NN. Urodynamic changes following hormonal replacement therapy in women with premature ovarian failure. Obstet Gynecol 1989;74:208–211.

105. Versi E, Cardozo L, Studd JWW. Long-term effect of estradiol implants on the female urinary tract during the climacteric. Int Urogynecol J 1990;1:87–90.

106. Salmon UJ, Walter RI, Geist SH. The use of estrogens in the treatment of dysuria and incontinence in postmenopausal women. Am J Obstet Gynecol 1941;42:845–851.

107. Bhatia NN, Bergman A, Karram MM. Effects of estrogen on urethral function in women with stress incontinence. Obstet Gynecol 1989;160:176–181.

108. Judge TG. The use of quinestradol in elderly women, a preliminary report. Gerontol Clin 1969;11:159–164.

109. Samsioe G, Jansson I, Mellstrom D, et al. Occurrence, nature and treatment of urinary incontinence in a 70 year-old female population. Maturitas 1985;7:335.

110. Wilson PD, Faragher B, Butler B, et al. Treatment with oral piperazine oestrone sulphate for genuine stress incontinence in postmenopausal women. Br J Obstet Gynecol 1987;94:568.

111. Fantl JA, Wyman JF, Anderson RL, et al. Postmenopausal urinary incontinence comparison between nonestrogen supplemented and estrogen-supplemented women. Obstet Gynecol 1988;41:823–826.

112. Fantl JA, Cardozo L, McClish DK, et al. Estrogen therapy in the management of urinary incontinence in postmenopausal women: a meta-analysis. First Report of the Hormone and Urogenital Therapy Committee. Obstet Gynecol 1994;83:12–18.

113. Fantl JA, Bump RC, Robinson D, et al. Efficacy of estrogen supplementation in the treatment of urinary incontinence. Obstet Gynecol 1996;88:745–749.

114. Ek A, Andersson KE, Gullberg B, et al. Effects of oestradiol and combined norephedrin and oestradiol treatment on female stress incontinence. Zentralbl Gynekol 1980;102:839.

115. Kinn AC, Lindskog M. Estrogens and phenylpropanolamine in combination for stress urinary incontinence in postmenopausal women. Urol 1988;32:273.

116. Ahlstrom K, Sandahl B, Sjoberg B, et al. Effect of combined treatment with phenylpropanolamine and estriol compared with estriol treatment alone in postmenopausal women with stress urinary incontinence. Gynecol Obstet Invest 1990;30:37.

6

Alterations in Cognitive Function in Menopause

Laura J. Tivis, PhD

Contents

INTRODUCTION: SPECIAL CONCERNS OF POSTMENOPAUSAL WOMEN

More than ever before, women are taking charge of their own health. In today's world of high-tech information supersystems, women are gaining access to information that has previously been available only to a select few. Media attention to government-sponsored health research projects and the rising popularity of the Internet have provided women with a substantial amount of information about their own health, as well as opportunities to question commonly held beliefs.

More specifically, women of today are learning about menopause. The National Women's Health Resource Center has suggested that women will spend about one-third of their lives in the postmenopausal state *(1)*. Whereas once "the change" was discussed only among mature women and associated only with the end of the childbearing years, it is now the topic of women's health seminars, support groups, and women's magazines. Concerns about menopause and the changes that accompany the reduced level of estrogen are, more than ever before, on the minds of women.

Physical symptoms such as hot flushes and vaginal dryness are common menopausal complaints, and are fairly responsive to hormone replacement therapy (HRT). Psychological or emotional symptoms are also distressing, but unlike the physical symptoms that are directly and clearly linked to low levels of estrogen, the cause of menopausal emo-

From: *Contemporary Endocrinology: Menopause: Endocrinology and Management*
Edited by: D. B. Seifer and E. A. Kennard © Humana Press Inc., Totowa, NJ

tional symptoms such as depression, mood swings, irritability, and fatigue are not well understood. Cognitive symptoms such as poor memory and inability to concentrate are also reported among menopausal women. Anderson et al. reported that as many as 75% of their menopause clinic patients reported problems with memory loss, and 82% experienced problems with concentration (2). Many others have also identified memory loss as one of the most common clinical complaints among postmenopausal women (3–9). Complaints of cognitive problems such as memory loss are frequently assumed to be related to emotional or psychological symptoms, primarily because changes in cognition can be linked to affective disturbances, such as depression and anxiety. Whereas affective disturbances may well be the reason some women experience memory and concentration problems, other possible factors such as changes in brain structure and function, as well as changes in neurotransmitter activity, are currently being explored.

The primary aim of this chapter is to review the available literature on cognition and menopause. Specifically, it will explore whether low estrogen levels, characteristic of the postmenopausal state, result in impaired performance on tests that measure cognitive functioning. Two types of studies will be reviewed: experimental studies in which cognitive performance is assessed when exogenous estrogen or placebo is administered to postmenopausal women, and quasi-experimental studies in which cognitive performances of women who do not use use exogenous estrogen are compared to women who use no hormone replacement therapy. Finally, confounding variables will be addressed and future directions for research will be considered.

OVERVIEW OF COGNITIVE FUNCTIONING AND AGING

Kolb and Whishaw (10) define cognition as "a general term used to refer to the processes involved in thinking." "Cognitive functions" can refer to any number of mental operations such as reaction time, memory, learning, abstraction, problem solving, concept formation, and visual-spatial processing.

Although the aging process is certainly considered to be a risk factor for cognitive decline (11), most elderly individuals remain within normal limits on tests of neuropsychological function (12). Even so, some significant differences in cognitive functioning from one age group to another have been reported. A recent population-based study of nearly 400 men and 1000 women revealed that cognitive performance declined as a function of age on a wide variety of neuropsychological tasks (11).

Halbreich et al. point out that for women, cognitive decline may be accelerated with the onset of menopause (13). To test their hypothesis, correlation coefficients were computed between cognitive performance scores and age in groups of premenopausal and postmenopausal women. Halbreich et al. found that age was significantly positively correlated with several aspects of cognition in postmenopausal women, but not in premenopausal women. Several possible explanations have been suggested as to why menopause would influence cognition, including modifications of psychosocial roles, alterations in affective stability, and changes in the hormone milieu.

COGNITION AND HORMONAL INFLUENCES

Over the years, many studies have been conducted with respect to gender differences in cognition (14). Traditionally, males have been found to excel on spatial tasks, whereas females excel on verbal tasks. Several studies have focused on hormonal influences on task performance. Specifically, these studies have assessed relationships between levels of sex steroids and cognition (15–24). Most have used women in various phases of the menstrual cycle; a convenient method for assessing hormonal influences on cognition. Hampson and Kimura (14) provide an excellent review of the most methodologically sound studies, summarizing some thought-provoking findings. For instance, higher estrogen levels (preovulatory estrogen surge and midluteal rise) have been associated in several studies with poorer performance on spatial tasks. Studies of verbal abilities suggest that higher levels of estrogen may enhance *simple* output tasks, such as speed and accuracy of verbal performance (e.g., speeded counting, reading aloud, speech fluency). Similarly, motor task performance may be facilitated by higher levels of estrogen. Studies of hormonal influences on other cognitive tasks have yielded inconsistent results, i.e., the relationships between sex steroids and reaction time, complex verbal abilities, and perceptual speed are, as yet, less well understood (14).

The menstrual cycle studies support the idea that at least some cognitive functions may be influenced by estrogen levels. Because postmenopausal women are, by definition, estrogen deficient, the findings are intriguing. These data suggest that postmenopausal women who do not use estrogen replacement therapy (ERT) may be impaired, compared to their ERT-using peers, with respect to certain cognitive functions.

Animal studies also lend strong support to the idea of an estrogen/cognition relationship. For example, McEwen et al. found that administration of estrogen to ovariectomized female rats is linked to increased spine density on dendrites of hippocampal pyramidal neurons; the hippocampus plays a major role in learning and memory functions. Furthermore, this group found that in intact female rats, dendritic spine density fluctuates with the estrous cycle, with a positive relationship between spine density and circulating levels of estrogen (25–29). These data indicate that estrogen may modulate hippocampal structure and provide important implications for hippocampal function. Whether or not dendritic spine formation/destruction processes are directly responsible for cognitive changes in humans, remains to be seen.

A separate line of research has explored the possibility that the postmenopausal state of estrogen deprivation may contribute to the development of Alzheimer's disease. The rationale for this work stems from animal studies indicating that administration of estradiol increases choline acetyl transferase activity, and from human studies linking Alzheimer's disease to deficits in central cholinergic transmitter activity (30). Studies have also indicated that other neurotransmitter systems (in addition to the cholinergic system) are involved in Alzheimer's disease, and are affected by estrogen (30–31). Additionally, estrogen is thought to improve cerebral blood flow in women with vascular disease; vascular disease is thought to be associated with the pathogenisis of Alzheimer's disease (32). Other possible mechanisms by which estrogen may effect the disease process include reduction of free-radical formation through alterations in MAO activity (33), stimulation of the expression of nerve growth factor (NGF) and brain-derived neurotrophic factor (34,35), and by decreasing serum amyloid P concentrations, thereby preventing deposits of the amyloid P component in the brain (36). Several recent reviews of these mechanisms are available (37–41).

Clinical studies have shown that some women with Alzheimer's-type dementia may improve on tests of cognition when given exogenous estrogen. In a small sample of female Alzheimer's patients (n = 7), Fillit et al. observed that patients who improved their cognitive performance and were thus thought to have responded to estradiol therapy, scored higher on baseline cognitive measures than nonimprovers. These data suggest that response to estradiol therapy may be dependent on baseline measures. In addition, they found that estrogen "responders" scored higher than "nonresponders" on a baseline measure of depression, suggesting that estradiol therapy may be most helpful to individuals with associated affective disorders (30). Similarly, Honjo et al. found statistically significant improvement on the Japanese New Screening Test for Dementia among six of seven Alzheimer patients who underwent estrogen therapy. Improvement was not observed in the nontreatment group (42).

Recently, Doraiswamy et al. (43) assessed cognition scores in a large group of Alzheimer's patients who had formerly participated in a multicenter clinical drug-trial study. Cognitive functioning was assessed as part of the original study with several instruments including the Alzheimer's Disease Assessment Scale-cognition subscale. Information regarding use of ERT was obtained from all female study participants. The authors found that concurrent use of estrogen was a significant predictor of cognitive functioning, i.e., estrogen users were less impaired than their nonusing peers.

The effects of estrogen therapy in combination with Tacrine, an acetylcholinesterase inhibitor that has been found to be helpful in improving cognitive performance among Alzheimer's patients, has also been assessed (44). Schneider et al. examined cognitive performance in a large number of patients who had participated in a recent multicenter study of Tacrine therapy. The authors found that women who took estrogen in combination with Tacrine performed significantly better at follow-up than those who received placebo or Tacrine therapy alone.

Several epidemiological studies have also been conducted to assess the possible protective effects of estrogen against development of Alzheimer's disease. From these, it has been suggested that women who eventually develop Alzheimer's disease are less likely to have used estrogen replacement therapy, lending support to the hypothesis that ERT may reduce the relative risk of developing Alzheimer's disease (31,40,45). A complete discussion of this literature is beyond the scope of this chapter; the interested reader is referred to Henderson (39) for a more comprehensive review of the available data.

In summary, there is some compelling evidence suggesting that at least some cognitive functions are associated with estrogen level in normal, cycling women, and in women diagnosed with dementia of the Alzheimer type. In the next section, we will review the available literature on cognitive functioning in nondemented postmenopausal women. The primary objective behind the studies that comprise this literature is to evaluate the effect of estrogen deficiency on cognition among normal, healthy, aging women and the potentially beneficial effect of HRT on cognitive functioning.

COGNITION, MENOPAUSE, AND ESTROGEN REPLACEMENT THERAPY

The risks and benefits of estrogen replacement therapy are currently receiving well-deserved attention (46–48). One possible benefit of ERT that has, however, received relatively little attention, is improved cognitive functioning. Two types of studies have addressed this issue. The first type, *experimental*, examines cognition among women who have been given controlled doses of estrogen therapy over a specific period of time, usually 3–6 mo. These studies typically have administered a placebo pill or injection during the same period of time to a control group and then compared pretreatment baseline scores with posttreatment scores in both groups. The second study type, *quasi-experimental*, examines cognitive functioning among postmenopausal women from the community who, at the time of the study, regularly use ERT. These studies generally compare the cognitive test performances of women using ERT to a control group of postmenopausal women who are not currently using estrogen preparations.

EXPERIMENTAL STUDIES

As early as the 1950s the effects of hormone treatment on the cognitive processes of postmenopausal women were of interest to clinicians. In a study designed to explore revitalization of tissue in postmenopausal women, Kountz *(49)* and Caldwell, Watson, and Kountz *(50)* isolated a subgroup of women to investigate hormonal influences on their "psychological behavior." Using a double-blind study design, 30 postmenopausal women, age 54–88, were chosen for study *(51)*. Following an initial period of estradiol stimulation, 2 mg/wk of estradiol benzoate were given to 15 of the women, along with a varying dose (5–10 mg over a period of 1–3 d per cycle) of progesterone to stimulate uterine bleeding. The remaining 15 participants received a placebo injection (sesame oil only; no progesterone).

Several neuropsychological tests including the Wechsler–Bellevue Intelligence Test and the Wechsler Memory Scale were administered prior to the initiation of hormone therapy and again following 6 mo of treatment. No changes were evident for either group on verbal IQ, performance IQ, or full-scale IQ. However, the experimental group showed significant improvement on the Wechsler Memory Scale total score; for the placebo group there was no significant change.

Although these findings were intriguing, relatively few investigators initiated additional studies of cognitive functioning among postmenopausal women over the next two decades. In the mid-70s, two studies were conducted, but provided little support for the earlier work. Rauramo, Lagerspetz, Engblom, and Punnonen *(52)* studied three groups of women: 1) patients who had undergone bilateral salpingo-oophorectomy and hysterectomy, but who would receive no HRT, 2) patients who had undergone the same procedure, but who would receive 2 mg/d of estradiol valerate beginning one month after surgery, and 3) patients who had undergone hysterectomy, but retained both ovaries. Reaction time, performance speed, memory, and logical thinking were assessed in all women prior to surgery. Tests were conducted 1 and 6 mo postsurgery. No significant differences were found on reaction time, speed, or memory, and only a slight improvement among the oophorectomy patients in logical thinking. The estrogen group did not improve on any measure, nor did they demonstrate at any time, superior performance compared to their nonestrogen receiving peers.

The lack of improvement in memory scores among the estrogen receiving group is surprising in light of the significant improvement on the Wechsler Memory Scale reported by Caldwell and Watson *(51)*. However, the differences in the choice of neuropsychological instruments of the two studies is noteworthy. The Wechsler Memory Scale is a well-known battery of subtests that measures both verbal and visual immediate memory and delayed recall. Rauramo et al., used as their measure of memory function, the Integration Memory Test, which requires the subject to memorize a set of instructions read only once, and to then carry them out. Although some aspects of memory are certainly necessary for this task, it is perhaps most reflective of organization and problem solving skills. As the authors point out, other tests of memory may have yielded quite different results.

In a double-blind study, Vanhulle and Demol (53) randomly assigned nuns living in a religious community to two study groups. The experimental group consisted of 11 women with an average age of 57 yr. They were each given 4 mg of estriol per d. Fifteen nuns with an average age of 59 yr made up the control group. They were each given a daily placebo treatment.

Several neuropsychological tests designed to measure visual and auditory memory, concentration, learning, reaction time/vigilance, and work tempo/attention were administered prior to beginning treatment and again following 3 mo of treatment. The groups did not differ on the pretreatment tests. Only the test measuring attention revealed a significant posttreatment group difference; the placebo group was significantly poorer than the estrogen group. Furthermore, the improvement in attention (from pretreatment to posttreatment) in the estrogen group was significantly greater than the placebo group's improvement. However, no differences between the groups were found on any of the other tasks.

Several additional studies were completed within the next few years, once again suggesting that estrogen may exert a positive effect on mental functioning. Using a double-blind design, Hackman and Galbraith (54,55) randomly assigned postmenopausal women to experimental and control groups. Half of them received 1.5 mg of piperazine estrone sulphate, twice daily. The remaining half were each given a placebo. Treatment was cyclic; 21 d on, 7 d off, for 6 mo.

All participants were given the Guild Memory Test (GMT) prior to beginning and at the end of treatment. The GMT is a six-part test that measures several aspects of memory function. Total scores (across the six memory components) revealed a statistically significant improvement of the average memory score for the estrogen-treated group. The average score of the placebo group was slightly (although not significantly) poorer at posttreatment testing. The authors report that for five of the six component scores, the estrogen group had either a larger improvement or a smaller deterioration than the placebo group, although these differences were not significant.

Subjective assessment of menopausal symptomatology, including memory and concentration abilities, was also collected before and after treatment. Interestingly, of the nine experimental patients, only four reported improved memory and only three reported improved concentration abilities. Within the control group, four reported improved memory and five reported improved concentration. At least for this group of women, estrogen therapy did not appear to affect *perceived* memory and concentration abilities, despite the observed improvement in GMT scores.

Fedor-Freybergh (56) treated postmenopausal women for 3 mo with either 2 mg daily of estradiol-17-valerianate, or placebo tablets. Neuropsychological tests were administered to all patients prior to treatment and after three months. Fedor-Freybergh found significant improvement among the estrogen-treated women, relative to their placebo-treated peers, on all tasks. Furthermore, for all cognitive tests, difference scores (posttreatment score minus pretreatment score) were significantly larger among the estrogen-treated women, suggesting significantly greater improvement on all tests.

The Campbell and Whitehead study (57) is unique to the early literature in that it incorporated a double-blind crossover design (i.e., each participant receives a placebo trial *as well as* an estrogen trial). Two studies were conducted, a short study (4 mo) in which women with severe menopausal symptoms participated, and a long study (12 mo) for women with less severe symptoms. In both studies, participants were randomly assigned to a treatment or placebo condition and then "crossed over" to the other condition at the midpoint.

For the estrogen trial, each participant received 1.25 mg of conjugated equine estrogen daily for 21 d. D 22–28 were therapy free. An identical regimen was followed for the placebo trial. The Graphic Rating Scale was completed by all participants along with other questionnaires designed to assess affective functioning, personality characteristics, and general health. Women in both the short and long studies reported significant improvements in memory function during the estrogen trials, as compared to the placebo trials.

The Campbell and Whitehead studies did not employ objective assessments of cognitive functioning; no standardized neuropsychological tests were used, only self-report questionnaires. Nevertheless, the quality of their design make these studies an important contribution to the literature.

In the tradition of Rauramo et al. (52) and Campbell and Whitehead (57), Sherwin et al. conducted a series of studies in the late 1980s and early 1990s that have provided strong support for the hypothesis that estrogen preserves cognitive functioning in postmenopausal women. Sherwin (58) recruited premenopausal women scheduled for gynecological surgery. Prior to surgery, all participants were randomly assigned to one of four groups: estrogen treatment, androgen treatment, estrogen+androgen treatment, or placebo. A fifth group was also recruited: hysterectomy only. Following surgery, hormone replacement therapy was begun according to group assignment. Injections of either estradiol valerate (10 mg), testosterone enanthate (200 mg), a combination comprised of testosterone enanthate benzilic acid hydrozone (150 mg), estradiol dienanthate (7.5 mg), and estradiol benzoate (1.0 mg), or a placebo were administered at 28 d intervals, for the first 3 mo (Treatment 1). In the fourth month, placebo was administered to all participants (Placebo Phase). As in the Campbell and Whitehead study (57), they were then randomly "crossed over" to another treatment condition for an additional 3 mo (Treatment 2). Cognitive functioning was assessed preoperatively and at three postoperative intervals.

Sherwin found that women treated with hormones (estrogen, androgen, or a combination) performed significantly better on all cognitive tests than did placebo treated women at Treatment 1 and Treatment 2. Furthermore, during the placebo phase, mean test scores of the hormone-treated women fell significantly lower on all cognitive measures compared to Treatment 1 and Treatment 2 scores. There were no significant cognition changes detected over time for the control women (hysterectomy only).

The inclusion of an androgen-only group was a unique feature and the results warrant continued investigation. Sherwin suggested that the improved performances of women who received androgen-only might be attributed to testosterone's aromatization to estradiol. Little is known of androgen's relationship to cognition.

In an attempt to replicate Sherwin's data with a more comprehensive battery of memory tests, Sherwin and Phillips (59) administered cognitive tests to premenopausal women scheduled for hysterectomy and bilateral salpingo-oophorectomy. Following surgery, subjects received either 10 mg of estradiol valerate or 1 mL of placebo, one time per month for two months. Neuropsychological tests were readministered following the second treatment injection.

Several well-known memory tasks were used in this study and scores on the individual tests revealed that the groups did not differ prior to surgery. At the second testing, estrogen-treated women scored significantly higher than those who received placebo on paired associates and immediate paragraph recall. No differences were observed on immediate or delayed visual recall, however, suggesting that not all aspects of memory are improved with administration of estrogen.

Additional support for this idea was provided by Phillips and Sherwin (60). Using a double-blind design, women undergoing hysterectomy with bilateral salpingo-oophorectomy were assigned to either an estrogen treatment or placebo group. Tests of cognitive function were administered prior to surgery and again two months postsurgery. A total of three monthly injections were given; women in the estrogen group received 10 mg of estradiol valerate or 1 mL of placebo. Several subtests from the Wechsler Memory Scale were administered. The groups did not differ on tests administered prior to surgery. Post-hoc comparisons indicated that the estrogen group improved significantly from baseline to posttreatment on immediate paragraph recall, whereas the placebo group's performance did not change. Interestingly, the estrogen group's performance did not change on any of the other subtests, however, the placebo group performed significantly poorer at posttreatment, relative to baseline, on immediate and delayed paired associates. No changes were evident for visual reproduction or digit span. Plasma sex steroid levels were measured throughout the study period to assess specific hormone concentrations between and within groups. Correlations indicated that immediate paired associate scores were positively and significantly correlated with plasma estrone and estradiol levels. These data have provided yet stronger support for the hypothesis that at least some areas of cognition are linked to estrogen levels.

Ditkoff, Crary, Cristo, and Lobo (61) examined short-term memory function in women who had previously undergone gynecological surgery. Initial testing indicated that all participants had estradiol levels below 20 pg/mL, confirming their postmenopausal status. All women were of Hispanic ancestry, making this one of the few studies to examine estrogen's influence on cognition in nonCaucasian women. Another unique feature of this study pertains to menopausal symptomatology; all of the women in this study were required to have no significant vasomotor symptoms, defined by the authors as fewer than five hot flush episodes within a given 2-wk period as assessed with a daily symptom-count diary.

All qualifying participants were randomly assigned to receive either 0.625 or 1.25 mg of conjugated equine estrogen or placebo 25 d/mo for a total of 3 mo. Participants were tested prior to beginning, and during the final week of treatment, with the Digit Span and the Digit Symbol test from the Wechsler Adult Intelligence Scale. These tests were chosen for their ability to assess some aspect of memory, as well as attention and concentration. The groups did not differ on their initial test scores, nor did they differ at the end of the study period (i.e., following treatment). The authors suggest (as have others) that improved test scores may be related to relief of menopausal symptoms rather than to a direct effect of estrogen on cognition.

QUASI-EXPERIMENTAL STUDIES

Quasi-experimental studies have dominated the most recent literature on cognitive functioning in postmenopausal women. Perhaps, in part, this is because of a recognized lack of information regarding long-term changes in cognition associated with the continued use (or nonuse) of HRT. Whatever the reason, the last decade's studies on cognition in postmenopausal women have focused on obtaining larger numbers of women, some of whom have had many years of ERT experience.

In the early 1990s, Barrett-Connor and Kritz-Silverstein *(62)* accessed cognitive functioning in a large community sample of older women who had, several years previously, participated in an epidemiological study on heart disease risk. During the early part of the study (1972–1974) information on the use of HRT was obtained; the majority of those who used HRT took conjugated equine estrogen. Cognitive functioning was assessed in 800 women age 65 and older, during follow-up clinic visits (1988–1991). The battery consisted of a test of memory storage and retrieval, immediate and delayed visual reproduction, the Mini-Mental State Examination, a task of mental control (naming the months of the year backward), a test of visuomotor tracking and attention, and a test of category fluency.

When the scores were adjusted for age and education differences, the authors found that women who had never used ERT did not score significantly poorer than "ever" users or "current" users on any test measure. To analyze the data for possible cognitive differences based on dosages and/or length of time used, the authors combined the "ever" and "current" users. One measure of short-term recall (from the visual reproduction test) yielded significant differences, but not in the hypothesized direction; women who had used ERT for longer periods of time scored poorer than those who had used it for shorter periods. This finding is interesting in light of previous studies finding that nontreated women performed as well as ERT-treated women on tests of visual memory *(53,59,60,62)*.

Only scores on category fluency (a measure of verbal fluency that requires set-shifting flexibility) were supportive of an association between estrogen and cognition: women who had used estrogen for 20 or more years scored significantly higher than women who had never used it. However, the superior performance of the long-term ERT women, although statistically significant, reflected only a one-point difference in group scores. This study provided no supporting evidence to indicate that exogenous estrogen use could provide a *substantial* benefit to cognitive functioning in postmenopausal women.

On a smaller scale, Kampen and Sherwin *(63)* recruited 71 postmenopausal women from the general community. At the time of testing, 28 were taking ERT (most frequently conjugated equine estrogen). Neuropsychological tests given included immediate and delayed paragraph recall, immediate and delayed paired associates, and the same test of memory storage and retrieval as given in the Barrett-Connor and Kritz-Silverstein study (the Buschke–Fuld Selective Reminding test).

Analyses indicated that estrogen users performed significantly better than nonusers on immediate and delayed paragraph recall. As in the Barrett-Connor and Kritz-Silverstein study, no differences were found for the test of memory storage and retrieval. Furthermore, in contrast to past studies from their own laboratory, they were unable to detect group differences in paired associate learning.

To ensure that the addition of progestin in some of the participants' hormone regimens was not affecting the results, test scores of women who took combination hormones were compared in a separate analysis to those of women taking only estrogen. No significant differences were found, suggesting that differences in paragraph recall, and the lack of differences in paired associate learning, were probably not linked to progestin.

Robinson et al. *(64)* administered verbal recall tests to age and education matched postmenopausal women. Analyses indicated that estrogen users (the majority took conjugated equine estrogen) scored significantly higher than nonusers on proper name recall, but not on general word recall.

Finally, Kimura *(65)* recruited postmenopausal women who took either no HRT or took conjugated equine estrogen (0.625 mg/d or greater). Five women took progestin in combination with estrogen on d 16–25. All of the participants took no hormones from d 26 through the end of the month. Testing was conducted on two occasions; the first session was held at a time when women who received HRT would be taking estrogen only (i.e., no progestin for the women using a combination therapy), and again at the end of the month when women who used hormones had not done so for several d. Ten cognitive tests were chosen because of their known ability to be "sexually dimorphic," i.e., favoring either males or females. Types of tests included measures of perceptual speed, spatial ability, motor function, and verbal fluency. A repeated measures analysis indicated that overall (across tests), estrogen users scored significantly higher than nonusers, once again lending some support to the hypothesized link between cognition and estrogen.

CONFOUNDING VARIABLES

Through the years, many tests of cognitive functioning have been administered to postmenopausal women within a variety of study designs and experimental contexts. Although several studies have found some degree of cognitive impairment among women not using ERT, others have not. There are several methodological issues that may help to explain some of the discrepancies in study results.

Several of these methodological problems involve subject selection. For instance, relatively few studies report that potential subjects were screened and excluded for health problems that could affect their neuropsychological test performance such as having a history of head injury, stroke, alcoholism, epilepsy, heart attack, psychiatric illness, or current use of hypnotics or mood altering medications. Furthermore, few studies matched groups for age and education levels; failure to do so may impact study results. Finally, only one study assessed socioeconomic status (SES). It is possible that women choose not to use estrogen replacement therapy for reasons related to lower SES and cost. This could be a serious confound; an asymmetrical distribution of these women into the "no-ERT" group could result in cognitive differences due to differences in SES.

Another methodological problem concerns the choices of neuropsychological tests. While several researchers have used well-known and well-researched tests, others have failed to do so. This practice may be the reason that many inconsistencies with regard to specific deficits in cognitive functioning can be seen throughout the literature.

A final methodological problem concerns the limited number of studies that control for *current* affective disturbances. Both depression and anxiety can negatively impact scores on neuropsychological tests. Recent research indicates that even subclinical levels of depression, as measured by the Beck Depression Inventory, are associated with poorer cognitive abilities in older adults *(66)*. Both depression and anxiety are common complaints among peri- and postmenopausal women. Sherwin *(67)* suggests that women who have undergone a surgical menopause may, in fact, be more vulnerable to depressive symptoms than women who have had a natural menopause. Thus, in studies that do not select participants based on type of menopause, an assessment of current affective functioning is imperative. A thorough discussion of menopause and depression can be found elsewhere in this text.

Simple variations from one study to another may also account for some of the discrepancies in findings. For instance, differences in types of estrogen preparations, dosing schedules, and estrogen blood levels might also contribute to data inconsistencies.

SUMMARY AND CONCLUSIONS

In summary, it appears that low levels of estrogen, which are characteristic of menopause, may be responsible for at least some deficits in certain aspects of cognition. Most studies have measured some facet of memory function, many with subtests of the Wechsler Memory Scale (WMS, 68; WMS-R, 69); a well-known highly researched instrument. Of these, most have reported deficits in various aspects of verbal memory, but not in visual memory. In some cases, deficits in other areas such as abstract reasoning, attention, and set-shifting flexibility have also been reported, however, these findings have not been consistent.

Methodological problems, such as failure to match groups on basic demographic characteristics, inadequate exclusionary criteria, and insufficient controls for affective disturbances are probably responsible, at least in part, for some of the contradictory findings. Despite the inconsistencies, the data suggest that at least some areas of cognition are vulnerable to estrogen deficiencies and that administration of exogenous estrogen may be beneficial.

The data suggest that impaired cognitive functioning is apparent, but subtle. Though differences are statistically significant, they are in many cases, a matter of only a few test points. Even so, the findings are intriguing, particularly in light of the link between administration of exogenous estrogen and dementia. Future studies are certainly warranted. For instance, although verbal memory is clearly more impaired than visual memory, relatively little is known about estrogen's influence on the specific aspects of various memory processes; memory is a broad, multifaceted function. Furthermore, few correlational studies have been conducted to assess the degree of association between blood levels of estrogen and specific aspects of cognitive functioning. Finally, variables that could potentially play interacting roles such as moderate alcohol consumption, hypertension, exercise, and diet could be explored.

REFERENCES

1. National Women's Health Resource Center. Risks vs. benefits: how does hormone replacement therapy measure up? National Women's Health Rep 1992;14:1–8.
2. Anderson E, Hamburger S, James BA, Liu JH, Rebar RW. Characteristics of menopausal women seeking assistance. Am J Obst Gynecol 1987;156:428–433.
3. Neugarten BL, Kraines RJ. Menopausal symptoms in women of various ages. Psychosom Med 1965;27:266–273.
4. Hackman BW, Galbraith D. Replacement therapy with piperazine oestrone sulphate ('Harmogen') and its effect on memory. Curr Med Res Opin 1976;4:303–306.
5. Fedor-Freybergh P. The influence of oestrogens on the wellbeing and mental performance in climacteric and postmenopausal women. Acta Obstet Gynaecol Scand 1977;64 (Suppl): 5–69.
6. Rauramo L, Lagerspetz K, Engblom P, Punnonen R. The effect of castration and peroral estrogen therapy on some psychological functions. Front Hormone Res 1975;3:94–104.
7. Phillips SM, Sherwin BB. Effects of estrogen on memory function in surgically menopausal women. Psychoneuroendocrinology 1992;17:485–495.
8. Hampson E, Kimura D. Sex differences and hormonal influences on cognitive function in humans. In: Becker JB, Breedlove SM, Crews, D, eds. Behavioral Endocrinology, 3rd ed. The Massachusetts Institute of Technology, Cambridge, MA, 1993.
9. Kampen DL, Sherwin BB. Estrogen use and verbal memory in healthy postmenopausal women. Obst Gynecol 1994;83:979–983.
10. Kolb B, Whishaw IQ. Fundamentals of human neuropsychology, 3rd ed. W.H. Freeman, New York, 1990.
11. Wiederholt WC, Cahn D, Butters NM, Salmon DP, Kritz-Silverstein D, Barrett-Connor E. Effects of age, gender and education on selected neuropsychological tests in an elderly community cohort. J Am Geriat Soc 1993;41:639–647.

12. Lezak MD. Neuropsychological Assessment, 3rd ed. Oxford University Press, New York, 1995.

13. Halbreich U, Lumley LA, Palter S, Manning C, Cengos G, Joe S. Possible acceleration of age effects on cognition following menopause. J Psych Res 1995;29:153–163.

14. Hampson E, Kimura D. Sex differences and hormonal influences on cognitive function in humans. In: Becker JB, Breedlove SM, Crews, D, eds. Behavioral Endocrinology, 3rd ed. The Massachusetts Institute of Technology, Cambridge, MA, 1993.

15. Klaiber EL, Broverman DM, Vogel W, Mackenberg EJ. Rhythms in cognitive functioning and EEG indices in males. In: Ferin M, Halberg F, Richart RM, Vande Wiele RL, eds. Biorhythms and Human Reproduction. Wiley, New York, 1974.

16. Wuttke W, Arnold P, Becker D, Creutzfeldt O, Langenstein S, Tirsch W. Circulating hormones, EEG, and performance in psychological tests of women with and without oral contraceptives. Psychoneuroendocrinology 1975;1:141–151.

17. Komnenich P, Lane DM, Dickey RP, Stone SC. Gonadal hormones and cognitive performance. Physiolog Psychol 1978;6:115–120.

18. Ward MM, Stone SC, Sandman CA. Visual perception in women during the menstrual cycle. Physiol Behav 1978;20:239–243.

19. Broverman DM, Vogel W, Klaiber EL, Majcher D, Shea D, Paul V. Changes in cognitive task performance across the menstrual cycle. J Compar Physiol Psychol 1981;95:646–654.

20. Gordon HW, Lee PA. A relationship between gonadotropins and visuospatial function. Neuropsychologia 1986;24:563–576.

21. Gordon HW, Corbin ED, Lee PA. Changes in specialized cognitive function following changes in hormone levels. Cortex 1986;22:399–415.

22. Hampson E, Kimura D. Reciprocal effects of hormonal fluctuations on human motor and perceptual-spatial skills. Behav Neurosci 1988;102:456–459.

23. Hampson E. Variations in sex-related cognitive abilities across the menstrual cycle. Brain Cognition 1990;14:26–43.

24. Hampson E. Spatial cognition in humans: possible modulation by androgens and estrogens. J Psych Neurosci 1995;20:397–404.

25. Gould E, Woolley C, Frankfurt M, McEwen BS. Gonadal steroids regulate dendritic spine density in hippocampal pyramidal cells in adulthood. J Neurosci 1990;10:1286–1291.

26. Woolley C, Gould E, Frankfurt M, McEwen BS. Naturally occurring fluctuation in dendritic spine density in hippocampal pyramidal cells in adulthood. J Neurosci 1990;10:4035–4039.

27. McEwen BS, Coirini H, Danielsson A, Frankfurt M, Gould E, Mendelson S, Schumacher M, Segarra A, Woolley C. Steroid and thyroid hormones modulate a changing brain. J Steroid Biochem Mol Biol 1991;40:1–14.

28. Woolley CS, McEwen BS. Estradiol mediates fluctuation in hippocampal synapse density during the estrous cycle in the adult rat. J Neurosci 1992;12:2549–2554.

29. McEwen BS, Woolley CS. Estradiol and progesterone regulate neuronal structure and synaptic connectivity in adult as well as developing brain. Experiment Gerontol 1994;29:431–436.

30. Fillit H, Weinreb H, Cholst I, Luine V, McEwen B, Amador R, Zabriskie J. Observations in a preliminary open trial of estradiol therapy for senile dementia-Alzheimer's type. Psychoneuroendocrinology 1986;11:337–345.

31. Paganini-Hill A, Henderson VW. Estrogen deficiency and risk of Alzheimer's disease in women. Am J Epidemiol 1994;140:256–261.

32. Gilligan DM, Quyyumi AA, Cannon RO. III Effects of physiologic levels of estrogen on coronary vasomotor function in postmenopausal women. Circulation 1994;89:2545–2551.

33. Chakravorty SG, Halbreich U. The influence of estrogen on monoamine oxidase activity. Psychopharmacol Bull 1997;33:229–233.

34. Singh M, Meyer EM, Simpkins JW. Ovariectomy reduces ChAT activity and NGF mRNA levels in the frontal cortex and hippocampus of the female Sprague-Dawley rats [abstract]. Soc Neurosci Astracts 514. 1994;11:1254.

35. Singh M, Meyer EM, Simpkins JW. The effect of ovariectomy and estradiol replacement on brain-derived neurotrophic factor messenger ribonucleic acid expression in cortical and hippocampal brain regions of female Sprague-Dawley rats. Endocrinology 1995;136:2320–2324.

36. Hashimoto S, Katou M, Dong Y, Murakami K, Terada S, Inoue M. Effects of hormone replacement therapy on serum amyloid P component in postmenopausal women. Maturitas 1997;26:113–119.

37. Birge SJ. The role of estrogen in the treatment of Alzheimer's disease. Neurology 1997;48(suppl 7):S36–S41.

38. Fillit H, Luine V. The neurobiology of gonadal hormones and cognitive decline in late life. Maturitas 1997;26:159–164.

39. Henderson VW. The epidemiology of estrogen replacement therapy and Alzheimer's disease. Neurology 1997;48(suppl 7):S27–S35.

40. Kawas C, Resnick S, Morrison A, Brookmeyer R, Corrada M, Zonderman A, Bacal C, Lingle DD, Metter E. A prospective study of estrogen replacement therapy and the risk of developing Alzheimer's disease: the Baltimore longitudinal study of aging. Neurology 1997;48:1517–1521.

41. Prelevic GM, Jacobs HS. New developments in postmenopausal hormone replacement therapy. Curr Opin Obst Gynecol 1997;9:207–212.

42. Honjo H, Ogino Y, Naitoh K, Urabe M, Kitawaki J, Yasuda J, Yamamoto T, Ishihara S, Okada H, Yonizawa T, Hayashi K, Nambara T. In vivo effects by estrone sulfate on the central nervous system-senile dementia (Alzheimer's type). J Steroid Biochem 1989;34:521–525.

43. Doraiswamy PM, Bieber F, Kaiser L, Krishnan KR, Reuning-Scherer J, Gulanski B. The Alzheimer's disease assessment scale: patterns and predictors of baseline cognitive performance in multicenter Alzheimer's disease trials. Neurology 1997;48:1511–1517.

44. Schneider LS, Farlow MR, Henderson VW, Pogoda JM. Effects of estrogen replacement therapy on response to tacrine in patients with Alzheimer's disease. Neurology 1996;46:1580–1584.

45. Henderson VW, Paganini-Hill A, Emanuel CK, Dunn ME, Buckwalter JG. Estrogen replacement therapy in older women. Arch Neurol 1994;51:896–900.

46. Ernster VL, Bush TL, Huggins GR, Hulka BS, Kelsey JL, Schottenfeld D. Benefits and risks of menopausal estrogen and/or progestin hormone use. Prevent Med 1988;17:201–223.

47. Grady D, Rubin SM, Petitti DB, Fox CS, Black D, Ettinger B, Ernster VL, Cummings SR. Hormone therapy to prevent disease and prolong life in postmenopausal women. Ann Internal Med 1992;117:1016–1037.

48. Barrett-Connor E. Risks and benefits of replacement estrogen. Ann Rev Med 1992;43:239–251.

49. Kountz WB. Revitalization of tissue and nutrition in older individuals. Ann Internal Med 1951;35:1055–1067.

50. Caldwell BM, Watson RI, Kountz WB. Psychologic effects of estrogen therapy in postmenopausal women. J Gerontol 1950;5:384.

51. Caldwell BM, Watson RI. An evaluation of psychologic effects of sex hormone administration in aged women. I. Results of therapy after six months. J Gerontol 1952;7:228–244.

52. Rauramo L, Lagerspetz K, Engblom P, Punnonen R. The effect of castration and peroral estrogen therapy on some psychological functions. Front Hormone Res 1975;3:94–104.

53. Vanhulle G, Demol R. A double-blind study into the influence of estriol on a number of psychological tests in postmenopausal women. In: van Keep PA, Greenblatt RB, Albeaux-Fernet M, eds. Consensus on Menopausal Research. MTP, London, England, 1976.

54. Hackman BW, Galbraith D. Replacement therapy with piperazine oestrone sulphate ('Harmogen') and its effect on memory. Current Med Res Opin 1976;4:303–306.

55. Hackman BW, Galbraith D. Six-month pilot study of oestrogen replacement therapy with piperazine oestrone sulphate and its effect on memory. Current Med Res Opin 1977;4,Suppl 21–28.

56. Fedor-Freybergh P. The influence of oestrogens on the wellbeing and mental performance in climacteric and postmenopausal women. Acta Obstet Gynaecol Scand 1977;64:1–69.

57. Campbell S, Whitehead M. Oestrogen therapy and the menopausal syndrome. Clin Obst Gynaecol 1977;4:31–47.

58. Sherwin B. Estrogen and/or androgen replacement therapy and cognitive functioning in surgically menopausal women. Psychoneuroendocrinology 1988;13:345–357.

59. Sherwin B, Phillips S. Estrogen and cognitive functioning in surgically menopausal women. Ann NY Acad Sci 1990;592:474–475.

60. Phillips S, Sherwin B. Effects of estrogen on memory function in surgically menopausal women. Psychoneuroendocrinology 1992;17:485–495.

61. Ditkoff EC, Crary WG, Cristo M, Lobo RA. Estrogen improves psychological function in asymptomatic postmenopausal women. Obst Gynecol 1991;78:991–995.

62. Barrett-Connor E, Kritz-Silverstein D. Estrogen replacement therapy and cognitive function in older women. JAMA 1993;269:2637–2641.

63. Kampen DL, Sherwin BB. Estrogen use and verbal memory in health postmenopausal women. Obst Gynecol 1994;83:979–983.

64. Robinson D, Friedman L, Marcus R, Tinklenberg J, Yesavage J. Estrogen replacement therapy and memory in older women. J Am Geriat Soc 1994;42:919–922.

65. Kimura D. Estrogen replacement therapy may protect against intellectual decline in postmenopausal women. Hormones Behav 1995;29:312–321.

66. Rabbitt P, Donlan C, Watson P, McInnes L, Bent N. Unique and interactive effects of depression, age, socioeconomic advantage, and gender on cognitive performance of normal healthy older people. Psychol Aging 1995;10:307–313.
67. Sherwin BB. Sex hormones and psychological functioning in postmenopausal women. Experiment Gerontol 1994;29:423–430.
68. Wechsler D. Manual for the Wechsler Memory Scale. Psychological Corporation, New York, 1945.
69. Wechsler D. Manual for the Wechsler Memory Scale-Revised. Psychological Corporation, New York, 1987.

7

Depression in Menopause

Bernard L. Harlow, PhD
and Melissa E. Abraham, MS

CONTENTS

INTRODUCTION

Considering that about one-third of an American woman's life expectancy occurs beyond the cessation of ovarian function, a proportionate amount of effort in terms of research and treatment should be directed toward affective disorders occurring during the peri- and postmenopausal periods *(1)*. Unfortunately, we have only recently moved beyond clinic-based studies and into community-based populations to better evaluate the true incidence and prevalence of mood disorders during this time period.

Although psychological and sociocultural events influence the presence and recurrence of affective illness (*see* Table 1), the accumulation of clinical studies suggest that endocrinological factors may underlie some of the psychological symptoms reported during the late reproductive and early postmenopausal periods. To better understand the relationship between depression and the climacteric period, we briefly describe how they may be associated and also their respective epidemiology.

DESCRIPTIVE EPIDEMIOLOGY

Menopause

Natural menopause is defined in the epidemiologic literature as the last menstrual period having occurred prior to 12 consecutive months of amenorrhea without an obvious intervening cause. The average age at a natural menopause has been estimated at between

From: *Contemporary Endocrinology: Menopause: Endocrinology and Management*
Edited by: D. B. Seifer and E. A. Kennard © Humana Press Inc., Totowa, NJ

Table 1
Suggested Further Reading on Social, Demographic, and Cultural Factors that May Be Associated with Both Menopause and Depression.

Cultural factors, culturally determined attitudes

Beyenne Y. Cultural significance and physical manifestations of menopause, a biocultural analysis. Cult Med Soc 1986;10:47–71.

Epidemiology of depression

Horwath E, Weissman MM. Epidemiology of depression and anxiety disorders. In: Tsuang MT, Tohen M, Zahner GEP, eds. Textbook in Psychiatric Epidemiology. Wiley, New York, 1995, pp. 317–344.

Social factors, social stressors

McKinlay JB, McKinlay SM, Brambilla D. The relative contributions of endocrine changes and social circumstances to depression in mid-aged women. J Health Soc Behav 1987;28:345–363.

Prior depression, health status

Dennerstein L. Well-being, symptoms and the menopausal transition. Maturitas 1996;23:147–157.

Family factors, life changes

Ballinger CB. Psychiatric aspects of the menopause. Br J Psych 1990;156:773–787.

Sex differences

Weissman MM, Klerman GL. Sex differences and the epidemiology of depression. Arch Gen Psych 1977;34:98–111.

Health care

Defey D, Storch E, Cardozo S, Diaz O, Fernandez G. The menopause: women's psychology and health care. Soc Sci Med 1996;42(10):1447–1456.

50 and 51 yr of age with little variation by ethnic and racial populations *(2–4)*. What little variation there is has been likely because of the large spectrum of methodologies used for the assessment of natural menopause ranging from comparison of means to life-table analyses. As shown in Fig. 1, a recent cross-sectional population-based study of women age 45–54 illustrates that less than 10% of nonsmoking women undergo a natural menopause before age 45, and less than 1% before age 40 *(4)*. Likewise, more than 95% of nonhysterectomized women will have undergone a natural menopause by age 55.

Depression

In the medical literature, the term "depression" can refer to an emotional state, a symptom of a number of disorders, or a clinical diagnosis, depending on the investigator's definition *(5)*. Because the incidence of depression is on the order from 1.4 to 2.7 times more common in women than men *(6–10)*, there are a number of theories involving ovarian steroid hormones and depression.

To what extent does the greatest incidence of depression coincide with the climacteric? In the National Comorbidity Survey (NCS) *(6)*, more than 8000 individuals were inter-

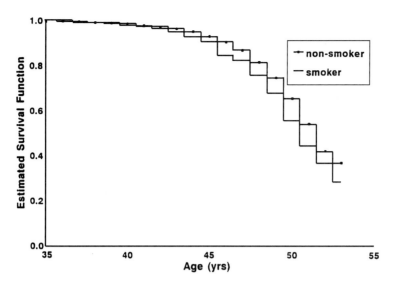

Fig. 1. Kaplan–Meier survival curves appled to age at menopause for women sampled in eastern Massachusetts and stratified by history of smoking.

viewed for psychiatric disorder. Prevalence estimates for lifetime major depressive disorder (MDD) in individuals age 45–54 ranged from 11.8% in men to 21.8% in women. The 1 mo prevalence estimate for the same age groups was 2.3% in men and 5.0% in women, with women overall at a risk 1.6 times higher than men for current (1 mo) major depressive episode *(6)*. Another large-scale community survey, the Epidemiologic Catchment Area (ECA) study, estimated the 1 mo prevalence of MDD to be 0.4% in men and 0.9% in women age 45–64 *(7)*. The differing rates for these two landmark studies, as well as for other studies in psychiatric epidemiology, are generally attributed to methodological issues, such as differing diagnostic criteria, interviewing techniques, and sampling methodology *(11,12)*. Although no consensus rate of major depression in women is available because of the variation in methods used in epidemiologic studies, all studies consistently show that the disorder is much more prevalent in women than men. Using data from the more conservative ECA study, the mean age of onset of major depression in women was 25, peaking at ages 15–19 *(13)*. This same study provided hazard rates, giving the probability that an individual who is free of MDD and enters the age interval, will develop MDD during the interval. These rates dropped dramatically around the time of the climacteric (ages 45–49, 0.0017; ages 50–54, 0.0008; ages 55–59, 0.0002) *(13)*. Another study found that 95% of women had the onset of a major depressive episode by age 43, with a mean age of 23.4 *(5)*.

FACTORS ASSOCIATED WITH EARLY AGE AT NATURAL MENOPAUSE AND DEPRESSION

Cigarette Smoking

One of the strongest and most clearly demonstrated risk factors for an early menopause is cigarette smoking *(14,15)*. In general, women who smoke are likely to undergo a natural menopause about 1 yr earlier than nonsmokers. The magnitude of this difference depends on the length and intensity of the smoking exposure. Investigators writing on the association between smoking and menopause have frequently cited the evidence that tobacco smoke contains polycyclic hydrocarbons, which may be toxic to ovarian germ cells and might lead to estrogen deficiency because of follicular exhaustion *(16)*. There is also good evidence that the alkaloid components of tobacco smoke, including nicotine and anabasine, may lower estrogen levels by interfering with its synthesis. Barbieri et al. demonstrated that cigarette smoke constituents inhibited granulosa cell aromatase, and other key enzymes in estrogen synthesis, to reduce estradiol production in vitro *(17)*. In addition, tobacco smoke components may cause a preferential shift of 2-hydroxylation over 16-hydroxylation of estrogen in smokers leading to less-active estrogens *(18)*. Finally, an effect of smoking on hypothalamic-pituitary function is also possible. In rats, tobacco smoke appeared to delay or blunt the surge of luteinizing hormone (LH) levels *(19)*. Currently, there is no evidence in humans that gonadotropins are lowered significantly enough to cause a subsequent decrease in estrogen production. Thus, smoking may affect age of natural menopause by lowering estrogen levels to a suboptimal level for the support of endometrial growth.

Many studies have shown a relationship between cigarette smoking and MDD *(20–22)*. Rates of smoking in depressed psychiatric patients exceeds that observed in the general population *(23)*, and smokers are known to have a significantly higher prevalence of major depression *(20,22)*. What continues to be less clear is whether major depression is a preceding risk factor for cigarette smoking, whether cigarette smoking increases the risk of major depression, or whether the association lacks a causal pathway. The antiestrogenic effect of cigarette smoking is well documented *(24,25)* and some studies have suggested that depression may be associated with low circulating endogenous estrogens *(26,27)*. Consistent with this theory are studies (discussed further in this chapter) that report success in treating mood disorder with high doses of estrogen *(28)*. Kendler et al. *(29)* in a study of 1566 adult female twins reported that, although an association between smoking and depression was evident, smoking did not cause women to develop major depression, nor did major depression cause women to begin smoking. Rather, the association was most likely mediated through genetic factors that influence the predisposition to both cigarette smoking and major depression. Studies that can pinpoint age at first smoking, first onset of mood disorder, and endocrinological profiles will have the best chance of sorting out this relationship.

Incessant Ovulation

The eventual cessation of menstrual periods is attributed to the loss of ovarian follicles. Although women begin menarche with about 500,000 primordial follicles, by age 40, perhaps only a few thousand remain *(30)*. Thus, it may seem logical to expect that the fewer the oocytes a woman has and the faster they are depleted, the sooner she will experience menopause *(31)*. By estimating total ovulatory years as the difference between age at menarche and menopause, less the number of years pregnant and/or on oral contraceptives, divided by the average menstrual cycle length, a trend of increasing likelihood of early menopause occurs with increasing numbers of ovulatory cycles *(31)*. Obviously, a model for menopause as a function of oocyte depletion is certainly simplistic and is not without limitations. For example, it is not known to what extent self-reported menstrual-cycle information serves as a reliable marker for ovulatory cycles and there is no known way to estimate the follicular number at the start of a woman's reproductive life.

As discussed later in this chapter, there is evidence to suggest that severe mood disorder may be associated with an early natural menopause. A mechanism by which such an association may operate could be through a precipitous decline in estrogen production as a consequence of a more rapid than normal depletion of oocytes. Certainly, mood disorder is associated with severe premenstrual symptomatology that is often a marker of normal ovulatory function. In addition (as previously discussed), incessant ovulation could lead to a premature decline in ovarian function *(31)*. Thus, in a cross-sectional analysis of women age 36–44 with and without major depression, factors that influence total ovulatory time were examined to see if they were associated with major depression *(32)*. For example, a menarche at age 10 or earlier was associated with a 2.3-fold increase in risk of current or past depression. Women with short menstrual cycles were more likely to have depleted ovarian function earlier than women with longer cycles and an increase in risk of depression among those with cycle lengths of less than 26 d was observed. The authors also observed less depression in women having had more than two livebirths. When all of these factors were assessed together as a continuous measure of total lifetime number of ovulatory cycles, there was an observed increase in risk of current or past depression in women with increasing number of ovulatory cycles with a statistically significant trend *(32)*.

REVIEW OF RESEARCH ON DEPRESSION IN MENOPAUSE

It is a common misconception that rates of depressive disorder increase as women enter the menopausal transition period. Kraepelin *(33)* in 1906 coined the term "involutional melancholia" as a condition predominately of women in their mid-40s that increases steadily with age and produces a state of agitation and hypochondriasis. Although this term was later discarded as having no scientific validity, scientists fostered the theory that physiological changes occurring at this time could add to women's vulnerability to psychiatric illnesses *(34)*. Much of this notion was based upon views related to clinical practice where women with the most severe menopausal symptoms sought treatment. In this section, we will discuss the results of epidemiological studies directed toward assessing the existence of such an association in the general population, endocrine hypotheses to explain such an association, and whether or not hormonal therapy has been effective in the treatment of depressive symptoms at the time of the climacteric and at other times.

Epidemiological Studies of Depression at the Time of Normal Natural Menopause

Systematic general population surveys initiated during the 1960s and 1970s provided better estimates of the prevalence of menopausal symptoms by avoiding the bias associated with clinic-based studies that were skewed toward patient populations more likely to seek medical care as a consequence of greater symptomatology. Cross-sectional surveys conducted in the United States, Britain, The Netherlands, and Australia all reported no evidence of a specific impact of the menopause on the prevalence of a wide variety of psychiatric symptoms at varying times across the pre-, peri-, or postmenopausal time period *(35–38)*. Although these studies were informative during their time, standardized measures for the assessment of psychiatric illness were lacking. With the advent of the *Diagnostic and Statistical Manual of Psychiatric Disorders* (*DSM*) *(39)*, studies could systematically distinguish major depressive disorder from depressed mood and depressed

Table 2
Population-Based Studies of the Association of Depression at the Time of Natural Menopause

Study	Number of participants	Depression instrument	Analysis	Association
Healthy Women's Study (40)	289	Beck Depression Inventory	Case-control	$p = 0.12$
Massachusettes Women's Health Study (41)	2565	Center for Epidemiology Studies Depression Scale (CES-D)	Repeated measures	$p = 0.16$
Manitoba Project (42)	1700	CES-D	Repeated measures	$p = 0.77$
South-East England Study (44)	47	Seven-Item Mood Assessment	Repeated measures	$p = 0.02$
Norwegian Menopause Project (45)	1886	Three-Point Scale of Symptoms	Cross-sectional	$p > 0.05$

symptoms. In Table 2, we highlight some recent population surveys that have assessed the prevalence of depression at the time of the normal menopausal transition.

The Healthy Women's Study (40) compared the changes in depression scores on the Beck Depression Inventory from study entry to reevaluation 12 mo later in a group of women who became menopausal during the interval, and a group of women who remained premenopausal during a similar interval of time. This case-control comparison revealed no association of a psychological response to the menopause. Longitudinal studies in Massachusetts (41) and Manitoba (42) used the CES-D (43) to assess depression symptomatology in a cohort of premenopausal women at baseline, and then repeated the assessment at defined intervals and compared the change in depression scores between those who did and those who did not make the transition through the climacteric. In both these large studies, no change in depression symptomatology was observed. A small study in England (44) did observe an increase in depressed mood as women entered the perimenopausal period. However, depression was assessed with a nonstandardized seven-item symptom scale and the authors acknowledge that their finding could be due to symptomatology associated with the menopause such as the change in vasomotor symptoms rather than the development of psychiatric illness. A large cross-sectional study of pre- and postmenopausal women in Norway (45) found no association between mood swings or irritability and chronological ovarian aging. These studies, and the evidence from the psychiatric epidemiological studies that show decreasing rates of depression after age 45, provide ample evidence that little or no association exists between depression occurring as a consequence of entering into the menopausal transition at a normal age.

Premenstrual Symptomatology and Depression at the Time of Menopause

Women who suffer regularly from premenstrual dysphoric disorder are at substantially greater risk of developing full-blown major depression (46,47). Of relevance for this review, however, is whether these women are also more likely to experience depression at the time of the climacteric compared to women with no such history of premenstrual symptomatology. Abraham et al. *(48)* studied 60 women during their premenopausal years and then 10 yr later during their postmenopausal period and reported that the severity of the menopausal symptoms experienced was directly proportional to their premenstrual symptomatology. Further research is needed to determine whether this association can be construed as evidence to support a greater risk of menopausal depression among women with a past history of severe premenstrual symptomatology.

ASSOCIATION OF DEPRESSION AND EARLY NATURAL MENOPAUSE

Virtually all community-based studies have shown the highest prevalence of major depression in women to be during the late premenopausal years between ages 35 and 45 *(6,49)*. As discussed above, an increase in depression following the menopause, a time period when circulating estrogens are already diminished, has not been clearly demonstrated. Thus, if there is any link between estrogen, depression, and menopause, it may be that depression occurs as a precursor to, or in association with, a premature cessation of menstrual cycles. Whether depression, or its treatment, is a preceding risk factor for a premature cessation of menstrual cycles, or whether it serves as a marker for a premature and precipitous decline in ovarian function, will be explored in the following sections.

Depression as a Cause of Early Natural Menopause

Emotional factors have been shown to influence the pituitary-ovarian axis at the level of the hypothalamus *(50)*. The best-known example is the link between environmental and endogenous stress and hypothalamic amenorrhea *(51)* thought to be a result from a deficiency in the pulsatile secretion of gonadotropin-releasing hormone (GnRH) *(52,53)*. There are, however, a few studies that link hypothalamic amenorrhea with risk of an early natural menopause, if any at all.

The mechanism by which depression may influence an early onset of menopause is a bit convoluted. Distinguishing an effect of the depression itself from an effect of therapy has yet to be accomplished. An earlier study of women with and without an early menopause noted that the association with depression was strongest for women pharmacologically treated for more than 3 yr *(54)*. Although this finding might be compatible with an effect of therapy, a long duration of treatment may also correlate with more severe emotional disturbance. The literature on adverse effects of antidepressants, particularly tricyclics, have focused on cardiovascular effects *(55)*, although a recently reported study by Grodstein et al. *(56)* suggested that the use of antidepressants or tranquilizers may increase the risk of ovulatory infertility. It is important for future studies to distinguish effects of the depression itself from the effects of treatment, especially because it is known that less than 50% of women with major depression seek therapy *(57)*.

Depression as a Marker for a Premature Decline in Ovarian Function

A second explanation for such an association may be that declining estrogen levels precede and predispose women to depression, rather than being the result of its presence or treatment. According to this interpretation, women with an early menopause may have a more precipitous or qualitatively different decline in endogenous estrogen levels compared to women destined to undergo a more normal transition to menopause.

Depression as a potential marker for ovarian dysfunction may be a clinically useful concept. For example, it may be appropriate to consider hormonal testing in premenopausal women with depression, or consider hormonal replacement therapy (HRT) in depressed women with evidence of an early menopause. Studies that have examined whether exogenous estrogen has an antidepressant effect are somewhat inconsistent (58–61) although the most recent study observed that a history of medically treated depression and early menopause declined with increasing length of oral contraceptive use (54).

ENDOCRINOLOGICAL HYPOTHESES

Aside from established social, demographic, and family risk factors, which may account for a diminished mood in older women (12,62,63), there are a number of plausible endocrinological mechanisms by which a depressed mood may be mediated (11,64,65) that may or may not be associated with menopausal changes.

Brain functioning is affected by gonadal hormones in a variety of ways, influencing different aspects of nerve-cell functioning (65). These hormones may also influence neurotransmitters and structural aspects of the brain that may be linked to depressive symptomatology (65).

Estrogen, in general, activates the central nervous system, whereas progesterone has inhibitory properties (66). It appears that the brain in women may depend on the presence of estrogen for particular aspects of functioning (67,68). Estrogen also increases serotonin-receptor concentration (69–71). Low levels of serotonin (5-HT) are associated with depressed mood (72), hence, the new class of effective antidepressants, the selective serotonin reuptake inhibitors (SSRIs) (73). When estrogen levels drop because of natural menopause, neuroamine levels including serotonin drop as well (74). In fact, exogenously administered estrogen has been demonstrated to have antidepressant qualities (75,76). Increased levels of estrogen have been associated with increases in 5-HT uptake, while progesterone has been shown to decrease 5-HT accumulation and reverse estradiol induced increase of 5-HT receptors (65). A recent study (77) has provided a potential mechanism by which estrogen therapy might be effective in treating depressive symptoms. The authors showed that estrogen increases the number of 5-HT_{2A} receptors in areas of the rat brain concerned with aspects of mood and behavior.

The class of antidepressants known as monoamine oxidase (MAO) inhibitors are thought to function by decreasing the activity of this enzyme, thereby increasing availability of central catecholamines that, if low, may be a cause of depression (78). Estrogen may function a bit like these antidepressant drugs. Because estrogen decreases MAO activity in the brain (79), the resulting decrease in catabolism of neuroamines increases their availability to the brain. Administration of estrogen to depressed outpatients significantly reduced "elevated plasma MAO activity" (78).

Progesterone has the opposite effect of estrogen in that it increases MAO activity and decreases the production of neuroamines (80,81). Allopregnenolone, a liver metabolite of progesterone, has anxiolytic effects as a GABA brain-receptor agonist (66). This is a potential mechanism by which the presence of progesterone exerts depressant effects (82).

HORMONAL THERAPY FOR DEPRESSION AT THE TIME OF MENOPAUSE

It is not unreasonable to hypothesize that reproductive hormones, given their effect on the neuroendocrine system, might be implicated in the pathogenesis of affective illness. Certainly the time of the menopause coincides with the greatest decline of estradiol levels. Therefore, if declining estradiol levels were responsible for the development of depressive symptomatology, one might expect therapeutic estrogen replacement therapy (ERT) to reduce the prevalence of affective disorders during the climacteric. Although the mechanism by which estrogen may exert its antidepressant influence is poorly understood, one theory suggests that estrogen is necessary for the reduction of serotonin-receptor binding sites and thus may influence affective illness via an interaction with thyroid hormones or antidepressant medications (83).

Although epidemiologic data suggests that depression is not more commonly observed during the climacteric, the efficacy of hormonal therapy in the treatment of climacteric depression has been addressed in a number of clinical studies.

Estradiol

Clinical studies and neuroendocrinological reviews suggest that estrogen has antidepressant characteristics. Proposed mechanisms for such an action include an effect on the adrenergic, serotonergic, and dopaminergic systems. Studies in mice suggested increased levels and bioavailability of norepinephrine following estradiol administration (84), and numerous laboratory studies demonstrated an effect of estrogen on serotonin- and dopaminergic-receptor binding sites (69,85). Recently, blood serotonin levels were increased to premenopausal levels in postmenopausal women after estrogen administration (86).

Armed with this laboratory data, investigators sought to test the hypothesis that postmenopausal estrogen therapy was efficacious in the treatment of climacteric depression. The inconsistency of the results from clinical trials is attributed to the lack of standardized depression inventories, sample size limitations, and self-selection of subjects attending menopausal clinics. Additionally, estrogen treatment of menopausal symptoms may contribute to a patient's comfort level and reduce affective symptoms. A large population-based cross-sectional study assessed differences in depression symptomatology between women receiving and not receiving HRT during various postmenopausal age categories. A substantially higher Beck Depression Inventory score was observed in women age 50–59 receiving HRT compared to untreated women. However, there were no differences in the age-adjusted measures of depressive symptoms across all age categories. The authors speculate that differences in the age-related patterns of depression between HRT treated and untreated women in their 50s may be because of a higher proportion of depressed climacteric women seeking HRT treatment for their menopausal symptoms (87).

Treatment trials carried out in menopausal clinics have examined the psychological consequences of HRT. Although a wide range of psychological symptoms and general well-being were improved, most studies reported a substantial placebo effect. For example, a recent double-blind placebo-controlled trial to assess the efficacy of transdermal estradiol therapy showed a significant improvement in depression symtomatology as assessed by HAM-D scores in both estrogen- and placebo-treated depressed postmenopausal women with no differences observed between the two treatment groups (86).

Adrenal Androgens

Whereas there is a clear understanding that estrogen declines as women make the transition through perimenopause, no clear relationship exists between adrenal androgens and menopause. Although studies suggest that adrenal androgens decline with aging, the levels of these hormones appear to be heavily influenced by external factors such as cigarette smoking, body mass, and nutritional correlates *(88,89)*. Nevertheless, the decline in adrenal androgens has been suggested to be associated with psychiatric illness. One randomized placebo-controlled trial of nightly oral DHEA adminstration over 6 mo in a small sample of men and women age 40–70 reported that DHEA levels returned to that seen in the second decade of life and that 82% of the women reported significant increases in energy, sleep, and overall mood compared to 10% of the placebo controls *(90)*. Although it is premature to speculate on a potential mechanism for such a positive effect on mood, there is evidence to suggest that DHEA acts as a memory enhancer and inhibitor of aggressive behavior in vivo, acting as a negative modulator to neuronal excitability by binding to the aminobutyric acid-A-receptor *(91)*. Studies to look at its specific effect on climacteric depression are needed.

Progesterone

Progesterone has been suggested to be linked to postpartum depression because of the massive changes in the hormonal environment after pregnancy *(92,93)*. It has also been used in the treatment of premenstrual syndrome with varied success. There are few, if any, studies that have adequately assessed its efficacy in the treatment of climacteric depression. The progesterone component of combined HRT may promote depression *(94)*. Synthetic progesterone preparations, such as medroxyprogesterone, may have less of a dysphoria promoting effect than natural progesterone *(95)*.

CONCLUSIONS

It is a fact that many women experience depression at the time of a natural menopause. However, rates of depression do not appear to be higher in women who experience a normal age of menopause compared to women not yet having entered the climacteric. The majority of menopausal women do not show signs of mood disorder and many of those who do can attribute their symptoms to factors other than those related to menopause such as health or social problems. Rates of depression may be higher in women who experience an early onset of natural menopause than similarly aged premenopausal women. Too few studies have been able to determine whether depression or its treatment is a preceding risk factor for an early onset of menopause, or whether depression is a marker for a premature decline in ovarian function that precedes the cessation of menstrual cycles. A new study *(32)* currently underway may help to disentangle the association of depression and early menopause by prospectively following premenopausal women with and without mood disorder and assessing the change in ovarian function through biannual menstrually timed hormonal assessments.

Understanding the molecular and genetic differences between women who do and do not suffer from depression during the menopausal transition is a challenge for future studies. The impact of various HRTs on not only depression symptomatology, but also on subsequent cardiovascular and other chronic disease conditions, is also an important area of study. We must also not forget to take into account cross-cultural differences, nutrition, social status, emotional function, and other social parameters because of their effect on both mood disorder and hormonal function. Thus, our studies of the future must integrate biological parameters with personal, social, and cultural nuances to obtain a full understanding of the health of women as they enter the menopausal transition.

REFERENCES

1. Sherwin BB. Impact of the changing horonal milieu on psychological functioning. In: Lobo RA, ed. Treatment of the Postmenopausal Woman. Basic and Clinical Aspects. Raven, New York, 1994, pp. 119–127.
2. Luoto R, Kaprio J, Uutela A. Age at natural menopause and sociodemographic status in Finland. Am J Epidemiol 1994;139:64–76.
3. Bromberger JT, Mathews KA, Kuller LH, et al. Prospective study of the determinants of age at menopause. Am J Epidemiol 1997;145:124–133.
4. Cramer DW, Harlow BL, Xu H, Fraer C, Barbieri RL. Cross-sectional and case-controlled analyses of the association between smoking and early menopause. Maturitas 1995;22:79–87.
5. Lehtinen V, Joukamaa M. Epidemiology of depression: prevalence, risk factors and treatment situation. Acta Psychiatr Scand Supp 1994;377:7–10.
6. Blazer DG, Kessler RC, McGonagle KA, Swartz MS. The prevalence and distribution of major depression in a national community sample: the National Comorbidity Survey. Am J Psych 1994;151(7):979–986.
7. Regier DA. Lifetime prevalence of specific psychiatric disorders in three sites. Arch Gen Psych 1984;41(10):949–958.
8. Weissman MM, Klerman GL. Sex differences in the epidemiology of depression. Arch Gen Psych 1977;34:98–111.
9. Kessler RC, McGonagle KA, Zhao S, Nelson CB, Hughes M, Eshleman S, Wittchen H, Kendler KS. Lifetime and 12-month prevalence of DSM-III-R psychiatric disorders in the United States. Arch Gen Psych 1994;51:8–19.
10. Weissman MM, Bland R, Joycd PR, Newman S, Wells JE, Wittchen HU. Sex differences in rates of depression: cross-national perspectives. J Affective Dis 1993;29(2–3):77–84.
11. Anthony JC, Aboraya A. The epidemiology of selected mental disorders in later life. In: Birren JE, Slane RB, Cohen GD, eds. Handbook of Mental Health and Aging, 2nd Edition. Academic, San Diego, CA, 1992, pp. 27–73.
12. Horwath E, Weissman MM. Epidemiology of depression and anxiety disorders. In: Tsuang MT, Tohen M, Zahner GEP, eds. Textbook in Psychiatry Epidemiology. Wiley, New York, 1995, pp. 317–344.
13. Burke KC, Burke JD, Regier DA, Rae DS. Age at onset of selected mental disorders in five community populations. Arch Gen Psych 1990;47(6):511–518.
14. McKinlay SM, Bifano NL, McKinlay JB. Smoking and age at menopause in women. Ann Intern Med 1985;103:350–356.
15. Midgette AS, Baron JA. Cigarette smoking and the risk of natural menopause. Epidemiology 1990;1:474–480.
16. Mattison DR, Thorgeirsson SS. Smoking and industrial polution, and their effects on menopause and ovarian cancer. Lancet 1978;i:187–188.
17. Barbieri RL, McShane PM, Ryan KJ. Constituents of cigarette smoke inhibit human granulosa cell aromatase. Fertil Steril 1986;46:232–236.
18. Michnovicz JL, Hershcopf RJ, Naganuma H, et al. Increased 2-hydroxylation of estradiol as a possible mechanism for the anti-estrogenic effect of cigarette smoking. N Engl J Med 1986;315:1305.
19. McLean BK, Rubel A, Nikitovitch-Winer MB. The differential effects of exposure to tobacco smoke on the secretion of luteinizing hormone and prolactin in the proestrous rat. Endocrinology 1977;100:1566–1570.
20. Glassman AH, Helzer JE, Covey LS, Cottler LB, Stetner F, Tipp JE, Johnson J. Smoking, smoking cessation, and major depression. JAMA 1990;264:1546–1549.
21. Anda RF, Williamson DF, Escobedo LG, Mast EE, Giovino GA, Remington PL. Depression and the dynamics of smoking. JAMA 1990;264:1541–1545.
22. Breslau N, Kilbey M, Andreski P. Vulnerability to psychopathology in nicotine-dependent smokers: an epidemiologic study of young adults. Am J Psych 1993;150:941–946.

23. Hughes JR, Hatsukami DK, Mitchel JE, Dahlgren LA. Prevalence of smoking among psychiatric outpatients. Am J Psych 1986;143:993–997.

24. Key TJ, Pike MC, Brown JB, Herman C, Allen DS, Wang DY. Cigarette smoking and urinary oestrogen excretion in premenopausal and post-menopausal women. Br J Cancer 1996;74:1313–1316.

25. Baron JA. Beneficial effects of nicotine and cigarette smoking: the real, the possible, and the spurious. Br Med Bull 1996;52:58–73.

26. Banger M, Hienke C, Knuppen R, Ball P, Haupt M, Weidmann K. Formation and metabolism of catecholestrogens in depressed patients. Biol Psych 1990;28:685–696.

27. Toren P, Dor J, Rehavi, Weizman A. Hypothalamic-pituitary-ovarian axis and mood. Biol Psych 1996;40:1051–1055.

28. Studd JWW, Smith RNJ. Estrogens and depression. Menopause: J North Am Menop Soc 1994;1:33–37.

29. Kendler KS, Neale MC, MacLean CJ, Heath AC, Eaves LJ, Kessler RC. Smoking and major depression. A causal analysis. Arch Gen Psych 1993;50:36–43.

30. Block E. Quantitative morphological investigations of the follicular system in women. Acta Anat 1952;14:108–123.

31. Cramer DW, Xu H, Harlow BL. Does "incessant" ovulation increase risk for an early menopause? Am J Obstet Gynecol 1995;172:568–573.

32. Harlow BL, Cramer DW. The Harvard study of moods and cycles: depression and factors related to menstruation and ovulation. Am J Epidemiol (Abstract) 1996;143:S6.

33. Kraepelin E. Lecture 1. Introduction: melancholia. In: Johnston T, ed. Lectures on Clinical Psychiatry. Bailliere, Tindall & Cox, New York, 1906.

34. Balinger CB. Psychiatric aspects of the menopause. Br J Psych 1990;156:773–787.

35. Neugarten BL, Kraines RJ. Menopausal symptoms in women of various ages. Psychosom Med 1965;27:266–273.

36. Dunnell K, Cartwright A. Medicine takers, prescribers, and hoarders. Routlege and Keegan Paul, London and Boston, 1972.

37. McKinlay SM, Jeffreys M. The menopausal syndrome. Br J Prev Med Soc Behav 1974;28:108–115.

38. Wood C. Menopausal myths. Med J Australia 1979;1:496–499.

39. Diagnostic and Statistical Manual of Mental Disorders. Am Psych Assoc, Washington DC.

40. Mathews KA, Kuller LH, Wing RR, Meilahn EN. Biobehavioral aspects of menopause: lessons from the Health Women Survey. Exper Gerontol 1994;29:337–342.

41. Avis NE, Brambilla D, McKinaley SM, Vass K. A longitudinal analysis of the association between menopause and depression. Results from the Massachussetts Women's Study. Ann Epidemiol 1994;4:214–220.

42. Kaufert PA, Gilbert P, Tate R. The Manitoba Project: a re-examination of the link between menopause and depression. Maturitas 1992;14:143–155.

43. Myers JK, Weissman MM. Use of a self-reported symptom scale to detect depression in a community sample. Am J Psych 1980;137:1081.

44. Hunter M. The South-East England longitudinal study of climacteric and postmenopause. Maturitas 1992;14:117–126.

45. Holte A. Prevalence of climacteric complaints in a representative sample of middle-aged women in Oslo, Norway. J Psychosom Obstet Gynecol 1991;12:303–317.

46. Halbreich U, Endicott J. Relationship of dysphoric premenstrual changes to depressive disorders. Acta Psychiatr Scand 1985;71:331–338.

47. Graze KK, Nee J, Endicott J. Premenstrual depression predicts future major depressive disorder. Acta Psychiatr Scand 1990;81:201–205.

48. Abraham S, Llewellyn-Jones D, Perz J. Changes in Australian women's perception of the menopause and menopausal symptoms before and after the climacteric. Maturitas 1994;20:121–128.

49. Weissman MM, Bruce ML, Leaf PJ, Florio LP, Holzer C. Affective disorders. In: Robins LN, Regier DA, eds. Psychiatric Disorders in America, The Free Press, new York, 1991, pp. 53–80.

50. Rivier C, Rivier J, Vale W. Stress-induced inhibition of reproductive functions: role of endogenous corticotropin-releasing factor. Science 1986;231:607–609.

51. Liu JH. Hypothalamic amenorrhea: clinical perspectives, pathophysiology, and management. Am J Obstet Gynecol 1990;163:1732–1736.

52. Khoury SA, Reame NE, Kelch RP, Marshall JC. Diurnal patterns of pulsatile luteinizing hormone secretion in hypothalamic amenorrhea: reproducibility and response to opiate-blockade and an alpha-2-adrenergic agonist. J Clin Endocrinol Metab 1987;64:755–762.

53. Quigley ME, Sheehan KL, Casper RF, Yen SSC. Evidence for increased dopaminergic and opioid activity in patients with hypothalamic hypogonadotropic amenorrhea. J Clin Endocrinol Metab 1980;50:949–954.

54. Harlow BL, Cramer DW, McGurk KM. The association of medically treated depression and age at natural menopause. Am J Epidemiol 1995; 141:1170–1176.

55. Preskorn SH, Irwin HA. Toxicity of tricyclic antidepressants—kinetics, mechanism, intervention: a review. J Clin Psychiatry 1982;43:151–156.

56. Grodstein F, Goldman MB, Ryan L, Cramer DW. Self-reported use of pharmaceuticals and primary ovulatory infertility. Epidemiology 1993;4:151–156.

57. Shapiro S, Skinner EA, Kessler LG, et al. Utilization of health and mental health services: three epidemiologic catchment area sites. Arch Gen Psych 1984;41:971–978.

58. Holsboer F, Benkert O, Demisch L. Changes in MAO activity during estrogen treatment of females with endogenous depression. Mod Probl Pharmacopsych 1983;19:321–326.

59. Klaiber EL, Broverman DM, Vogel W, Kobayashi T. Estrogen therapy for severe persistent depressions in women. Arch Gen Psych 1979;36:550–554.

60. Shapira B, Oppenheim G, Zohar J, Segal M, Malach D, Belmaker RH. Lack of efficacy of estrogen supplementation to imipramine in resistant female depressives. Biol Psych 1985;20:576–578.

61. Oppenheim G. Estrogen in the treatment of depression: neuropharmacological mechanisms. Biol Psych 1983;18:721–725.

62. McKinlay JB, McKinlay SM, Brambilla D: The relative contributions of endocrine changes and social circumstances to depression in mid-aged women. J Health and Soc Behav 1987;28:345–363.

63. Horwath E and Weissman MM: Epidemiology of depression and anxiety disorders. In: Tsuang MT, Tohen M, Zahner GEP, eds. Textbook in Psychiatric Epidemiology. Wiley, New York, 1995, pp. 317–344.

64. Coulam CB. Age, estrogens, and the psyche. Clin Obstet Gynecol 1981;24(1):219–220.

65. Halbreich U, Lumley LA. The multiple interactional biological processes that might lead to depression and gender differences in its appearance. J Affect Dis 1993;29(2–3):159–173.

66. Smith SS. Hormones, mood and neurobiology: a summary. In: Berg G, Hammar M, eds. The Modern Managment of the Menopause. Parthenon, New York, 1994, pp. 295–299.

67. Rauce NE. Hormonal influences on morphology and neuropeptide gene expression in the infundibular nucleus of postmenopausal women. Progr Brain Res 1992;93:221–235.

68. Barrett-Connor E and Kritz-Silverstein D. Estrogen replacement therapy and cognitive functions in older women. JAMA 1993;269:2637–2641.

69. Pfaff DW, McEwen BS. Actions of estrogens and progestins on nerve cells. Science 1983;219:808–814.

70. McEwen BS, Bigeon A, Fischette CT et al: Towards a neurochemical basis of steroid hormone action. In: Martini L, Ganong WF, eds. Frontiers of Neuroendocrinology. Raven, New York, 1984, pp. 1153–1176.

71. D'Amico JF, Greendale GA, Lu JK, et al. Induction of hypothalamic opioid activity with transdermal estradiol administration in postmenopausal women. Fertil Steril 1991;55:754–758.

72. Risch SC. Recent advances in depression research: from stress to molecular biology and brain imaging. J Clin Psychiatry 1997;58(suppl 5):3–6.

73. Petty F, Davis LL, Kabel D, Kramer GL. Serotonin dysfunction disorders: a behavioral neurochemistry perspective. J Clin Psychiatry 1996;57(suppl 8):11–16.

74. Gonzales GF, Carillo C. Blood serotonin levels in postmenopausal women: effects of age and serum oestraiol levels. Maturitas 1993;17:23–29.

75. Gregoire AJ, Kumar R, Everitt B, Henderson AF, Studd JW. Transdermal oestrogens for treatment of severe postnatal depression. Lancet 1996;347:930–933.

76. Klaiber EL, Broverman DM, Vogel W, Kobayashi Y. Estrogen therapy for severe persistent depression in women. Arch Gen Psych 1979;36:742–744.

77. Fink G, Sumner BE, Rosie R, Grace O, Quinn JP. Estrogen control of central neurotransmission: effect on mood, mental state, and memory. Cell Mol Neurobiol 1996;16(3):325–44.

78. Klaiber EL, Broverman DM, Vogel W, Kobayashi Y, Moriarty D. Effects of estrogen therapy on plasma MAO activity and EEG driving responses of depressed women. Am J Psych 1972;128:1492–1498.

79. McEwen BS, Rhodes JC. Gonadal hormone regulation of MAO and other enzymes in hypothalamic areas. Neuroendocrinology 1983;36:235–238.

80. Gereau RW, Kedzie KA, Renner KJ. Effect of progesterone on serotonin turnover in rats primed with estrogen implants into the ventromedial hypothalamus. Brain Res Bull 1993;32:293–300.

81. Holzbauer M, Yondon MBH. The oestrous cycle and monoamine oxidase activity. Br J Pharmacol 1973;48:600–608.

82. Majewska MD, Harrison NL, Schwartz RD, Barker JL, Paul SM. Steroid hormone metabolites are barbiturate-like modulators of the GABA receptor. Science 1986;232:1004–1007.

83. Backstrom J Oestrogen and progesterone in relation to different activities in the central nervous system. Acta Obstet Gyneaecol Scand 1977;66:1.

84. McGeer E, McGeer P. Neurotransmitter metabolism in the aging brain. In: Terry RD, Gershon S, eds. Neurobiology of Aging, vol 3. Raven, New York, 1976, pp. 389–391.

85. Saletu B, Brandstatter N, Metka M, et al. Double-blind, placebo controlled, hormonal, syndromal and EEG mapping studies with transdermal oestradiol therapy in menopausal women. Psychopharmacology 1995;122:321–329.

86. Parry BL. Reproductive factors affecting the course of affective illness in women. Psychiat Clin North Am 1989;12:207–220.

87. Palinkas LA, Barrett-Connor E. Estrogen and depressive symptoms in post-menopausal women. Obstet Gynecol 1992;80:30–36.

88. Bancroft J, Cawood EHH. Androgens and the menopause: a study of 40–60 year old women. Clin Endocrinol 1996;45:577–587.

89. Cawood EHH, Bancroft J. Steroid hormones, the menopause, sexuality and well-being of women. Psychol Med 1996;26:925–936.

90. Morales AJ, Nolan JJ, Nelson JC, Yen SC. Effects of replacement dose of dehydroepiandrosterone in men and women of advancing age. J Clin Endcorinol Metab 1994;78:1360–1367.

91. Wolkowitz OM. Reus VI, Roberts E, et al. Antidepressant and congnition-enhancing effects of DHEA in major depression. Ann NY Acad Sci 1995;774:337–339.

92. Harris B, Lovett L, Smith J, et al. Cardiff puerperal mood and hormone study. III Postnatal depression at 5 to 6 weeks postpartum, and its hormonal correlates across the peripartum period. Br J Psychiatry 1996;168:739–744.

93. de Lignieres B, Vincens M. Differential effects of exogenous oestradiol and progesterone on mood in post-menpausal women: individual dose/effect relationship. Maturitas 1982;4:67–72.

94. Sherwin BB. The impact of different doses of estrogen and progestin on mood and sexual behavior in post-menopausal women. J Clin Endocrinol Metab 1991;72:336–343.

95. Prior JC, Alojado N, McKay DW, Vigna YM. No adverse effects of medroxy-progesterone treatment without estrogen in post-menopausal women: double blind, placebo controlled, cross-over trial. Obstet Gynecol 1994;83:24–28.

8

Premature Ovarian Failure and Surgical Menopause

Roger P. Goldberg, MD and Alan S. Penzias, MD

CONTENTS

INTRODUCTION

Premature ovarian failure (POF) is commonly defined as the cessation of ovarian function accompanied by gonadotropin measurements in the menopausal range before age 40. This entity occurs in roughly 1% of women. Although for many patients, the etiology of their gonadal failure remains an enigma, others demonstrate convincing chromosomal, infectious, autoimmune, or iatrogenic risk factors. Elevated serum gonadotropin levels may reflect a total depletion of ovarian follicles in some patients; in others, increased follicle stimulating hormone (FSH) and luteinizing hormone (LH) may signify the resistance of primitive follicles to stimulation. In either case, major repercussions of premature ovarian failure can stem from both diminished ovarian estrogen production and the associated disease states responsible for the condition. Clinical sequelae

From: *Contemporary Endocrinology: Menopause: Endocrinology and Management*
Edited by: D. B. Seifer and E. A. Kennard © Humana Press Inc., Totowa, NJ

from occult gonadal failure range in severity, encompassing infertility, irregular menses, and moderately elevated gonadotropin levels, to frank ovarian endocrine failure with hypoestrogenemia and amenorrhea. Similar to the physiologic menopause, the rapidity of each woman's progress through this spectrum of ovarian demise is highly variable.

When fertility is a concern, as it often is for these women in the prime of their reproductive years, the precise etiology of the condition can have a major impact on the likelihood of achieving a pregnancy. Because the different causes of POF can have significant impact on reproductive capacity and the patients overall state of health, it is critical to perform a comprehensive evaluation on each patient. Although the incidence of some etiologies is low, the impact upon the patient's total health, and even her life, can be high. In caring for women with POF, one must address a broad range of endocrinologic, developmental, and long-term clinical issues, which vary according to each patient's developmental and reproductive stage.

INCIDENCE AND EPIDEMIOLOGY

Coulam et al. *(1)* reported the age-specific prevalence of POF among a cohort of over 1800 women, followed longitudinally. By age 30, the cumulative risk of ovarian failure reached 0.1% overall; interestingly, all cases occurred between ages 15–19, whereas none was found among 20–29-year-old women in the series. From age 30–39, incidence rates rose again to nearly 80/100,000. This bimodal incidence pattern seemingly reflects an initial subset of patients with primary ovarian failure presenting in adolescence, followed by patients with POF of heterogeneous autoimmune, infectious, and iatrogenic etiologies typically manifesting in the fourth decade. By the onset of the fifth decade, age 40, the cumulative risk of POF in the general population approaches 1%, according to several surveys *(2)*. Among women with primary amenorrhea, the prevalence of gonadal failure ranges from 10 to 28% *(3)*.

GONADAL FAILURE: CLINICAL SEQUELAE

Ovarian failure represents the single most common cause of delayed sexual development *(4)*, and a potentially damaging psychological burden for the adolescent female. Abnormal pubertal development occurs at a critical period of emotional, physical, and social development. For the clinician, delivering effective and appropriate treatment, education, and counseling represents a profound challenge.

Low levels of circulating estradiol, comparable to the postmenopausal range, accounts for the lack of secondary sexual development in girls with primary ovarian failure, and for most of the substantial long-term morbidity associated with POF presenting at any age. Among women meeting the diagnostic criteria for POF, however, the decline in endogenous hormone production may be partial or complete. Rebar et al. studied the endocrinologic characteristics of 26 POF patients, using serial blood assays. Nearly half of the sample demonstrated the classical postmenopausal profile of low-serum estradiol levels and elevated serum gonadotropins; the remaining patients demonstrated some cyclical rise in estradiol during their menstrual cycle *(5)*. Nevertheless, estrogen levels are sufficiently low to place women with gonadal failure at risk for osteoporosis and cardiovascular disease, and perhaps other recently proposed complications of prolonged hypoestrogenemia, such as Alzheimer's disease.

Prolonged estrogen deficiency in POF has been shown to result in significantly decreased bone mineral density, and increased spinal osteopenia, compared with matched control subjects. Untreated Japanese women with POF carry a 40% incidence of osteopenia, versus 0% of age-matched controls *(6)*. Whereas the decrease in bone mineral density results primarily from a decline in circulating estrogen, other alterations in POF may contribute. Prior et al. suggested that decreased progesterone production, resulting from shortened luteal phases and anovulatory cycles, contributes to the risk of osteoporosis *(7)*. In chromosomally abnormal forms of POF, genetic effects may further contribute to osteopenia, independent of estrogen levels.

Infertility invariably stands out as the prime concern among women with POF, often diagnosed in the midst of their reproductive life span. A comprehensive evaluation can be invaluable in providing accurate counseling for patients regarding their prognosis for spontaneous or pharmacologically induced pregnancy. Some women with seemingly irreversible forms of gonadal failure may conceive spontaneously or following different regimens of ovulation induction. These women invariably have a normal chromosome complement. For those with chromosomal causes of POF, oocyte donation provides an alternative with excellent success rates.

Identifying the presence of dysgenetic gonads and the associated risk for malignancy is of primary importance in the evaluation of a young patient with POF. Some patients with 45,X-cell lines may be mosaics for 46,XY. The detection of a Y-chromosome dictates gonadectomy *(8)*. Screening for autoimmune disorders known to accompany ovarian failure — most commonly of the thyroid and adrenal glands — is also of importance in addressing comprehensive health maintenance for the woman with ovarian failure, and may occasionally impact her treatment and prognosis for fertility. Effectively addressing the broad range of clinical problems associated with POF requires an understanding of its heterogeneous etiologies.

ETIOLOGY AND CLASSIFICATION

Ovarian failure may be broadly categorized into chromosomally normal and chromosomally abnormal forms. The majority of women with POF — up to 68% in some series — have the normal 46,XX karyotype *(9)*, though these estimates vary widely according to selection criteria for study populations. Other women with POF have detectable X-chromosome anomalies, the most common being 45,X mosaicism, and structural X-chromosome abnormalities.

KARYOTYPICALLY ABNORMAL POF

Normal ovarian function is dependent on the presence of two intact X-chromosomes during embryologic development. Although lionization or inactivation of one of the pair of X-chromosomes does occur later in development, two functional X-chromosomes are required initially. Deletion of an entire X-chromosome, or even a portion of it, can lead to primary gonadal dysgenesis, which is manifest at the onset (or lack thereof) of puberty or POF later in reproductive life.

DELETION OF X-CHROMOSOME MATERIAL

Deletion of ovarian-determinant genes from either X-chromosome may cause POF in sporadic and familial forms. Apart from monosomy and numerical anomalies, various deletions, duplications, and translocations of the X-chromosome have been reported in association with POF. Most abnormalities of the short arm (Xp) do not affect ovarian function, whereas deletions and translocations involving the long arm (Xq) do impact normal ovarian function. For instance, Powell et al. utilized fluorescence *in situ* hybridization (FISH) to analyze a balanced X-autosome translocation in a patient with POF. Disruption in the Xq13–q26 region appeared to play a role in the decline of ovarian function. Correlation between specific Xq mutations and the degree of clinical ovarian failure, however, has been inconsistent. Patients with similar deletions have been found to possess widely different phenotypes. Further studies, controlling for important factors such as mosaicism, may provide for more precise localization of the critical ovarian-determinant genetic loci.

Although nearly all documented cases of Xq anomalies are sporadic, familial cases with vertical transmission infrequently occur. Krauss et al. reported on a family in which women with POF from three successive generations shared an inherited interstitial deletion of the long arm of the X-chromosome *(10)*. A familial case of a mother and an infertile daughter with premature menopause at ages 31 and 28, respectively, has also been reported *(11)*. Karyotypes of these women revealed an identical small terminal deletion of the long arm of the X-chromosome; with the exception of short stature, neither woman demonstrated Turner's syndrome stigmata. The patient's sister, possessing a normal chromosome, had normal menses and had not yet undergone menopause by age 35.

TURNER'S SYNDROME

The best known cause of gonadal dysgenesis is Turner's syndrome, marked clinically by primary ovarian failure, streak gonads, and characteristic physical stigmata. Deletion of either X-chromosome may result in 45,X or a mosaic. The wide variety of Turner's syndrome phenotypes depends upon the specific chromosomal endowment and the degree of mosaicism present. For example, two women, each possessing a 45,X/46,XX karyotype can have widely discrepant phenotypes. If one of the women is euploid *(46,XX)* in 95% of her cells and aneuploid (45,X) in 5%, she will have fewer physical stigmata of the Turner phenotype than a woman who is 60% euploid and 40% aneuploid. However, both women will have physiologically irreversible infertility at the onset of their POF.

Rather than an inborn absence of ovarian follicles, the primary pathophysiologic mechanism underlying Turner's syndrome appears to be accelerated atresia of an initially full complement of primordial ovarian follicles. Consequently, it is unsurprising that although bilateral streak ovaries represent the classic anatomical finding, some residual follicular function characteristically exists. This feature also varies widely depending upon the degree of mosaicism that is present. Women who present with delayed puberty and elevated gonadotropin levels and are diagnosed as having full Turner's syndrome, pure 45,X, have already depleted their complement of germ cells and gonadal function of these women is not possible. However, nature occurs along a continuum rather than through discrete steps. Some women with Turner's syndrome may experience partial pubertal development and rare pregnancies can be seen among these women.

X-chromosome mosaicism is defined by one euploid cell line along with one or more aneuploid cell lines. Mosaicism is found in up to 8–15% of women with POF according to cytogenetic analyses *(12)*. Mosaicism accounts for a significant proportion of detected, and a large number of undetected, X-chromosome abnormalities. Patterns associated with POF include Turner mosaic (45,X/46,XX or 45,X/46,XY); triple-X syndrome

(46,XX/47,XXX), and more complex mosaicism. The reproductive performance of X-chromosome mosaicism is highly variable, and the ratio of mosaic cell lines does not appear to correlate well with the severity of gonadal failure.

KARYOTYPICALLY NORMAL POF

Genetically based POF in the presence of a 46,XX karyotype most commonly results from new mutations and chromosomal accidents; familial inheritance is rare. The mechanisms whereby euploid chromosomal abnormalities result in the depletion of ovarian function remain poorly understood. One theory suggests abnormal primordial germ cell proliferation or migration to the embryonic genital ridges. This hypothesis is supported by a transgenic mouse model. In this mouse model, a recessive insertional mutation confers early germ cell depletion and infertility.

MENDELIAN RECESSIVE POF

ODG Locus (Chromosome 2p) — FSH Receptor Gene Point Mutation

Abnormal FSH receptor structure or function has been implicated as a cause of familial POF, because of a mutation in the FSH-receptor (FSH-R) gene with Mendelian recessive inheritance. Matthews, et al. *(13)* reported a family with primary amenorrhea and infertility, with an apparent vertical Mendelian recessive inheritance, attributed to an isolated deficiency of FSH. The patient was found to be homozygous for a two-nucleotide frame shift deletion in the FSH beta-subunit gene; her mother and son were heterozygous for this mutation, which appears to impair binding and activation of the FSH receptor. Ovulation was induced using exogenous FSH therapy, which resulted in pregnancy. Aittomaki et al. identified 75 patients with 46,XX gonadal dysgenesis — that is, karyotypically normal POF accompanied by streak gonads — before age 20, and found their geneology and segregation ratios to be compatible with recessive inheritance *(14)*. The determinant locus for their ovarian dysgenesis, named ODG1, was mapped by linkage to chromosome 2p, consistent with previous cloning and mapping of the FSH-R gene to 2p. In 29% of cases, an identical C to T point mutation was identified as the cause of amino acid substitutions disabling the FSH-R protein *(15)*. Other investigators, including Whitney et al., failed to identify causative mutations within human FSH receptor in 21 women with POF. Nevertheless, it appears plausible that point mutations, by altering gonadotropin receptor function and via other unknown mechanisms, may account for rare sporadic and familial cases of POF.

As mentioned, the majority of women with POF, and an even higher percentage of those presenting with secondary amenorrhea, are karyotypically normal. Appropriate evaluation entails consideration of potential underlying autoimmune, environmental, and iatrogenic conditions. Particularly in younger women, the diagnosis of "idiopathic" POF should be assigned only after thorough exclusion of the significant possible comorbidities and risk factors.

AUTOIMMUNITY

Autoimmunity is believed to account for perhaps up to 20% of POF, after chromosomal, genetic, and environmental etiologies have been excluded. An important role for autoimmunity is supported by the apparent high prevalence of various circulating autoantibodies among women with POF, the frequency of other associated autoimmune disorders among women with POF, increased T-cell activation *(16)*, possible aberrant expression of class II major histocompatibility complex (MHC) antigens *(17)*, and lymphocytic infiltration in ovarian cells *(18)*.

Conway et al. *(19)* reported 34% of 135 patients diagnosed with "idiopathic" POF had at least one positive autoantibody titer, similar to the 39% reported by Alper et al. *(20)*. Antithyroid antibodies are the most commonly detected in conjunction with POF *(21–23)*. Obviously, the prevalence of detected autoantibodies may be expected to further rise along with increasing sensitivity and scope of available laboratory assays.

OVARIAN ANTIBODIES

Antibodies to ova cytoplasm were described in association with POF as early as 1966 *(24)*. Since then, the reported incidence of antibodies to ovarian antigens has varied widely, according to patient selection and sensitivity of the antigen-binding assay. Wheatcroft et al., using direct immunofluorescence, found a 24–60% prevalence in a sample of 45 POF patients, with a wide variation observed according to the specific ovary/antigen preparation used. Using ELISA, positivity for either antiovary or antioocyte antibodies have been reported in up to 70% of sera from women with POF *(25)*. Damenwood et al. *(26)* found a 100% incidence of antiovary antibodies in women with ovarian failure and Addison's disease. However, the presence of ovarian antibodies does not necessarily indicate an autoimmune etiology; they have been observed in patients with other known etiologies for ovarian failure, including 45,X gonadal dysgenesis, chemotherapy, pelvic irradiation, and perhaps nonspecific tissue injury. Because of their poor specificity, the presence of antiovarian antibodies confers no practical diagnostic or clinical significance.

Moderate titers of autoantibody to the zona pellucida — the glycoprotein matrix surrounding the oocyte — have been reported in at least two case reports of POF. The prevalence of these autoantibodies in normal fertile controls is uncertain, there is speculation that ZP antibodies may be associated with gonadal failure *(27)*. One proposed etiology involves sensitization of the immune system resulting from release of the products of oocyte destruction and follicular atresia, including the zona pellucida; alternatively, T-cell-mediated oophoritis may represent the primary etiology, secondarily triggering the production of autoantibodies. This latter hypothesis appears to be supported by a report of the sperm-binding peptide component of the zona pellucida (ZP3) inducing POF in a mouse model *(28)*. The primary mechanism of disease in this experiment appeared to be local T-cell-mediated oophoritis, and the production of autoantibodies represented a secondary response. Other autoimmune ovarian targets have been the subject of case reports, though none have been shown to be consistently elevated among POF patients in general.

Although antibodies for both LH and FSH have been detected, they appear to be present in a small percentage of patients with POF *(29)*. Nevertheless, various researchers have suggested that anti-FSH antibodies, which have been demonstrated to inhibit FSH receptors in vitro *(30)*, may account for the clinical FSH resistance postulated within the "resistant ovary" subset of POF cases.

Autoantibodies to adrenal steroidogenic enzymes, including 17-α-hydroxylase and 21-hydroxylase, were studied by Chen et al. in patients with various clinical autoimmune diseases. Although autoantibodies to 17-alpha-OH and P-450scc were prevalent among women with Addison's disease, none of the autoantibodies was detected in POF patients without any clinical evidence of adrenal failure *(31)*. Wheatcroft et al. similarly found that a significant proportion of women with autoimmune adrenal failure had circulating antibodies which reacted with steroid-synthesizing cells in both the adrenal and the ovary. Patients with POF associated with polyglandular autoimmune failure syndromes also have been shown to possess low titers of antisteroid cell antibodies *(32)*. The presence of autoantibodies to other steroid producing cells or the diagnosis of polyglandular autoimmune failure syndrome is particularly important to the well being of the patient with POF. In completing an evaluation of the patient presenting with POF it is incumbent upon the physician to make sure that the condition is not part of a larger autoimmune syndrome. Therefore, it is critical to rule out other endocrine autoimmune diseases such as hypothyroidism, hypoadrenalism, and hypoparathyroidism.

Indeed, the clinical diagnosis of POF is often made in conjunction with other clinically apparent autoimmune endocrinopathies. Thyroid and Hashimoto's disease represent the most common clinical autoimmune disorders accompanying ovarian failure. Addison's disease is strongly associated with POF; conversely, POF accompanies 10–20% of autoimmune adrenal insufficiency cases *(33)*. Other suspected POF-associated disorders include polyglandular autoimmume syndrome, Rheumatoid arthritis, systemic lupus erythematosis, myasthenia gravis, insulin dependent diabetes mellitus, and Crohn's disease.

Cell-mediated immune parameters may be altered in women with POF. Increased CD4+ and CD8+ blood T-cells have been demonstrated in POF patients *(34)*, similar to other autoimmune disorders including Graves' disease, Addison's disease, and type 1 diabetes mellitus. Some authors have hypothesized that MHC antigen expression activates the cascade via T-lymphocytes, interleuken-1, and various cytokines which then predispose to atresia of the developing follicle *(35)*. The number of CD 19+ B-cells were found to be significantly elevated in a series of women with POF, whereas NK cells were decreased. Delayed-type hypersensitivity towards candida is significantly more likely to be negative among POF patients, compared with controls *(36)*, and monocyte chemotaxis and macrophage function may also be impaired. Estrogen therapy has been shown to reduce the levels of some, but not all, subsets of T-cells.

Although increased expression of the HLA-DR3 locus was reported in an early series *(37)*, along with elevated levels of HLA-DR+ T-cells *(38)*, subsequent studies have failed to confirm consistently aberrant expression of MHC antigens in POF patients *(39)*. Although the effects of these abnormalities on ovarian function are not well understood, immune system dysregulation clearly may contribute to ovarian tissue damage. Histologically, an inflammatory cell infiltrate surrounding the developing and atretic follicles, in contrast to the primordial follicles, may suggest cell-mediated activity directed against granulosa cells, rather than oogonia. Further study is needed to understand the etiology of autoimmune ovarian failure.

ENVIRONMENTAL CAUSES

Acquired forms of POF may result from infectious, infiltrative, metabolic, and toxic gonadal insults. The mumps virus, even through subclinical infections, has been known to inflict gonadal damage, leading to ovarian failure during the fetal and pubertal periods *(40)*; pelvic tuberculosis may rarely lead to ovarian failure, typically later in the reproductive years. Among patients with thalassemia major, iron overload may result in an infiltrative form of POF. Galactosemia is another rare — but well described — etiology for acquired POF, due to the toxicity of galactose or its metabolites towards the ovarian parenchyma during the prenatal and neonatal period (41). Kaufman et al. documented eighteen 46,XX female patients with galactosemia and hypergonadotropic hypogonadism, with no evidence of underlying autoimmunity. Ovarian tissue was absent or diminished on ultrasound among these patients; the extent of ovarian failure appeared to correlate with delays in dietary treatment for galactosemia. However, even with optimal dietary treatment, galactosemic girls appear to carry a substantial risk of developing POF, owing to the exquisite sensitivity of ovarian tissue to galactose metabolites and galactose-1-phosphate in particular (42).

Pelvic radiation therapy in doses of 250–500 rads — far below the 4500 rad pelvic dose traditionally used to treat Hodgkin's disease — causes permanent ovarian failure in 66% of patients. With 800 rad treatment, 100% of women are affected, emphasizing the importance of gonadal shielding (43). Oophoropexy, or surgical transposition of the ovaries from the radiation field, may also provide effective protection, and a laparoscopic technique has been described (44). Using both maximal shielding and oophoropexy, the total dose received by the ovaries may be reduced to 8–15% of the pelvic node dosage (45). Nevertheless, ovarian ablation may occur despite these measures. Recent treatment regimens, particularly in pediatric oncology, have focused on the development of combined-modality therapy, in order to reduce radiation doses and thereby diminish late sequelae. In a series of 18 teenagers receiving pelvic radiation in a combined regimen for Hodgkin's disease, six developed ovarian failure during a follow-up of 4 yr, despite oophoropexy and maximal shielding; moreover, other reports have suggested a substantial risk of delayed ovarian failure, even many years after treatment (46).

Ovarian failure following chemotherapy is a common entity, appearing in both transient and permanent forms. Using multiagent regimens for Hodgkins disease, between 15–70% of women may develop POF (47,48). Predicting individual prognoses is difficult, however age of the patient appears to be significant. Women aged 30–35 or older are far more prone to develop ovarian failure during the postchemotherapy period; those younger than 30 tend to maintain normal ovulatory and menstrual patterns, though they appear to be at significant risk for undergoing premature menopause over the years following treament.

Hysterectomy with ovarian conservation has traditionally been thought not to affect the incidence of ovarian failure, or age of menopause, for most women postoperatively (49). A recent retrospective study of 90 women, however, revealed 34% of posthysterectomy patients suffered ovarian failure within 2 yr, with a significantly lower mean age of ovarian failure in hysterectomized compared with matched nonhysterectomized women (45.4 vs 49.5 yr). In total, nearly 45% of hysterectomized women had developed ovarian failure by age 45 vs only 13% of similar nonhysterectomized women by this age (50).

RESISTANT OVARY SYNDROME

The "insensitive ovary syndrome," or "resistant ovary syndrome," was described as early as 1960, in patients with amenorrhea, elevated gonadotropins, and demonstrable ovarian follicles on histologic biopsy (51,52). This histological distinction was viewed as a means to identify women with the most capacity for ovulation and conception, from among those satisfying the diagnostic criteria for POF (53). Ovarian biopsy was recommended by some investigators, to differentiate this subgroup (54).

Rebar et al. (1982) studied a series of 18 karyotypically normal women less than age 35, with idiopathic POF based on amenorrhea or menstrual irregularities and FSH levels >40 mIU/mL. Of nine women consenting to ovarian biopsy, four had viable oocytes retrieved; 50% of patients had hormonal evidence of ovarian follicular function. More recent studies have reported up to 65% of karyotypically normal POF patients demonstrate potential ovarian follicle function as determined by serial estrogen measurement *(55)*, with actual ovulation occurring in roughly 20% of women, and occasional pregnancies observed. Nelson et al. (1995) confirmed ovarian follicular activity in 50% of 65 women with POF, and biopsies revealed luteinized Graafian follicles in all women. Serum progesterone reached ovulatory levels, however, in only 16% of patients. Vaginal ultrasound has identified subsets of POF patients in whom follicular activity is present. Initial studies identified ultrasonographically identifiable follicles in 46% of patients *(56)*. Using pelvic ultrasonography, Conway et al. detected follicular activity in 60% of 135 women with idiopathic POF *(57)*.

The distinction between resistant ovary syndrome and POF is presently of no practical diagnostic or prognostic value in predicting fertility. The two entities appear to reside along a clinical continuum, and sporadic pregnancies occur both in the presence or absence of identifiable follicles on biopsy *(58)*. Furthermore, the precision of ovarian biopsy is poor, and its validity in determining the presence or absence of follicular activity appears to be uncertain at best. Immature follicles are likely to be more prevalent in POF patients than ovarian biopsy would suggest, as a result of the inherent inaccuracy of the procedure. As a result, ovarian biopsy should not be included in the workup of POF. The utility of ultrasound, for the identification of follicular activity in planning ovulation induction, is unsettled at present.

OCCULT OVARIAN FAILURE

Frank POF likely represents an extreme form of a broad clinical spectrum of ovarian dysfunction and demise. However, subtler forms of "occult" ovarian failure may present in women with regular menses, infertility, and elevated gonadotropin levels. Cameron et al. (1988) studied ten women with regular menses, infertility, and elevated levels of FSH, who had demonstrated a poor response to ovulation induction during attempted IVF *(59)*. Among them, plasma levels of estradiol, progesterone, and inhibin were normal, suggesting a compensated state of reduced granulosa cell function. The presence of circulating antithyroid, ovary, or adrenal autoantibodies in 50% of the patients suggested a possible connection with POF. A similar series of women with "occult" ovarian failure was reported by Ebbiary et al. *(60)* with slowed follicular growth, smaller follicle diameter, and decreased luteal-phase salivary progesterone, compared to age-matched controls with normal FSH. Whether occult ovarian failure represents exaggerated oocyte atresia or ovarian resistance to gonadotropin stimulation, remains uncertain. Continued prospective follow-up of women with occult ovarian failure will hopefully enable the prediction of ovarian reserve, and of the probability of progression from an occult elevated FSH and infertility to frank ovarian failure.

SURGICAL MENOPAUSE VS NATURAL MENOPAUSE

There are several major differences between surgical and natural menopause, namely, the rapidity with which hormonal withdrawal occurs and the substantial decrease in

Table 1
Minimum tests for the patient with premature ovarian failure

Test	Reason
FSH	Confirmation of gonadal dysfunction.
Ca^{2+}, Phos, Albumin	Evaluate parathyroid function.
TSH, thyroxine	Evaluate thyroid function.
Fasting blood sugar	Evaluate pancreatic function.
Cortisol	Evaluate adrenal reserve. If >18 mcg/dL, good adrenal reserve is assured. If < 3 mcg/dL, the diagnosis of adrenal compromise is made. For levels in between a Cortrosyn stimulation test may be indicated.
Complete blood count	Rule out megaloblastic anemia which may be due to malabsorption of Vitamin B12 as a consequence of autoimmune destruction of intrinsic factor producing cells.
Antinuclear antibody	Assess for the possibility of systemic lupus erythematosis
Karyotype	Rule out privation syndromes with deletion of X-chromosome material.

androgen levels following castration. The rapid decline in circulating levels of estradiol, testosterone, and androstenedione may impact physiologically and psychologically. Pansini et al. *(61)* compared HDL, LDL, total cholesterol, and triglyceride levels in women who underwent spontaneous and surgical menopause. They reported that the atherogenic metabolic risk observed in surgical menopause is higher than in spontaneous menopause. However, conservation of the ovaries at hysterectomy seems to only partially protect against such an increase. Concern over the emotional changes relating to sudden menopause exist, though it is not well studied. One study of 2000 Australian women concluded that current health status and psychological and lifestyle variables, rather than endocrine changes, are the dominant contributors to the well-being of middle-aged women *(62)*.

Hughes et al. *(63)* reported a 50% decrease in testosterone and androstenedione levels in postmenopausal women undergoing bilateral oophorectomy for malignancy. Sherwin and Gelfand *(64)* reported a prospective, double-blind crossover design comparing patients who received either a combined estrogen-androgen or androgen alone to patients who received either estrogen alone or placebo. They found that the energy level, well-being, and appetite levels were higher in the androgen or estrogen-androgen compared to estrogen alone or placebo. Furthermore, patients taking the androgen containing preparations also reported lower somatic, psychological, and total scores on the menopausal scale. The authors concluded that the reduced levels of circulating testosterone subsequent to bilateral oophorectomy may play a role in development of physical and psychological symptoms that are frequent sequalae of bilateral gonadectomy.

SUMMARY

Premature ovarian failure (POF) is a devastating diagnosis to present to a young woman. Gonadal failure poses a threat to the woman's health because of the absence of estrogen. Health risks may also be imparted by one or more medical conditions that led to the ovarian failure. The etiology of POF can be chromosomal, including Turner's syndrome and its mosaic variants. Women with a normal chromosome complement may still harbor a genetic etiology, such as an FSH gene point mutation. More commonly, however, autoimmunity is to blame. Associated autoimmune conditions can also lead to failure of the thyroid, parathyroid, pancreas and adrenal glands. Occult ovarian failure represents a major diagnostic challenge as its causes still remain elusive. Whether this syndrome is because of accelerated oocyte atresia or ovarian resistance to gonadotropin stimulation remains uncertain (Table 1). If a woman loses gonadal function following surgery, the added consequences include a substantial and rapid decrease in androgen production. Replacement of estrogen in cases of POF is essential in most women, but replacement of androgens remains controversial. Regardless of the etiology, the significance of POF necessitates a comprehensive evaluation and close examination for associated disease states. Prompt diagnosis, accurate counseling, and appropriate treatment can improve the patient's well-being and quality of life.

REFERENCES

1. Coulam CB, Adamson SC, Annegers JF. Incidence of premature ovarian failure. Obstet Gynecol 1986;67:604.
2. Krailo MD, Pike MC. Estimation of the distribution of age at natural menopause from prevalence data. Am J Epidemiol 1983;117:356.
3. Alper MM, Garner PR. Premature ovarian failure: its relationship to autoimmune disease. Obstet Gynecol 1985;66:27.
4. Reindollar RH, Byrd JR, McDonough PG. Delayed sexual development: a study of 252 patients. Am J Obstet Gynecol 1981;140:371.
5. Rebar RW, Erickson GF, Yen SSC. Idiopathic premature ovarian failure: clinical and endocrine characteristics. Fertil Steril 1982;37:35.
6. Kurabayashi T, Yasuda M, Fujikmaki T, et al. Effect of hormone replacement therapy on spinal bone mineral density and T lymphocyte subsets in premature ovarian failure and Turners syndrome. Int J Gynecol Obstet 1993;42(1):25.
7. Prior JC, et al. Spinal bone loss and ovulatory disturbances. N Engl J Med 1990;323:1221.
8. Reindollar RH, McDonough PG. Delayed sexual development: common causes and basic clinical approach. Pediatric Annals 1981;10:5.
9. Castillo S, Lopez F, Tobella L, et al. Citogenetica de la falla ovarica prematura. Rev Chil Obstet Ginecol 1992;57(5):341.
10. Krauss CM, Turksoy RN, Atkins L, et al. Familial premature ovarian failure due to an interstitial deletion of the long arm of the X chromosome. N Engl J Med 1977;117:125.
11. Veneman TF, Beverstock GC, Exalto N, et al. Premature menopause because of an inherited deletion in the long arm of the X-chromosome. Fertil Steril 1991;55(3):631.
12. Wu RC, Kuo PL, Lin SJ, et al. X-Chromosome mosaicism in patients with recurrent abortion or premature ovarian failure. J Formos Med Assoc 1993;92(11):953.
13. Matthews CH, Borgato S, Beck-Peccoz P, et al. Primary amenorrhea and infertility due to a mutation in the beta-subunit of FSH. Nat Genet 1993;5(1):83.
14. Aittomaki K. The genetics of XX gonadal dysgenesis. Am J Hum Genet 1994;54:844–851.
15. Aittomaki K, Herva R, Stenman UH, et al. Clinical features of primary ovarian failure caused by a point mutation in the FSH receptor gene. J Clin Endocrinol Metab 1996;81(10):3722.
16. Rabinowe SL, Ravnikar VA, Dib SA, et al. Premature menopause: monoclonal antibody define T lymphocyte abnormalities and antiovarian antibodies. Fertil Steril 1989;51:450.
17. Hill JA, Welch WR, Faris HMP, et al. Induction of class II major histocompatibility complex antigen expression in human granulosa cells by interferon gamma: a potential mechanism contributing to autoimmune ovarian failure. Am J Obstet Gynecol 1990;162:534.
18. Sedmak DD, Hart WR, Tubbs RR. Autoimmune Oophoritis: a histopathologic study of involved ovaries with immunologic characterization of the mononuclear cell infiltrate. Int J Gynecol Pathol 1987;6:73.
19. Conway GS, Kaltsas G, Patel A, et al. Characterization of idiopathic premature ovarian failure. Fertil Steril 1996;65(2):337.

20. Alper MM, Garner PR. Premature ovarian failure: its relationship to autoimmune disease. Obstet Gynecol 1985;66:27.
21. Rebar, RW, Connolly HV, et al. Clinical features of young women with hypergonadotropic amenor-rhea. Fertil Steril 1990;53:804.
22. Alper MM, Garner PR. Premature ovarian failure: its relationship to autoimmune disease. Obstet Gynecol 1985;66:27.
23. Vasquez AM, Kenny FM. Ovarian failure and antiovarian antibodies in association with hypoprarathyroidism, moniliasis, and Addison's and Hashimoto's Diseases. Obstet Gynecol 1973;41:414.
24. Vallotton MB, Forbes AP. Premature menopause in autoimmune diseases. Lancet 1969;1(586):156.
25. Luborsky, JL, Visintin J, Boyers S, et al. Ovarian antibodies detected by immobilized antigen immu-noassay in patients with premature ovarian failure. J Clin Endocrinol Metab 1990;70:69.
26. Damewood MD, Zacur HA, Hoffman GJ, et al. Circulating antibodies in premature ovarian failure. Obstet Gynecol 1986;68:850.
27. Smith, S, Hosid S. Premature ovarian failure associated with autoantibodies to the zona pellucida. Int J Fertil 1994;39(6):3 16,
28. Rhim SH, Millar SE, Robey F, et al. Autoimmune disease of the ovary induced by a ZP3 peptide from the mouse zona pellucida. J Clin Invest 1992;89:28.
29. Tang VW, Faiman C. Premature ovarian failure: a search for circulating factors against gonadotropin receptors. Am J Obstet Gynecol 1983;146:816.
30. Chiauzzi V, Cigorraga S, Escobar ME, et al. Inhibition of follicle-stimulating hormone receptor binding by circulating immunoglobulins. J Clin Endocrinol Metab 1982;54:1221.
31. Chen S, Sawicka J, Betterle C, et al. Autoantibodies to steroidogenic enzymes in autoimmune polyglan-dular syndrome, Addison's disease, and POF. J Clin Endocrinol Metab 1996;81(5):1871.
32. Ahonen P, Miettinen A, Perheentupa J. Adrenal and steroid cell antibodies in patients with autoim-mune polyglandular disease type I and risk of adrenocortical and ovarian failure. J Clin Endocrinol Metab 1987;64:494.
33. Winqvist O, Gebre-Medhin G, Gustafsson J, et al. Identification of the main gonadal autoantigens in patients with adrenal insufficiency and associated ovarian failure. J Clin Endocrinol Metab 1995;80(5):1717.
34. Ho PC, Tang GWK, Fu KH, et al. Immunologic studies in patients with premature ovarian failure. Obstet Gynecol 1988;71:622.
35. Fox, H. The pathology of premature ovarian failure. J Pathol 1992;167:357.
36. Hoek A, van Kasteren Y, de Haan-Meulman M, et al. Analysis of peripheral blood lymphocyte subsets, NK cells, and delayed type hypersensitivity skin test in patients with premature ovarian failure. Am J Reprod Immunol 1995;33:495.
37. Walfish PG, Gottesman IS, Shewchuk AB, et al. Association of premature ovarian failure with HLA antigens. Tiss Antig 1983;21:168.
38. Rabinowe SL, Ravnikar VA, Dib SA, et al. Premature menopause: monoclonal antibody defined T lymphocyte abnormalities and antiovarian antibodies. Fertil Steril 1989;51:450.
39. Jaroudi KA, Arora M, Sheth KV, et al. Human Leukocyte antigen typing and associated abnormalities in premature ovarian failure. Human Reproduct 1994;9(11):2006.
40. Morison JC., et al. Mumps oophoritis: A cause of premature menopause. Fertil Steril 1975;26:255.
41. Kaufman FR, Kogut MD, Donnell GN, et al. Hypergonadotropic hypogonadism in female patients with galactosemia. N Engl J Med 1982;304:994.
42. Gitzelman R, Steinmann B. Galactosemia: how does long-term treatment change the outcome? Enzyme 1984;32(1):37.
43. Cohen I, Speroff L. Premature ovarian failure: update. Obstetr Gynecolog Surv 1991;46(3):156.
44. Williams RS, Mendenhall N. Obstet Gynecol 1992;80(3):541.
45. Le Floch O, Donaldson SS, Kaplan HS. Pregnancy following oophoropexy and total nodal irradiation in women with Hodgkin's disease. Cancer 1976;38:2263.
46. Byrne J, Fears TR, Gail MH, et al. Early menopause in long-term survivors of cancer during adoles-cence. Am J Obstet Gynecol 1992;166(3):788.
47. Whitehead E, Shalet SM, Blackledge G, et al. The effect of combination chemotherapy on ovarian function in women treated for Hodgkin's disease. Cancer 1983;52:988.
48. Horning SJ, hoppe RT, Kaplan HS, et al. Female reproductive potential after treatment for Hodgkin's disease. N Engl J Med 1981;304:1377.

49. Dippel AL. The role of hysterectomy in the production of menopausal symptoms. Am J Obstet Gynecol 1939;37:111.
50. Siddle N, Sarrel P, Whitehead M. The effect of hysterectomy on the age at ovarian failure: identification of a subgroup of women with premature loss of ovarian function and literature review. Fertil Steril 1987;47(1):94.
51. Hertz R, Vallee CA. Control of Ovulation. Perganon Press, New York, 1961, p. 221.
52. Jones GS, DeMoraes-Ruehsen M. A new method of amenorrhea in association with hypergonadotropism and apparently normal follicular apparatus. Am J Obstet Gynecol 1969;104:597.
53. Rebar RW, Erickson GF, Coulam CB. Premature Ovarian Failure. In: Gondos B, Riddrek D, eds., Pathology of Infertility. Thieme Medical, New York, 1987, pp. 123–141.
54. Goldenberg RL, Grodin JM, Rodbard D, et al. Gonadotropins in women with amenorrhea. The use of plasma follicle stimulating hormone to differentiate women with and without ovarian follicles. Am J Obset Gynecol 1973;116:1003.
55. Anasti JN, Kimzey LM, Defensor RA, et al. A controlled study of danazol for the treatment of karyotypically normal spontaneous premature ovarian failure. Fertil Steril 1994;62(4):726.
56. Mehta AE, Matwijiw I, Lyons EA, et al. Noninvasive diagnosis of resistant ovary syndrome by ultrasonography. Fertil Steril 1992;57(1):56.
57. Conway GS, Kaltsas G, Patel A, et al. Characterization of idiopathic premature ovarian failure. Fertil Steril 1996;65(2):337.
58. Rebar RW, Erickson GF, Yen SSC. Idiopathic premature ovarian failure: clinical and endocrine characteristics. Fertil Steril 1982;37:35.
59. Cameron IT, O'Shea FC, Rolland JM, et al. Occult ovarian failure: a syndrome of infertility, regular menses, and elevated follicle-stimulating hormone concentrations. J Clin Endocrinol Metab 1988;67:1190.
60. Ahmed Ebbiary NA, Lenton EA, Salt C, et al. The significance of elevated basal follicle stimulating hormone in regularly menstruating infertile women. Hum Reproduct 1994;9(2):245.
61. Pansini F, Bonaccorsi G, Calisesi M, Campobasso C, Franze GP, Gilli G, Locorotondo G, Mollica G. Influence of spontaneous and surgical menopause on atherogenic metabolic risk. Maturitas 1993;17:181.
62. Dennerstein L, Smith AM, Morse C. Psychological well-being, mid-life and the menopause. Maturitas 1994;20:1.
63. Hughes CL Jr, Wall LL, Creasman WT. Reproductive hormone levels in gynecologic oncology patients undergoing surgical castration after spontaneous menopause. Gynecol Oncol 1991;40:42.
64. Sherwin BB, Gelfand MM. Differential response to parenteral estrogen and/or androgen administration in the surgical menopause. Am J Obstet Gynecol 1985;151:153.

9   Hormone Replacement Therapy

Elizabeth A. Kennard, MD

INTRODUCTION

Hormone replacement therapy (HRT) has been available for years, but there are still many areas of exciting advances in this field. The endocrine basis for this replacement, and for the variable tissue effects of estrogens, is only now being completely elucidated. Knowledge of estrogen receptors, their mechanism of action, and its modulation is continually expanding. Although the concept of replacing estrogen after the ovary has ceased production is not new, some of the health benefits of this treatment are just beginning to come to light. Concerns about the risks of hormone replacement therapy continue to plague those who care for women and problems with compliance abound. This chapter will provide a brief overview of both estrogen replacement therapy (ERT) and combined HRT.

Mechanism of Action of Estrogen

Estrogen is a steroid hormone that acts via an intracellular receptor. The conformation of the estrogen receptor can be altered by coligands and there is more than one type of estrogen receptor. Once an estrogen has bound its receptor, it modulates tissue function by effects on gene transcription. Coactivators can also change the effect of a given estrogen.

From: *Contemporary Endocrinology: Menopause: Endocrinology and Management*
Edited by: D. B. Seifer and E. A. Kennard © Humana Press Inc., Totowa, NJ

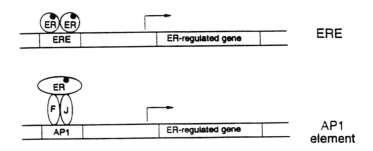

Fig. 1. Estrogen-receptor complex binding to DNA.

Estrogen enters a cell by simple diffusion. The estrogen receptor is normally bound to heat-shock proteins. The hormone binds to its receptor and this induces a conformational change. This change results in release from the heat-shock proteins and exposure of an area of the receptor that allows the formation of a dimer with another receptor-hormone complex. This dimer binds to the target gene in the area of DNA termed the hormone response element (HRE). Transcriptional activation of the target gene is mediated through transactivation domains of the receptor termed AF-1 and AF-2 *(1)*.

Estrogens can also exert their effect through the AP1 enhancer element. This is a separate area of DNA from the HRE. Transcriptional activation from this area of the DNA requires the presence of transcription factors Fos and Jun *(see* Fig. 1). These transcription factors interact with the hormone-receptor complex and the DNA, acting as a sort of bridge between the complex and the DNA. Therefore, there are at least two separate ways for the estrogen-receptor complex to bind to the DNA.

The structure of the estrogen receptor's ligand binding domain is such that it requires the ligand to have an aromatic ring, but can accommodate a variety of side groups *(2)*. For example, the side chains on estradiol help direct the activation domain of the receptor away from inhibitory proteins, thus freeing them to interact with coactivators which promote transcription. Differently configured estrogens or estrogen-like compounds will bind the same receptor and have a different effect because of the conformational changes caused by their side groups.

In 1996, the exciting discovery of a second type of estrogen receptor further explained the variety of tissue effects found with estrogens *(3)*. The two types of estrogen receptors are termed ERα and ERβ and are present in different tissues (Table 1). Investigators have found that ERα and ERβ respond differently to the same ligand *(4)*. A possible third distinct type of estrogen receptor was recently identified in rat tissues and named ERβ2 *(5)*. Estrogen receptors can also bind auxiliary proteins or can be modified by phosphorylation after they have bound the ligand *(1)*. These properties diminish or enhance the activity of the hormone-receptor complex.

In summary, in addition to at least two possible DNA binding mechanisms, there are at least two and possibly three distinct types of estrogen receptors, and multiple modifiers that can alter the effects of any given estrogen-like compound in any cell type. This begins to explain the varied effects of estrogen compounds in different tissues and different conditions.

ENDOCRINOLOGY OF MENOPAUSE

During the climacteric and after, there is a decline in ovarian hormone production. Specifically, there are declines in serum estradiol, estrone, and inhibin levels, reflecting

Table 1
Distribution of Estrogen Receptors

Alpha Receptors	Beta Receptors	Alpha and Beta Receptors
Breast	Blood vessels	Ovary
Liver	Bone	CNS
Uterus	Lungs	
	Urogenital tract	

the exhaustion of the granulosa cell pool. Postmenopausal estradiol and estrone levels are around 18 pg/mL and 30 pg/mL. Simultaneously, the serum follicle stimulating hormone (FSH) and luteinizing hormone (LH) levels rise as the hypothalamic-pituitary-ovarian axis tries to compensate for the lower estradiol level. FSH also rises because of a lack of inhibin. The levels of other pituitary hormones, such as prolactin, cortisol, and growth hormone, do not change in the menopause. Adrenal steroid hormone production is also unaltered by the menopause.

ENDOCRINOLOGY OF HORMONE REPLACEMENT

Using exogenous estrogens, the serum levels of estrogens are measurably increased. Oral estradiol products are largely converted to estrone during a first past effect through the liver. Using oral estradiol products, estradiol and estrone levels will average around 75 and 330 pg/mL. With transdermal estradiol products, the plasma estradiol and estrone levels average 50 and 42 pg/mL. This difference in estrone levels demonstrates the first past effect of the oral route. Estropipate is a preparation of estrone conjugated to piperazine and leads to elevations of serum estrone levels. Conjugated equine estrogens and esterified estrogens are prepared from the urine of pregnant mares and contain mostly estrone sulfate with a small amount of equilin sulfate and other equine estrogens. These preparations result in plasma estradiol levels of 45–50 pg/mL as well as increases in estrone and the equine estrogens.

The serum FSH and LH levels will decrease in postmenopausal women on HRT. The amount of effect appears to vary directly with the time since menopause, with elderly women having increased FSH and LH suppression in response to estradiol (6). However, HRT usually does not result in a normalization of FSH levels to the premenopausal range because of the continued absence of inhibin production.

Hormone Replacement Regimens

Estrogen is given to menopausal women in a variety of forms and doses. In women who have had a hysterectomy, there is no need to prescribe progestins, and estrogen should be prescribed continuously. Table 2 lists types of estrogens available. Used alone, in traditional doses of conjugated estrogens 0.625 mg or its equivalent, estrogen will result in an 11%/yr incidence of endometrial hyperplasia in women who retain their uterus (7). Usually, progestins are added to the regimen to reduce the incidence of hyperplasia and cancer. Table 3 lists progestins available in the United States. When estrogens are combined with progestins, there are a variety of regimens available following two basic types: sequential and continuous combined. In the sequential regimen, estrogens are used with progestins for a portion of the cycle. In the continuous combined regimens, estrogens are

Table 2
Estrogen Preparations Available in the United States

Brand	Estrogen	Available doses/frequency
Oral:		
Estrace	17β Estradiol	0.5 or 1.0 mg daily
Estratab	Esterified estrogens	0.3, 0.625, 1.25, or 2.5 mg daily
Menest	Esterified estrogens	0.3, 0.625, 1.25, or 2.5 mg daily
Ogen .625, Ogen 1.25, Ogen 2.5	Estropipate	0.75, 1.5, or 3 mg daily
Ortho-Est .625, Ortho-est 1.25	Estropipate	0.75, or 1.5 mg daily
Premarin	Conjugated estrogens	0.3, 0.625, 0.9, 1.25, or 2.5 mg daily
Transdermal:		
Alora	17β Estradiol	0.05 mg per day in twice a week patch
Climara	17β Estradiol	0.05 or 0.1 mg per day in weekly patch
Estraderm	17β Estradiol	0.05 or 0.1 mg per day in twice a week patch
Vivelle	17β Estradiol	0.0375, 0.05, 0.075, or 0.1 mg per day in twice a week patch

Table 3
Progestin Tablets Available in the United States

Brand	Progestin
Amen	10 mg medroxyprogesterone acetate
Cycrin	5 or 10 mg medroxyprogesterone acetate
Micronor	0.35 mg norethindrone
Provera	2.5, 5.0, or 10 mg medroxyprogesterone acetate

combined with daily progestins. Table 4 lists different regimens for HRT. There are also medications available that combine estrogen with other compounds for a variety of indications (*see* Table 5).

The incidence of hyperplasia in the continuous combined regimens is the same or lower than the sequential ones *(7)*. The dose of progestin necessary to prevent an increase in uterine cancer in the sequential regimens is a matter of debate. Studies that show a decreased risk of cancer used 10 mg of medroxyprogsterone acetate. However, the Menopause Study Group showed no difference in endometrial hyperplasia in the group that received 5 mg as opposed to 10 mg of medroxyprogsterone acetate *(8)*. The length of time of progestin use is another variable. Use of progestins for 12 d/mo is less likely to result in hyperplasia than use for shorter intervals *(9)*. Many clinicians prescribe progestins for 14 d to allow for easier dosing instructions. More recently, investigators have proposed that progestins need only be given on a quarterly basis while maintaining a low incidence of hyperplasia *(10)*. However, in a letter to the editor, Scandinavian

Table 4
Hormone Replacement Regimens

Regimen	Medication
Continuous: 1. Take estrogen and progestin on daily basis 2. As above, but omit Saturday and Sunday of each week	Estrogens: 0.625 mg conjugated or esterified estrogens or 1 mg oral estradiol or 0.75 mg estropipate, or 0.05 mg transdermal estradiol Progestins: 2.5 mg medroxyprogesterone acetate or 0.35 mg norethindrone acetate
Sequential regimens: 1. Take estrogen daily, add progestin for 10–14 d of month 2. Take estrogen daily for first 25 d of month add progestin for 10–14 d of month Up to 6 d without hormones 3. Take estrogen daily, use progestin for 14 d every 3 mo	Estrogens: 0.625 mg conjugated or esterified estrogens or 1 mg oral estradiol or 0.75 mg estropipate, or 0.05 mg transdermal estradiol Progestins: 5 or 10 mg medroxyprogesterone acetate

Table 5
Estrogen Combination Medications Available in the United States

Brand	Preparation	Dose/frequency
Estratest	1.25 mg Esterified estrogens and 2.5 mg Methyltestosterone	Once daily
Estratest H.S.	0.625 mg Esterified estrogens and 1.25 mg Methyltestosterone	Once daily
PMB 200,400	0.45 mg conjugated estrogens with 200 or 400 mg Meprobamate	Once daily Seldom used estrogen combined with tranquilizer
PremPhase	0.625 mg conjugated estrogens alone and combined with 5 mg medroxyprogesterone acetate	2 wk of estrogens alone followed by 2 wk of combined tablets
PremPro	0.625 mg conjugated estrogens and 2.5 mg or 5 mg medroxyprogesterone acetate	Once daily

authors reported an 11% incidence of hyperplasia in a quarterly withdrawal regimen after 3 yr of therapy (11). Although this was not a peer-reviewed publication, it is concerning and annual endometrial biopsies should probably be performed on women using this regimen.

There are estrogen preparations that are approved for the treatment of urogenital atrophy and vasomotor symptoms. These products produce low serum levels of estradiol and are not expected to provide all the proven benefits of HRT (see Table 6).

Mortality Among Hormone-Replacement Users

Studies have repeatedly shown that users of estrogen or combined estrogen and progestin HRT have greatly decreased mortality. One such study is the Leisure World

Table 6
Estrogen Products Approved for Treatment of Atrophy[a]

Brand	Dose/frequency	Estrogen
Estring	One ring placed vaginally for 90 d	17b Estradiol
Fempatch	0.025 mg patch, once per week	17b Estradiol
Estrace Vaginal Cream	2–4 g daily for 2 wk then tapered to 1 g 1–3 times per week	17b Estradiol
Ogen Vaginal Cream	2–4 g daily	Estropipate
Ortho Dienestrol Cream	1 applicator daily	Dienestrol 0.1%
Premarin Vaginal Cream	0.5–2 g. daily	Conjugated estrogens

[a]These products will not necessarily provide all the benefits of the estrogen doses available in HRT.

study of 8881 postmenopausal women in a retirement community. The authors described a reduced risk of all-cause mortality in women who used HRT (12). Another large cohort study, the Nurse's Health Study enrolled more than 120,000 registered nurses in 1976. Death registry data was obtained and each death was matched with 10 controls from the cohort. A total of more than 34,000 women provided information as controls for the 3637 deaths. The relative risk of death among hormone users was 0.63 compared to nonusers (13). These are but two examples of several large published studies showing the survival benefit of HRT. Since cardiovascular deaths are the leading cause of death in postmenopausal women, any effect in this area would provide a large advantage to hormone users (14).

HEALTHY USER EFFECT

Skeptics of HRT trials have argued that they are usually observational and that users of hormone replacement are less likely to have adverse health events, particularly cardiovascular events, because they are healthier than controls when therapy is begun (15). Indeed this may explain some of the benefits found in large cohorts such as the Leisure World study and National Health and Nutrition Examination Survey (NHANES) (12,16). Analysis of characteristics of women enrolled in these types of studies has been conflicting. Derby et al. found that estrogen users were leaner and of higher socioeconomic status and less likely to smoke prior to starting HRT (17). In contrast, there was no difference between users and nonusers in measures of cholesterol and blood pressure prior to beginning therapy. A review of the Rancho Bernardo trial, another retirement community cohort of 909 women, seemed to indicate that there were no differences at baseline, but that these appeared over time. Women using HRT decreased smoking, increased exercise, and modified their diet. The authors proposed this might have been a result of increased contact with the health care system (18). A recent study from Finland demonstrated that there were no differences in diet, smoking, and exercise between users and nonusers. However users of estrogen were more likely to be from a higher socioeconomic group and had higher education (19). The results of the ongoing prevention trials should help answer this question.

Cardiovascular Effects of Hormone Replacement

A strongly decreased risk of cardiovascular disease and death is one of the most consistently reported benefits of HRT. A recent review of all studies showed a 50% reduced risk of cardiovascular disease in women receiving HRT *(20)*. Estrogen clearly decreases the concentration of low density lipoprotein (LDL) and raises the level of high density lipoprotein (HDL) *(21,22)*. This profile has been associated with decreased risk for cardiovascular disease. Progestins will attenuate some of the benefits on the lipid profile. However, recent reviews have attributed only about 20% of the cardiovascular protection to lipid effects *(23)*. This explains how the addition of progestins to estrogen replacement therapy has not negated the cardiovascular advantage *(24,25)*.

In addition to lipid effects, hormone replacement has several other beneficial effects on the cardiovascular system. Estrogens enhance vasodilatation of blood vessels. This appears to be a direct effect on the endothelium. The magnitude of this effect is similar in women who are taking estrogen alone or estrogens with progestin therapy *(26)*. Elegant studies in primates by Clarkson have shown that hormone replacement stops formation of atherosclerotic plaques and decreases LDL uptake by blood vessel walls, even in the face of high-fat diets *(27)*. Estrogen reduces plasminogen activator inhibitor type-1 (PAI-1) by 50%, causing a decrease in an antagonist of fibrinolysis *(28)*. Trials have shown a decrease in fibrinogen levels in women using estrogens combined with different progestins *(7)*. Estrogen decreases thromboxane A2 and increases prostacyclin formation, which would be expected to decrease the thrombotic tendency as well *(29)*. Insulin sensitivity also improves on HRT, a known marker for decreased risk *(30,31)*. A more extensive review of the cardiovascular effects of HRT is provided in Chapter 3.

USE OF HRT IN WOMEN WITH CARDIOVASCULAR DISEASE

One issue that deserves special attention is the reluctance of general physicians to prescribe HRT to women with cardiovascular disease. Reluctance to prescribe medications for this group seems to stem from contraindications to the use of oral contraceptives in women with cardiovascular disease. However, there are several studies that support the use of HRT in this group of women.

The Nurse's Health Study calculated the relative risk of mortality for women with and without coronary risk factors. They found a much more significant reduction, to a relative risk of 0.51, in hormone users who had coronary risk factors compared to women with no risk factors *(12)*. The National Health and Nutrition Examination Survey (NHANES) found that survival was higher in women with cardiovascular disease who were hormone users *(16)*. The Leisure World study also demonstrated that women with established cardiovascular disease who were placed on hormone replacement had approx 50% less risk of recurrence or death from cardiovascular disease *(32)*. A study of 726 women hospitalized for acute MI between 1980 and 1991 found the relative risk of reinfarction was 0.5 for current estrogen users *(33)*.

These results are supported by reports of angiography in postmenopausal women. A multicenter trial followed women who had anterioplasty for cardiovascular disease and found less progression of lesion size in women who took HRT after the intervention *(34)*. In addition, O'Keefe et al. followed women after angioplasty and found fewer myocardial infarctions in users of hormones compared with nonusers *(35)*. These studies are consistent with a study of 90 postmenopausal women with chest pain, which found that present users of HRT had an odds ratio of 0.13 of having angiographically documented coronary artery disease compared to those who were nonusers of HRT *(36)*. Sullivan et al. reported on 2000 women who under went arteriography of whom 200 were estrogen users. A 10-yr follow-up showed that women with no disease did well whether or not they took HRT. In contrast, those with severe disease had a markedly increased survival if they were taking HRT *(37)*. The Nurse's Health Study data confirmed this, with the biggest reduction in risk of death found in women with multiple risk factors for coronary disease *(12)*. Women with angina, hypertension, and a past history of cardiovascular disease should be strongly considered for HRT. Currently, ongoing trials to further assess the benefit of HRT in women with cardiovascular disease will be completed in the next few years.

Stroke and HRT

Most studies show a decreased risk of stroke in women who receive HRT although the data are not as consistent as the protection against cardiovascular disease. This probably reflects the varying etiologies of stroke. Both the NHANES study and the Leisure World study demonstrated a decreased risk of stroke and stroke mortality in estrogen users *(38,39)*. A cohort study from Sweden also described a 30% decreased risk of stroke in users of combined HRT *(40)*. Finally, a review of studies that used death from stroke as the endpoint showed 20–60% reduction of risk in estrogen users *(41)*.

There are reports that do not demonstrate protection against stroke with HRT. The Nurses' Health Study has failed to demonstrate a reduced risk of stroke, although the cardiovascular risk is clearly reduced in hormone-replacement users *(42)*. A literature review by Paganini-Hill did not find consistency between studies in the risk of incident stroke *(41)*. For unclear reasons, the Framingham Study alone reports an increase in the incidence of stroke with postmenopausal hormone use *(43)*. With all other studies showing protection or no effect of hormone use and stroke, we conclude that although HRT may not protect against stroke, it probably does not significantly increase the risk of stroke in the postmenopausal woman.

Osteoporosis Prevention

Estrogens are FDA-approved for two uses, the prevention of osteoporosis and the mitigation of symptoms of estrogen withdrawal, such as hot flashes. The data on osteoporosis prevention are overwhelming and HRT should be the first and most commonly used treatment for this debilitating condition *(44–46)*.

Several studies have examined the issue of whether bone protection continues after HRT is stopped. The consensus is that protection is lost after HRT is discontinued. Cauley et al. prospectively studied 9704 women age 65 and older *(47)*. The average age at which past-users had discontinued HRT was 55.5 yr. They found that those who discontinued HRT after as much as 10 yr of use, had low bone densities and the same fracture risk as never-users. The Rancho Bernardo study of more than 900 women, showed that past users of HRT had the same bone mineral density levels as nonusers *(48)*. This is explained by work demonstrating that discontinuation of HRT leads to "catch-up" bone loss *(49,50)*. Current concerns about prolonged HRT use and breast cancer need to be balanced with the knowledge that discontinuing HRT will result in bones just as osteoporotic as those of a women who never used these preparations at all.

The practitioner is often faced with clinical questions regarding the usefulness of HRT if it is initiated several years after menopause. There is some evidence that women may gain benefit from starting HRT even 10 years after menopause *(48,51)*. However, the data in this area are limited. Fracture is dependent on low bone density combined with trauma and type-II osteoporosis is age related and not impacted by estrogen replacement. One might also consider the cardiovascular and other benefits prior to initiating HRT in the elderly.

Patients will also ask about the usefulness of calcium supplementation to prevent osteoporosis. At best, calcium will retard bone loss, but certainly not prevent it. A placebo-controlled randomized trial of calcium supplementation showed that a total intake of 1750 mg of calcium slowed, but did not prevent bone loss compared to a baseline intake of 750 mg calcium *(52)*. A separate trial comparing calcium with and without hormone replacement showed a similar effect; retardation, but not prevention of bone loss in the calcium-only group *(53)*. For a more detailed discussion of this aspect of menopause and HRT, *see* Chapter 4.

COLON CANCER

Several studies have shown a decreased risk of colon cancer in hormone users. Newcomb et al. performed a case control study of Wisconsin women with a diagnosis of colorectal cancer *(54)*. They found a relative risk of 0.5 of colon cancer in current users and of 0.7 in ever-users. This reduced risk was found even after controling for dietary differences, age, weight, exercise, family history, and frequency of screening sigmoidoscopy. Similar protection was found for users of both ERT and HRT. Equivalent decreases have been found in several other studies *(55–58)*. In addition, at least one study appears to show a dose-response effect. Calle et al. studied mortality from colon cancer stratified by years of use. They found a decreasing risk with increased years of use of hormone replacement *(58)*. However, there are studies that do not show this benefit, and the subject remains controversial *(59,60)*. If nothing else, the yearly pelvic exam required to continue HRT might reasonably be expected to lead to increased early detection of colorectal cancer because of increased fecal occult blood testing and rectal exams.

ALZHEIMER'S DISEASE

Several studies have demonstrated a decrease in Alzheimer's disease in women receiving HRT *(61–63)*. The relative risk was usually found to be approx 0.5, and in most of the studies, the women were receiving unopposed estrogen replacement. The Leisure World Study also found that increased duration of use provided increased protection against Alzheimer's disease, an apparent dose-response effect *(61)*.

Investigators have demonstrated many different in vitro effects of estradiol on cultured neuronal cells. This includes prevention of hypoglycemia-induced neuronal death, an increase in dendritic spine density, and an increase in synapses in estrogen-exposed neurons *(64–66)*. Small studies also show some improvement in Alzheimer's disease during treatment with estrogen *(67)*. Other investigators have found decreased serum levels of amyloid P, the glycoprotein present in the neurofibrillary tangles of Alzheimer's disease, when oral estrogens were administered *(68)*. Studies in normal aging women have sometimes shown subtle improvements in memory and other cognitive functions. This exciting area of research is further explored in Chapter 6.

RISKS OF HRT

Breast Cancer

The myriad studies addressing the issue of breast cancer risk and hormone replacement are a testament to both the overriding fear of breast cancer among patients and the difficulty in discerning the actual risk attributable to the use of hormone replacement.

There is no consensus as to the presence or amount of increased breast cancer risk when using HRT. One can clearly state that if there is increased risk, it is small and difficult to detect. Several meta-analyses seem to show an increased incidence with a relative risk of about 1.2 *(69–72)*. There is much less data surrounding the risk associated with the addition of progestins to estrogen replacement. The largest study to address this was the Nurse's Health study that showed an increase in breast cancer risk on long-term (greater than 10 yr) estrogen therapy with no effect on this risk with the addition of progestins *(71)*. However, discontinuing HRT after 10 years of use out of fear of breast cancer will negate the osteoporosis-prevention effect. It may also remove any cardiovascular protection. For a more comprehensive discussion of this area, *see* Chapter 11.

Most studies show that survival with breast cancer appears to be improved among those who were taking HRT at the time of diagnosis *(73–75)*. One study showed that tumors of similar size and receptor status were more likely to be lower grade in HRT users as compared to nonusers *(76)*. The Nurse's Health study is one notable exception to this general finding of increased survival in HRT users *(71)*. There are varied explanations for the survival benefit demonstrated by most studies. The "healthy-user effect" would come into play with HRT, because these women are more likely to have breast cancer surveillance in the form of mammograms and exams. In addition, women with a higher risk for breast cancer may be discouraged from receiving HRT. There are also theories that estrogens may selectively suppress growth of more virulent tumors. There is much more research to be done in this area.

Use of HRT in Breast Cancer Survivors

Because HRT has generally been considered contraindicated in breast cancer patients, there is little clinical data in this area. Two small case-control studies show no increased risk of recurrence or mortality in breast cancer survivors placed on HRT. Bonnier et al. treated 90 patients who had a recurrence-free 5-yr survival with HRT and matched them with 180 controls. The relative risk or recurrence during HRT was 0.40 *(75)*. DiSaia et al. also reported no change in the recurrence risk or survival rate in a group of 41 patients who received HRT after surviving breast cancer *(77)*. Some of DiSaia's patients also received treatment with tamoxifen, which may have confounded the data analysis. Further research is needed in this area. In particular, selective estrogen-receptor modulators such as raloxifene may warrant consideration for use by breast cancer survivors.

PULMONARY EMBOLISM AND VENOUS THROMBOEMBOLISM

There may be a very slight increase in the risk of thromboembolism in hormone users. However, it must be remembered that the incidence of these disorders is very low. The risk of deep vein thrombosis in HRT users is estimated at no more than 3 per 10,000 women-years, which represents a two- to threefold increase over nonusers. Because of

Table 7
Laboratory Screening for Patients
with History of Thromboembolism

- Protein C
- Protein S
- Antithrombin III
- Factor V Leiden

the rarity of this condition, the studies which address it are case control and therefore fraught with potential for bias *(78,79)*. Others have not been able to demonstrate an increased risk *(80)*.

The risk of pulmonary embolism may also be slightly increased in women using hormone replacement *(81)*. Again, the incidence of this occurrence is rare and hormones are estimated to have a negligible increase in this disease.

It is recommended that women with a history of unexplained venous thromboembolism undergo screening for abnormalities of the coagulation pathway to determine if they have a hereditary thrombotic tendency (*see* Table 7). It may be possible to use HRT in women who have a thrombotic tendency who are properly anticoagulated.

COMPLIANCE ISSUES

According to an analysis of a nationally representative sample of 6341 office visits to primary care physicians in 1993–1994, HRT is grossly underutilized. Stafford et al. showed only 8% of women were receiving HRT *(82)*. Some of this is because of decreased prescription by family practitioners and internists, who accounted for 69% of the office visits. Several other studies have shown that nongynecologists are far less likely to recommend HRT *(83–85)*. This would imply that further efforts need to be made to alert physicians outside of gynecology to the benefits of HRT.

A second and equally important reason for the underutilization of HRT is that women are reluctant to take the preparations. The Massachusetts Women's Health Survey showed that more than 40% of women surveyed either did not fill their hormone replacement prescription or discontinued it in less than 9 mo *(83)*. Fear of breast cancer is the most commonly cited reason *(86)*. Some women are also wary of interfering with a "natural" state of menopause *(87)*. Discontinuation after starting the medication is most commonly because of side effects, particularly vaginal bleeding (Table 8).

FACTORS ENHANCING COMPLIANCE

The two factors most important in enhancing patient compliance with medications are patient education and use of a simple regimen. In the case of HRT, education seems to be the most important component because simple regimens are available. In a survey of 274 women, physician recommendation and education was the most important reason for initiating and continuing HRT *(88)*. This was followed by relief of hot flashes as the second-most common reason for continuing prescribed therapy. Underscoring the need for physician education, this investigator also found that of the 125 women who had never taken HRT, 64% claimed that their physician had never discussed it. Nachtigall also showed that improved patient education and counseling led to discontinuation rates of 5–

Table 8
Reasons for Noncompliance with HRT

• Fear of cancer
• Wish to avoid bleeding
• Fear of weight gain
• Not "natural"
• Breast tenderness

Table 9
Risks and Benefits of Hormone Replacement Therapy (HRT)

Benefits	Relative Risk	Reference
Decrease in mortality from CVD	0.5	12,16,20,32,33
Decrease in osteoporosis	0.38–0.68	44–46
Decrease in/improvement in Alzheimer's disease	0.5	61–63
Decrease in colon cancer	0.5–0.7	54–58

Risks	Relative Risk	Reference
Increase in breast cancer	1.2	69–72
Increased thromboembolism	2–3	78,79

7%, far lower than the national average *(89)*. It was hoped that bone densitometry might help improve compliance with HRT. However, this is a seldom researched area. Ryan et al. sent follow-up questionnaires to 400 women seen for bone densitometry in their clinic. Referring doctors were sent letters recommending HRT to 105 of these women. Between 6 and 12 mo after the bone scan 39% of women whose physicians were advised to prescribe estrogens were not taking estrogens. Compliance was not affected by age, class, or family history of osteoporosis *(90)*. This study has been criticized because the advice was given to the referring doctors, not to the patients, and no assessment was made of whether the patients were actually prescribed HRT. In a second study by Torgerson et al., women were randomly invited to have bone densitometry performed and 685 were advised to have HRT if there were no contraindications. After one year, only 49% of women were continuing to take the prescribed treatments. Compliance was 59% in women who had undergone hysterectomy and were not prone to vaginal bleeding in response to HRT *(91)*. These were disappointing results and illustrate how complicated the issue of compliance is. In contrast, a recent randomized trial of bone desitometry showed that there was a higher rate of compliance with HRT among the 93 women who underwent bone densitometry compared to 43 control women *(92)*. Even then, compliance in the group who had the testing was only 63.4% after one year. At present, bone densitometry should be used only in selected cases where it might help the patient make her decision about initiating or continuing HRT because it has not been clearly demonstrated to enhance compliance when applied to large groups.

Patient involvement in decision making and treatment monitoring, simplification of the treatment regimen, and reduction of side effects are important in any prescription *(93)*. With HRT, the public is inundated with myths and misinformation. The benefits of the prescribed treatment must be emphasized. Table 9 lists the benefits and risks of HRT. Common side effects should be reviewed along with the availability of options to correct these problems. In this way, patients who might discontinue the therapy are encouraged to consult with their caregiver for other options prior to stopping the medication.

SUMMARY

Estrogen is a multisystem hormone that has receptors in many tissues. The systemic effects of HRT are still being discovered. It appears that most women will benefit from increased life expectancy and quality-of-life if they replace the ovarian hormones lost after menopause. However, the risks of this therapy are also a concern and compliance issues are a continuing problem. Despite the development of a variety of medications and treatment regimens, the perfect HRT has not been described. We may be able to use lower doses of estrogen or alternative delivery systems to optimize therapy. Ongoing trials and the development of new medications continually advance this exciting area of medical care.

REFERENCES

1. Tsai MJ, O'Malley BW. Molecular mechanisms of action of steroid/thyroid receptor superfamily members. Ann Rev Biochem 1994;63:451–486.
2. Brzozowski AKM, Pike AC, Dauter Z, et al. Molecular basis of agonism and antagonism in the oestrogen receptor. Nature 1997;389:753–758.
3. Mosselman S, Polman J, Dijkema R. ERβ: identification and characterization of a novel human estrogen receptor. FEBS Lett 1996;392:49–53.
4. Paech K, Webb P, Kuiper G, et al. Differential ligand activation of estrogen receptors ERα and ERβ at AP1 sites. Science 1997;277:1508–1511.
5. Petersen D, Tkalcevic GT, Koza-Taylor PH, et al. Identification of estrogen receptor β2, a functional variant of estrogen receptor β expressed in normal rat tissues. Endocrinol 1998;139:1082–1092.
6. Santoro N, Banwell T, Tortoriello D, et al. Effects of aging and gonadal failure on the hypothalamic-pituitary axis in women. Am J Obstet Gynecol 1998;178:732–741.
7. The writing group for the PEPI trial. Effects of estrogen or estrogen/progestin regimens on heart disease risk factors in postmenopausal women. JAMA 1995;273:199–208.
8. Woodruff JD, Pickar JH, for the Menopause Study Group. Incidence of endometrial hyperplasia in postmenopausal women taking conjugated estrogens (Premarin) with medroxyprogesterone acetate or conjugated estrogens alone. Am J Obstet Gynecol 1994;170:1213–1223.
9. King RJB, Whitehead MI. Assessment of the potency of orally administered progestins in women. Fertil Steril 1986;46:1062–1066.
10. Ettinger B, Selby J, Citron JT, et al. Cyclic hormone replacement therapy using quarterly progestin. Obstet Gynecol 1994;83:693–700.
11. Cerin A, Heldaas K, Moeller B. Adverse endometrial effects of long-cycle estrogen and progestogen replacement therapy. NEJM 1996;334:668–669.
12. Henderson BE, Paganini-Hill, Ross R. Arch Int Med 1991;151:75–78.
13. Grodstein F, Stampfer MJ, Colditz GA, et al. Postmenopausal hormone therapy and mortality. N Engl J Med 1997:336;1769–1775.
14. National Center for Health Statistics. Vital Statistics of the United States, 1992. Vol. II-Mortality Part. DHHS pub no 96–1101. Public Health Service, Washington, 1996.
15. Matthew KA, Kuller LH, Wink RR, et al. Prior to use of estrogen replacement therapy are users healthier than nonusers? Am J Epidemiol 1996;143:971–978.
16. Wolf PH, Madans JH, Finucane FF, et al. Reduction of cardiovascular disease-related mortality among postmenopausal women who use hormones: evidence from a national cohort. Am J Obstet Gynecol 1991;164:489–494.
17. Derby CA, Hume AL, McPhillips JB, et al. Prior and current health characteristics of postmenopausal estrogen replacement therapy users compared to non-users. Am J Obstet Gynecol 1995;173:544–550.

18. Barrett-Connor E. Postmenopausal estrogen and prevention bias. Ann Intern Med 1991;115:455–456.

19. Luoto R, Mannisto S, Vartiainen E. Hormone replacement therapy and body size: how much does lifestyle explain? Am J Obstet Gynecol 1998;178:66–73.

20. Grodstein F, Stampfer MJ. The epidemiology of coronary heart disease and estrogen replacement in postmenopausal women. Prog Cardiovasc Dis 1995;18:199–210.

21. Samaan SA, Crawford MH. Estrogen and cardiovascular function after menopause. J Am Coll Cardiol 1995;26:1403–410.

22. Wild RA. Estrogen: effects on the cardiovascular tree. Obstet Gynecol 1996;87(suppl):27s–35s.

23. Clarkson TB. Estrogens, progestins and coronary heart disease in cynomolgus monkeys. Fertil Steril 1994;62(suppl 2):147s–151s.

24. Grodstein F, Stampfer M, Manson J, et al. Postmenopausal estrogen and progestin use and risk of cardiovascular disease. N Eng J Med 1996;335:453–461.

25. Psaty B, Heckbert S, Atkins D, et al. The risk of myocardial infarction associated with the combined use of estrogens and progestins in postmenopausal women. Arch Intern Med 1994;154:1333–1339.

26. McCrohon JA, Adams MR, McCredie RJ et al. Hormone replacement therapy is associated with improved arterial physiology in healthy postmenopausal women. Clin Endocrinol 1996;45:435–441.

27. Clarkson TB, Shively CA, Morgan TM, et al. Oral contraceptives and coronary artery artherosclerosis of cynomolgus monkeys. Obstet Gynecol 1990;75(2):217–222.

28. Koh KK, Mincemoyer R, Bui M, et al. Effects of hormone-replacement therapy on fibrinolysis in postmenopausal women. NEJM 1997;336:683–690.

29. Fogelberg M, Vesterqvist O, Diczfalusy U, et al. Experimental atherosclerosis: effects of oestrogen and atherosclerosis on thromboxane and prostacyclin formation. Eur J Clin Invest 1990;20(1):105–110.

30. Barrett-Connor E, Laakso M. Ischemic heart disease risk in postmenopausal women: effects of estrogen use on glucose and insulin levels. Arteriosclerosis 1990;10(4):531–534.

31. Stevenson JC, Crook D, Godsland EF, et al. Hormone replacement therapy and the cardiovascular system. Drugs 1994;47(suppl 2):35–41.

32. Henderson BE, Paganini-Hill A, Ross RK. Decreased mortality in users of estrogen replacement therapy. Arch Intern Med 1991;151:75–78.

33. Newton KM, LaCroix AZ, McKnight B, et al. Estrogen replacement therapy and prognosis after first myocardial infraction. Am J Epidemiol 1997;145:269–277.

34. O'Brien JE, Peterson ED, Keeler GP, et al. Relation between estrogen therapy and restenosis after percutaneous coronary interventions. J Am Coll Cardiol 1996;28:1111–1118.

35. O'Keefe JH, Jr, Kim SC, Hall RR, et al. Estrogen replacement therapy after coronary angioplasty in women. J Am Coll Cardiol 1997;29:1–5.

36. Hong MK, Ronin PA, Reagan K, et al. Effect of estrogen replacement therapy on serum lipid values and angiographically defined coronary artery disease in postmenopausal women. Am J Cardiol 1992;69:176–178.

37. Sullivan JM, Vander Zwaag R, Hughes JP, et al. Estrogen replacement and coronary artery disease. Effect on survival in postmenopausal women. Arch Intern Med 1990;150:2557–2562.

38. Finucane FF, Madams JH, Bush TL, et al. Decreased risk of stroke among postmenopausal hormone users. Results from a national cohort. Arch Intern Med 1993;153:73–79.

39. Paganini-Hill A, Ross RK, Henderson BE. Postmenopausal oestrogen treatment and stroke: a prospective study. BMJ 1988;297:519–522.

40. Falkeborn M, Persson I, Terent A, et al. Hormone replacement therapy and the risk of stroke. Follow-up of a population-based cohort in Sweden. Arch Intern Med 1993;153:1201–1209.

41. Paganini-Hill A. Estrogen replacement therapy and stroke. Prog Cardiovasc Dis 1995;38:223–242.

42. Grodstein F, Stampfer MJ, Manson JE, et al. Postmenopausal estrogen and progestin use and the risk of cardiovascular disease. N Engl J Med 1996;335:453–461.

43. Wilson PW, Garrison RJ, Castelli WP. Postmenopausal estrogen use, cigarette smoking, and cardiovascular morbidity in women over 50. The Framingham Study. N Engl J Med 1985;l313:1038–1043.

44. Lindsay R, Bush TL, Grady D, et al. Therapeutic controversy. Estrogen replacement in menopause. J Clin Endocrinol Metab 1996;81:3829–3838.

45. Ettinger B, Genant HK, Cann CE. Postmenopausal bone loss is prevented by treatment with low-dose estrogen and calcium. Ann Intern Med 1987;106:40–43.

46. Prince Rl, Smith M, Dick IM, et al. Prevention of postmenopausal osteoporosis. A comparative study of exercise, calcium supplementation and hormone replacement therapy. NEJM 1991;325:1189–1195.

47. Cauley JA, Seeley DG, Ensrud K, et al. Estrogen replacement therapy and fractures in older women. Ann Int Med 1995;122:9–16.

48. Schneider DL, Barrett-Connor EL, Morton DJ. Timing of postmenopausal estrogen for optimal bone mineral density. The Rancho Bernardo Study. JAMA 1997;277:541–547.

49. Erdtsieck RJ, Pols HAP, Van Kuijk C, et al. Course of bone mass during and after hormonal replacement therapy with and without addition of nandrolone decanoate. J Bone Miner Res 1994;9:277–283.

50. Christiansen C, Christiansen MS, Transbol I. Bone mass in postmenopausal women after withdrawal of oestrogen/gestagen replacement therapy. Lancet 1981;1:459–461.

51. Marx, CW, Kailey GE, Cheney C, et al. Do estrogens improve bone mineral density in osteoporotic women over age 65? J Bone Min Res 1992;7:1275–1279.

52. Reid IR, Ames RW, Evans MC, et al. Effect of calcium supplementation on bone loss in postmenopausal women. N Engl J Med 1993;328:460–465.

53. Aloia JF, Vaswani A, Yeh JK, et al. Calcium supplementation with and without hormone replacement therapy to prevent postmenopausal bone loss. Ann Int Med 1994;120:97–103.

54. Newcomb PA, Storer BE. Postmenopausal hormone use and risk of large-bowel cancer. J Natl Cancer Inst 1995;87:1067–1071.

55. Jacobs EJ, White E, Weiss NS. Exogenous hormones, reproductive history, and colon cancer (Seattle, WA) Cancer Causes Contr 1994;5:359–366.

56. Furner SE, Davis FG, Nelson RL, et al. A case-control study of large bowel cancer and hormone exposure in women. Cancer Res 1989;49:4936–4940.

57. Gerhardsson de Verdier M, London S. Reproductive factors, exogenous female hormones, and colorectal cancer by subsite. Cancer Causes Contr 1992;3:355–360.

58. Calle EE, Miracle-McMahill HL, Thun MJ, Heath CW, Jr. Estrogen replacement therapy and risk of fatal colon cancer in a prospective cohort of postmenopausal women. J Natl Cancer Inst 1995;87:517–523.

59. Bostick RM, Potter JD, Kushi LH, et al. Sugar, meat and fat intake, and non-dietary risk factors for colon cancer incidence in Iowa women (United States). Cancer Causes Contr 1994;5:538–552.

60. Chute CG, Willett WC, Colditz GA, et al. A prospective study of reproductive history and exogenous estrogens on the risk of colorectal cancer in women. Epidemiol 1991;2:201–207.

61. Paganini-Hill A, Henderson VW. Estrogen replacement therapy and risk of Alzheimer's disease. Arch Intern Med 1996;156:2213–2217.

62. Tang M-X, Jacobs D, Stern Y, et al. Effect of oestrogen during menopause on risk and age at onset of Alzheimer's disease. Lancet 1996;348:429–432.

63. Morrison A, Resnick S, Corrada M, et al. A prospective study of estrogen replacement therapy and the risk of developing Alzheimer's disease in the Baltimore longitudinal study of aging. Neurol 1996;46(suppl 2);A435–A436.

64. Simpkins JW, Singh M, Bishop J. The potential role for estrogen replacement therapy in the treatment of the cognitive decline and neurodegeneration associated with Alzheimer's disease. Neurobiol Aging 1994;15:S195–S197.

65. McEwen BS, Wooley CS. Estradiol and progesterone regulate neuronal structure and synaptic connectivity in adult as well as developing brain. Exper Gerontol 1994;29:431–436.

66. Woolley CS, Wenzel HJ, Schwartzkroin PA. Estradiol increases the frequency of multiple synapse boutons in the hippocampal CA1 region of the adult female rat. J Compar Neuro 1996;373:108–117.

67. Ohkura T, Isse K, Akazawa K, et al. Low-dose estrogen replacement therapy for Alzheimer's disease in women. Menopause 1994;1:125–130.

68. Hashimoto S, Katou M, Dong Y, et al. Effects of hormone replacement therapy on serum amyloid P component in postmenopausal women. Maturitas 1997;26:113–119.

69. Steinberg KK, Thacker SB, Smith SJ, et al. A meta-analysis of the effect of estrogen replacement therapy on the risk of breat cancer. JAMA 1991;265:1985–1990.

70. Sillero-Arenas M, Delgado-Rodriguez M, Rodigues-Canteras R, et al. Menopausal hormone replacement therapy and breast cancer: a meta-analysis. Obstet Gynecol 1992;79:286–294.

71. Colditz GA, Hankinson SE, Hunter DJ, et al. The use of estrogens and progestins and the risk of breast cancer in postmenopausal women. N Engl J Med 1995;332:1589–1593.

72. Grady D, Rubin SM, Petitti DB, et al. Hormone therapy to prevent disease and prolong life in postmenopausal women. Ann Intern Med 1992;117:1016–1037.

73. Bergkvist L, Adami HO, Persson I, et al. The risk of breast cancer after estrogen and estrogen-progestin replacement. N Engl J Med 1989;321:293–297.

74. Willis DB, Calle EE, Miracle-McMahill HL, Heath CW, Jr. Estrogen replacement therapy and risk of fatal breast cancer in a prospective cohort postmenopausal women in the United States. Cancer Causes Contr 1996;7:449–457.

75. Bonnier P, Romain S, Giacalone PL, et al. Clinical and biologic prognostic factors in breast cancer diagnosed during postmenopausal hormone replacement therapy. Obstet Gynecol 1995;85:11–17.

76. Harding C, Snow WF, Faragher EB, et al. Hormone replacement therapy and tumour grade in breast cancer: prospective study in screening unit. Br Med J 1996;312:1646–1647.

77. Disaia PJ, Grosen EA, Kurosaki T, et al. Hormone replacement therapy in breast cancer survivors: a cohort study. Am J Obstet Gynecol 1996;174:1494–1498.

78. Daly E, Vessey M, Hawkins M, et al. Risk of venous thromboembolism in users of hormone replacement therapy. Lancet 1996;348:977–980.

79. Jick H, Derby L, Myers M, et al. Risk of hospital admission for idiopathic venous thromboembolism among users of post-menopausal oestrogens. Lancet 1996;348:981–983.

80. Devor M, Barrett-Connor E, Renvall M, et al. Estrogen replacement therapy and the risk of venous thrombosis. Am J Med 1992;92:275–282.

81. Grodstein F, Stampfer M, Goldhaber S, et al. Prospective study of exogenous hormones and risk of pulmonary embolism in women. Lancet 1996;348:983–987.

82. Stafford RS, Saglam D, Causino N, Blumenthal D. Low rates of hormone replacement in visits to United States primary care physicians. Am J Obstet Gynecol 1997;177:381–387.

83. Ravnikar VA. Compliance with hormone therapy. Am J Obstet Gynecol 1987;156:1332–1334.

84. Stouthamer N, Visser AP, Oddens BJ, et al. Dutch general practitioners' attitudes towards the climacteric and its treatment. Eur J Obstet Gynecol Reprod Biol 1993;50:147–152.

85. Grisso JA, Baum CR, Turner BJ. What do physicians in practice do to prevent osteoporosis? J Bone Miner Res 1990;3:213–220.

86. Salamone LM, Pressman AR, Seeley DG, Cauley JA. Estrogen replacement therapy. A survey of older women's attitudes. Arch Intern Med. 1996;156:1293–1297.

87. Hammond CB. Women's concerns with hormone replacement therapy—compliance issues. Fertil Steril 1994;62(suppl 2):157s–160s.

88. Ferguson KJ, Hoegh C, Johnson S. Estrogen replacement therapy. A survey of women's knowledge and attitudes. Arch Int Med 1989;149:133–136.

89. Nachtigall, LE. Enhancing patient compliance with hormone replacement therapy at menopause. Obstet Gynecol 1990;75(s):77s–83s.

90. Ryan PJ, Harrison R, Blake GM, Fogelman I. Compliance with HRT after screening for postmenopausal osteoporosis. Br J Ob Gyn 1992;92:325–28.

91. Torgerson DJ, Donaldson C, Russell IT, Reid DM. Hormone replacement therapy: compliance and cost after screening for osteoporosis. Eur J Obstet Gynecol Reprod Biol 1995;59:57–60.

92. Silverman SL, Greenwald M, Klein RA, Drinkwater BL. Effect of bone density information on decisions about hormone replacement therapy: a randomized trial. Obstet Gynecol 1997:89;321–325.

93. Sclar D. Improving medication compliance: a review of selected issues. Clin Ther 1991;13:436–440.

10   Cancer Risk Associated with Hormone Replacement

Daniel W. Cramer, MD, ScD

CONTENTS

INTRODUCTION

When a woman is considering whether or not to use estrogen replacement therapy (ERT), concerns about cancer risks often weigh heavily against the decision. In an attempt to address these concerns in a knowledgeable manner, the clinician is confronted by a vast and conflicting literature. This chapter will summarize epidemiologic information on cancer risk associated with ERT. The types of studies related to cancer and ERT will be discussed; the evidence relating ERT to particular kinds of cancer reviewed, and the need to balance risks and benefits emphasized.

TYPES OF STUDIES OF ERT AND CANCER

Information about cancer risks and menopausal hormones largely comes from observational studies that either have examined ERT use in women who did or did not have a particular type of cancer or that record cancer occurrence in follow-up of women who used or did not use ERT. Before discussing these studies, it is worthwhile to review potential problems in defining ERT. Studies often rely on the woman's recall of the specific type of estrogen, its dose, and whether a progestagen was concomitantly used. This may lead to imprecise information about the exposure, particularly because the history may date back over a 20-yr period. Prescribing habits have also varied over the

From: *Contemporary Endocrinology: Menopause: Endocrinology and Management*
Edited by: D. B. Seifer and E. A. Kennard © Humana Press Inc., Totowa, NJ

years. Before 1970, menopausal therapy was, almost exclusively, conjugated equine estrogen and was prescribed in an unopposed fashion. Today there is a greater choice of estrogen therapies and these are generally prescribed with a progestagen to women who have not had a hysterectomy. This combination therapy is sometimes referred to as hormone replacement therapy (HRT) and may be given in a sequential or continuous manner with varying dosages or types of progestagens. Our use of the term ERT will encompass, not exclude, combination therapy and studies including opposed therapy will be distinguished.

The Case-Control Study

Probably the most frequent type of epidemiologic study of ERT and cancer is the case-control study. In a case-control study, the starting population is defined by the presence or absence of a particular illness. Case women with breast cancer, for example, are identified and questioned about their use of menopausal hormones prior to the cancer. Control women who did not have breast cancer are also questioned about hormone use. The odds that cases used hormones divided by the odds that controls used hormones provides a measure of association between illness and exposure called the exposure–odds ratio that is equivalent to the rate ratio (*see* the discussion of cohort studies). In an unbiased study, an exposure–odds ratio significantly greater than one indicates that exposure is associated with increased risk for the disease.

There are three principal types of biases that must be addressed in case-control studies: selection, recall, and confounding. Selection bias may occur if exposed cases were more likely to come to diagnosis than nonexposed cases. This could occur if, compared to nonexposed cases, exposed cases were more likely to have screening tests leading to a cancer diagnosis. This type of bias, also called surveillance bias, was proposed in case-control studies of ERT and endometrial cancer. Women using estrogen might have irregular bleeding and come to endometrial sampling more frequently than nonexposed women and, hence, have greater opportunity for diagnosis of endometrial cancer. Similarly, women using ERT might be more likely to have mammograms and, hence, come to a breast cancer diagnosis sooner than nonexposed women. Selection bias also might occur if disease associated with exposure was more likely to have a favorable outcome leading to longer survival and greater opportunity for study than nonexposed cases might have. Recall bias occurs when individuals with a particular illness are more likely to remember or admit to a particular exposure; e.g., the link between induced abortion and breast cancer may be attributed to the likelihood that cases with breast cancer are more willing than controls to share history of an induced abortion with the researcher. Confounding occurs when a variable is associated with both exposure and illness and an imbalance in the distribution of that variable between cases and controls leads to a biased odds ratio. If socioeconomic status is associated with likelihood of using hormones and a greater risk for cancer, then socioeconomic status may be a confounder. Confounding can be controlled, in the design phase, by matching or, in the analytic phase, by techniques such as multivariate analysis.

The Cohort Study

In a cohort study, the starting populations are identified by the presence or absence of a particular exposure. Cohort members are followed and disease occurrence recorded. The rate of disease in exposed divided by the rate of disease in nonexposed is called the rate ratio or relative risk—a result significantly greater than one indicates an increased risk for disease associated with the exposure. Cohort studies can be prospective in nature (i.e., the exposure is assessed by the investigator who must then wait for outcomes of interest to occur) or retrospective if the study can be conducted from medical records that record prior exposures and subsequent illnesses that have already occurred. In general, cohort studies are less likely to suffer from selection or recall bias but may be subject to confounding similar to case-control studies.

Experimental Studies

Experimental studies are prospective cohort studies that include randomized assignment of treatment, blindness of subjects and investigators to therapy, and objective assessment of outcome. These features minimize bias and provide strong evidence on the benefits (or risks) of an exposure. Although a clinical trial solely designed to study whether a drug caused cancer would be unethical, cancer, as an adverse outcome, might be observed in an experimental study of an exposure believed to be beneficial. Randomized studies of ERT have been undertaken and a few of these are now yielding data about potential benefits as well as risks, including cancer or cancer precursors. The largest of these, the Woman's Health Initiative, is still underway

Meta-Analysis

The meta-analysis is not a distinct type of study, but rather an analytic technique for combining results from independent studies examining the same exposure (or treatment) and outcome so that a more precise estimate of the effect and powerful statistical test can be conducted. As part of the process of conducting a meta-analysis, investigators will often grade studies by their quality and omit those not meeting certain standards. A weighted average of the exposure–odds ratios or relative risks from each of the selected individual studies is calculated with the weight inversely proportional to the variance of the association. This means that larger studies will contribute greater weight to the summary relative risk. A meta-analysis may also determine whether heterogeneity exists, i.e., whether individual study results are inconsistent with the summary relative risk. Significant heterogeneity might imply either that dissimilar exposures were being assessed or that factors other than ERT were causing variation in the association.

With this background on the types of epidemiologic studies, we will now review the evidence regarding ERT and risk for those cancers thought to be estrogen dependent including breast, endometrial, and ovarian cancer.

BREAST CANCER AND ERT

Case-Control Studies

Because of the large number of case-control studies of breast cancer, we will restrict our attention to major studies *(1–5)* completed within the last 10 yr (Table 1). In these studies, ERT exposure has generally been categorized as ever or current use of unopposed conjugated estrogen and ever-use of opposed therapy. Statistically significant risk estimates would be indicated by the presence of a 95% confidence interval that did not include the value one. A "dose-response" indicates the presence of increasing (or decreasing risk) for longer durations of the exposure and is often cited as evidence for a biologically plausible association between exposure and disease. As is evident from

Table 1
Major Recent Case-Control Studies of Breast Cancer and ERT

Reference	Number of subjects		Findings	
	Cases	Controls	Descriptors of use	rr (95% C.L.)
(1) Kaufman et al. (1991)	1686	2077	Ever	1.2 (1.0–1.4)
			Current	1.2 (0.8–1.8)
			Opposed	1.7 (0.9–3.6)
			Dose-response	No
(2) Palmer et al. (1991)	607	1214	Ever	0.9 (0.6–1.2)
			Current	0.9 (0.4–1.9)
			Opposed	0.6 (0.2–1.9)
			Dose-response	No
(3) LaVecchia et al. (1990)	2569	2588	Ever	1.2 (0.9–1.5)
			Current	0.8 (0.5–1.4)
			Opposed	1.6
			Dose-response	Yes
(4) Newcomb et al. (1995)	3130	3698	Ever	1.05 (0.93–1.18)
			Current	0.88 (0.72–1.08)
			Opposed	1.01 (0.78–1.31)
			Dose-response	No
(5) Sanford et al. (1995)	537	492	Ever	0.9 (0.6–1.1)
			Current	0.9 (0.7–1.3)
			Opposed	0.9 (0.7–1.3)
			Dose-response	No

Table 1, the majority of these studies, including the very large study by Newcomb et al. (4) found no increased risk for breast cancer associated with ERT. A dose response was observed in only one study (13) and no significantly increased risk with opposed regimens was observed. In none of these studies was an increased risk for breast cancer from ERT found for women with a history of benign breast disease or those with a family history of breast cancer.

Cohort Studies

Table 2 shows risk for breast cancer associated with ERT from recent cohort studies (6–9). As opposed to the case-control studies, all of the cohort studies show an elevated risk for breast cancer associated with current or ever-use of ERT with relative risks from 1.1 to 1.67. A dose response was also observed in these studies. In the Nurses Health Cohort (9), current use of unopposed ERT was associated with a 30% increase in risk for breast cancer, rr = 1.31 (1.14, 1.54) and current use of an opposed ERT regimen was associated with a 40% increase in risk for breast cancer rr = 1.41 (1.15, 1.74). The opposed regimen generally involved sequential use of 10 mg of medroxyprogesterone acetate (mpa). Bergkvist et al. (6) emphasized an increased risk of 4.4 (0.9, 22.4) associated with six or more years of use of an opposed regimen, despite its lack of significance. Not reviewed in this table are an earlier analysis of the Nurses Health data based on four years of follow-up that did not find an increase in risk for breast cancer (10) and a cohort study of women with benign breast disease that found no increased risk for breast cancer associated with ERT (11).

Table 2
Major Recent Cohort Studies of Breast Cancer and ERT.

Reference	Cohort size	Follow-up		Findings	
		Beginning	Average	Descriptors of use	rr (95% C.L.)
(6) Bergvist et al. (1989)	23,244	1977	6 yr	Ever	1.1 (1.0–1.3)
				Current	Not stated
				Opposed	4.4 (0.9–21.4) of > 6 yrs of use
				Dose-response	Yes
(7) Mills et al. (1989)	20,341	1976	6 yr	Ever	1.67 (1.17–2.39)
				Current	2.53 (1.62–3.98)
				Opposed	Not available
				Dose-response	Yes
(8) Risch et al. (1994)	32,790	1976	14 yr	Ever	1.33 (1.11–1.59)
				Current	Not available
				Opposed	"Not significant"
				Dose-response	Yes
(9) Colditz et al. (1995)	69,586	1978	14 yr	Ever	Not stated
				Current	1.32 (1.14–1.54)
				Opposed	1.41 (1.15–1.74)
				Dose-response	Yes

Meta-Analyses

Table 3 shows the results of five meta-analyses related to breast cancer and ERT (12–16). It is somewhat discouraging that, even when largely similar lists of studies are reviewed and subjected to formal meta-analysis, the conclusions of experts may differ somewhat. The conclusion of four of these studies is that there is no overall increase in breast cancer risk associated with ever-use of ERT. Only one study (14) found evidence for a dose response such that use of ERT for 15 or more years was associated with a summary relative risk of 1.3(1.2–1.6). This same study emphasized an increased risk for breast cancer associated with ERT in women with a family history of breast cancer based on five studies completed before 1987 and not including the studies cited in Table 1, which did not identify women with a family history of breast cancer as a high risk group. In two of the meta-analyses, a tendency for higher relative risks to be observed in cohort, compared to case-control studies, was found (15,16). Significant heterogeneity among individual case-control or cohort studies was observed in all meta-analyses that tested for this. The meta-analyses in Table 3 did not include some of the studies in Tables 1 and 2, but it is unlikely that the conclusions would differ much since the two recent cohort studies citing an increased risk would appear to be more than offset by the three recent case-control studies finding no association.

Summary — Breast Cancer and ERT

What seems apparent, even from our brief review, is that case-control studies generally find little or no association between ERT and breast cancer, whereas cohort studies are more likely to report increased risk for breast cancer associated with ERT including the presence of a dose-response. One potential bias of the cohort studies is that women who

Table 3
Meta-Analyses of Breast Cancer and ERT

Reference	Studies included	Decriptors of use	Findings	
			rr (95% C.L.)	Heterogeneity
(12) Armstrong et al. (1988)	23	Ever	1.01 (0.95–1.08)	Yes
		Current	Not stated	
		Opposed	Not stated	
		Dose-response	Not stated	
(13) Dupont et al. (1991)	28	Ever	1.08 (0.96–1.2)	Yes
		Current	Not stated	
		Opposed	Not stated	
		Dose-response	No	
(14) Steinberg et at (1991)	25	Ever	"Not significant"	Yes
		Current	Not stated	
		Opposed	Not stated	
		Dose-response	Yes, after 15 yr of use 1.3 (1.2–1.6)	
(15) Sillero-Arenas et al. (1992)	37	Ever	1.06 (1.0–1.12)	Yes
		Current	1.23 (1.12–1.35)	
		Opposed	0.99 (0.94–1.14)	
		Dose-response	No	
(16) Colditz et al. (1993)	31	Ever	1.02 (0.93–1.12)	Not addressed
		Current	Not stated	
		Opposed	1.13 (0.78–1.64)	
		Dose-response	No	

use ERT are more likely to have screening mammography performed, which suggests that users may come to a breast cancer diagnosis sooner than women in the nonexposed cohort. Indeed, at least two studies found that survival after breast cancer appears to be better for the women who used ERT prior to diagnosis *(17,18)*. In addition, cohort studies typically adjust for fewer potential confounding variables than case-control studies. According to Newcomb et al. women who use ERT are more likely than nonusers to report a history of biopsied benign breast disease, to be nulliparous or of low parity, to consume alcohol, to be lean, to report a surgical menopause, and to have higher educational attainment *(4)*. Newcomb et al. considered these potential confounding factors and adjusted the odds ratio for them in their study. None of these variables were considered in three of the cohort studies which adjusted only for age *(6–8)*. Even in the Nurses Health Cohort *(9)*, body mass, alcohol consumption, and education were not considered in risk adjustment. Thus, although cohort studies are generally considered to be less biased than case control studies, a failure to consider all pertinent confounding variables might represent a bias in the cohort studies.

Regarding breast cancer and ERT, the author believes the following conclusions are possible:

1. The weight of epidemiologic evidence from case-control studies favors no significant association between breast cancer and ERT use and no dose-response for greater risk with longer duration of use.

2. Although the increased risk for breast cancer found in the cohort studies is concerning, these studies have not been rigorous in controling for potential confounders that may correlate with likelihood of using ERT and risk for breast cancer.

3. Studies finding a positive association with unopposed therapy also find it with opposed therapy and studies finding no association with unopposed therapy also fail to find it for opposed therapy. Thus, it seems unlikely there will be major differences in breast cancer risk by whether or not the ERT regimen includes a progestagen.

4. There is no basis, from either case-control or cohort studies, to propose that women with a personal history of benign breast disease or a family history of breast cancer will have greater risk for breast cancer with ERT use.

5. The lack of consistency between case-control and cohort studies and heterogeneity among studies of similar types suggests that ERT is, at worst, a weak risk factor for breast cancer that should not drive the decision process to use or not use estrogen. Nevertheless, ERT users should be encouraged to adhere to the recommended schedule for mammographic screening and self-breast examination.

ENDOMETRIAL CANCER AND ERT

According to a meta-analysis by Grady et al. as of 1994, there were 27 published case-control studies of ERT and endometrial cancer; and a significant association was found in 23 of these (19). The summary rr for ever-use of ERT was 2.3 (2.1–2.5). A dose-response was evident in the combined summary estimates with a rr of 1.4 (1.0–1.8) for less than one year of use and 9.5 (7.4–12.3) for 9–10 yr of use. Unlike the association for breast cancer and ERT, there is agreement between the case-control studies and the cohort studies with a significant association between endometrial cancer and ERT found in both types of studies. Despite the potential "surveillance" bias proposed by Horowitz and Feinstein (20), there is little doubt that a real and, likely, causal association between unopposed ERT and endometrial cancer risk exists. The only issue the author feels compelled to address is, to what extent, the increased risk for endometrial cancer associated with ERT has been eliminated by opposed regimens.

Table 4 shows the results of five recent studies addressing risk for endometrial cancer with use of opposed ERT regimens (21–25). Several of these studies had generally poor information about the specific dose, type, and number of days each month that a progestagen was taken. Nevertheless, in all of theses studies no significant elevation in risk for endometrial cancer associated with ERT use was found with the exception of the study by Beresford et al., which reported an elevated risk associated with regimens including less than 10 days each month of a progestagen (25). However, they found no increased risk for endometrial cancer in women using a progestagen for at least 10 days each month. Thus epidemiologic data suggest that use of an opposed ERT regimen is unlikely to be associated with an increased risk for endometrial cancer when it includes at least 10 days of a progestagen each month. Case-control or cohort data on use of regimens involving continuous estrogen and progestagen is lacking, but is unlikely to be associated with any less protection than that seen with the sequential regimens including at least 10 days of a progestagen.

The conclusions of these observational epidemiologic studies are supported by prospective studies that have monitored endometrial features or rates of endometrial hyperplasia in women receiving unopposed or various opposed regimens. Whitehead et al. (26) found that unopposed estrogen was associated with a significant increase in nuclear

Table 4
Recent Studies of Opposed ERT Regimens on Endometrial Cancer Risk

Reference	Type of study	Findings
(21) Persson et al. (1989)	Cohort — 23,244 Followed — 1977–1980	"Opposed" regimens (generally 7–10 d of progestagens) associated with rr of 0.9 (0.4–2.0)
(22) Voigt et al. (1991)	Case-Control 158 Cases, 182 Controls	Opposed regimens with <10 d progestagen month rr = 2.4 (0.6,9.3). Opposed with > 10 d of progestagen rr = 1.1 (0.4–3.6)
(23) Brinton et al. (1993)	Case-Control 300 Cases, 207 Controls	Opposed regimens (not further clarified) rr = 1.8 (0.6–4.9)
(24) Jick et al. (1993)	Case-Control 172 Cases, 172 Controls	Opposed regimens (generally sequential with 10 mg mpa) rr = 1.3 (0.5–3.4)
(25) Beresford et al. (1997)	Case-Control 1154 Cases, 1526 Controls	Opposed regimens < 10 d progestagen monthly rr = 3.1 (1.7–5.7) Opposed regimen with > 10 d monthly rr = 1.3 (0.8–2.2)

estradiol receptor levels (a presumed signal for proliferation) that could be counteracted by 6–10 d of exposure to the progestogen, norethindrone, or norgestrel. In a randomized study known as the postmenopausal estrogen/progestogen interventions (PEPI) trial, the occurrence of simple, complex, or atypical hyperplasia occurred almost exclusively in women assigned to the unopposed estrogen regimen (27). Over the three years of follow-up, about 62% of the subjects receiving unopposed therapy developed hyperplasia, compared to about 5% of women who received 10 mg of MPA or 200 mg of micronized progesterone for 12 d. Notably, only 1 (1%) of the women assigned continuous therapy with 2.5 mg of MPA developed hyperplasia, and this was characterized as a simple hyperplasia.

Regarding endometrial cancer and ERT, the author believes the following conclusions are possible.

1. There is unequivocal evidence for an increased risk for endometrial cancer associated with unopposed ERT such that women can expect a threefold increase in risk when they are on this regimen for 1–5 yr, a sixfold increase when they are on this regimen for 5–10 yr, and more than a 10-fold increase in risk when they are on unopposed ERT for more than 10 yr.
2. Use of a sequentially opposed regimen (generally, 10 mg of MPA for at least 10 days per month) is associated with no increased risk for endometrial cancer.
3. As inferred from experimental studies with hyperplasia as an endpoint, women on a continuous opposed regimen (2.5 mg of MPA on a daily basis) can expect to have the lowest risk for endometrial cancer.

OVARIAN CANCER AND ERT

It is reasonable to suppose that ERT might be related to ovarian cancer, but there is conflicting biologic data to indicate which direction the association would take. Would ERT act more like oral contraceptives, which have a clear protective effect on the disease,

Table 5
Studies of Ovarian Cancer and ERT

Reference	Type of Study	Finding	
		Descriptors of Use	RR (95% C.L.)
(28) Weiss et al. (1982)	Case-Control 207 Cases, 613 Controls	Ever	1.3 (0.9–1.8)
		Dose-response	No
		Opposed	Not available
(29) Cramer et al. (1982)	Case-Control 173 Cases, 173 Controls	Ever	1.6 (0.9–2.9)
		Dose-response	Yes
		Opposed	Not available
(30) Tzonou et al. (1984)	Case-Control 112 Cases, 188 Controls	Ever	"Not Significant"
(31) Booth et al. (1989)	Case-Control 156 Cases, 293 Controls	Ever	1.5 (0.9–2.6)
		Dose-response	Not stated
		Opposed	Not available
(32) Kaufman et al. (1989)	Case-Control 377 Cases, 2030 Controls	Ever	1.1 (0.8–1.6)
		Dose-response	No
		Opposed	0.7 (0.2–1.8)
(33) Whittimore et al. (1992)	Case-Control 315 Cases, 1633 Controls (hospital based)	Ever	0.9 (0.7–1.3)
		Dose-response	No
		Opposed	Not available
	624 Cases, 2425 Controls (population based)	Ever	1.1 (0.9–1.4)
		Dose-response	No
		Opposed	Not available
(34) Parazzini et al. (1994)	Case-Control 953 Cases, 2503 Controls	Ever	1.6 (1.2–2.4)
		Dose-response	Yes
		Opposed	Not available
(35) Rodrigues et al. (1995)	Cohort of 240,073 followed from 1982 to 1989. Outcome death from ovarian cancer	Ever	1.15 (0.94–1.42)
		Dose-response	Yes
		Opposed	Not available
(36) Purdie et al. (1996)	Case-Control 824 Cases, 856 Controls	Ever	2.81 (1.45–5.4)
		Dose-response	Not stated
		Opposed	Not stated
(37) Risch (1996)	Case-Control 367 Cases, 564 Controls	Ever (all nonmucinous)	1.32 (0.9–1.95)
		Dose-response	Yes
		Opposed	Not significant

or would it act to stimulate the Mullerian-like and (presumably) estrogen-sensitive tissue that comprise the majority of "epithelial" ovarian cancers? Table 5 summarizes the results of epidemiologic studies addressing the question of ERT and ovarian cancer (28–37). Ever-use of ERT (mostly unopposed estrogen) is associated with risk ratios greater than one but, generally, with confidence intervals overlapping one except for two studies finding significantly elevated risk (34,37). A dose response was found in at least two studies. A formal meta-analysis has not been performed but would likely suggest that, taken as a whole, use of ERT is associated with an increased risk for ovarian cancer. Dose response was addressed in six studies and observed in three. At least three studies (28,29,34) also suggest that ERT use is more likely to be associated with increased risk for a particular histologic type of ovarian cancer: endometrioid and clear cell cancer — types of ovarian cancer that share some histologic and epidemiologic features with endometrial cancer *(38)*. Only two studies have addressed risk associated with opposed therapy and these found lower risk for ovarian cancer compared to unopposed therapy *(32,37)*.

Based on this limited epidemiologic data, the author believes the following conclusions are possible.

1. The fact that a majority of studies find odds ratios greater than one suggest that (unopposed) ERT may increase risk for ovarian cancer, particularly for endometrioid and clear cell histologic types.
2. Only a few studies have addressed opposed therapy and these suggest that risk may be lower than that observed for unopposed ERT. Given the clear and consistent protection against ovarian cancer seen with oral contraceptive use, it is reasonable to predict that opposed therapy (particularly continuous regimens) may have a protective effect.

OTHER CANCERS AND ERT

Epidemiologic studies have generally focused on risk for breast and genital tract neoplasms associated with ERT. Several recent studies have address the risk for colon cancer and ERT and have reported a protective effect *(39–41)*. These studies have included both case-control and cohort designs and found a decreased risk for colon cancer occurrence or death associated with ERT use with relative risks between 0.5 and 0.6. A dose response was observed. In the study by Newcomb et al. *(41)*, protection was seen with both opposed and unopposed regimens. Because colon cancer is the third leading cause of cancer death in women, a protective effect from ERT for this neoplasm has important public health implications.

ERT AND THE CANCER SURVIVOR

ERT therapy is generally discouraged for breast cancer survivors. A recent article by Cobleigh et al. called for a re-evaluation of this policy after a review of the evidence *(42)*. As mentioned, two studies found that women who were using ERT around the time of their breast cancer diagnosis had more favorable survival than women who were nonusers of ERT or used it more remotely *(17,18)*. In particular, Bergkvist et al. reported a 40% reduction in excess mortality from breast cancer in recent users *(18)*. More favorable survival also appeared to be associated with recent use of oral contraceptives for premenopausal breast cancer in one study *(43)*.

The proscription against estrogen use is curious since estrogen has been and is used as a treatment for breast cancer. Although the dosage is often greater than would be employed in ERT, more modest dosage using oral contraceptives has been tried with apparent success *(44)*. At least three observational studies of ERT use after a diagnosis of breast cancer have been published and have shown no adverse effects *(45–47)*. These studies are small and their nonrandomized nature limit the strength of their conclusions. However, these studies do provide a clinical basis for initiating randomized control trials of ERT among breast cancer survivors, as well as for prescribing ERT to the properly informed breast cancer survivor who wishes to use it.

Because of the firmer biologic and epidemiologic basis that links estrogen and endometrial cancer, there may be greater concern about the use of ERT in the woman who

Table 6
Cohort Studied of Mortality in ERT Users and Nonusers

Reference	Number of subjects		Findings, users vs nonusers	
	Cohort size	Follow-up	Mortality	rr (95% C.L.)
(49) Criqui et al. (1988)	1868	12 yr	All causes	0.69 (0.55–0.87)
			IHD[a]	0.75 (0.45–1.24)
			All cancers	0.73 (0.44–1.22)
(50) Hunt et al. (1990)	4544	5 yr	All causes	0.56 (0.41–0.68)
			IHD	0.41 (0.20–0.61)
			All cancers	0.70 (0.55–0.85)
(51) Henderson et al. (1991)	8881	7.5 yr	All causes	0.80 (0.70–0.87)
			IHD	0.79 (not significant)
			All cancers	0.82 (not significant)
(52) Grodstein et al. (1997)	34,625	16 yr	All causes	0.63 (0.56–0.70)
			IHD	0.35 (0.25–0.49)
			All cancers	0.71 (0.62–0.81)
(53) Schairer et al. (1997)	23,246	8.6 yr	All causes	0.77 (0.73–0.8)
			IHD	0.61 (0.55–0.69)
			All cancers	0.85 (0.78–0.92)

[a]Ischemic heart disease.

has had endometrial cancer; but no studies could be found that have addressed the use of ERT in women with early stage and localized endometrial cancer. Use of ERT in the premenopausal patient who has undergone oophorectomy for ovarian cancer appears not to have generated the same degree of controversy as breast cancer and ERT. In an analysis of women who had received ERT after surgery for ovarian cancer, survival was better even after adjustment for stage at diagnosis and differentiation of the tumor (48).

RISKS AND BENEFITS

Ultimately the decision about whether to use ERT will rest on the balance of risks and benefits. Evaluating this balance can be difficult particularly if individual studies addressing single diseases are relied upon. Such studies yield odds ratios or relative risks, which may not readily translate into absolute or attributable risks. If the relative risk for breast cancer associated with 15 yr of ERT use is 1.3, how does this compare with a relative risk of 0.5 or 0.6 for coronary heart disease or osteoporosis? Clearly, coronary heart disease accounts for more deaths in women than breast cancer and should translate into lower overall mortality.

Studies that compare mortality rates in ERT users and nonusers offer a good approach to assessing the balance of risks and benefits. Table 6 shows the results of studies that have examined mortality rates by ERT use (49–53). These studies consistently demonstrate lower mortality rates for ERT users compared to nonusers. The relative risk for mortality from any cause in ERT users ranged from 0.56 to 0.80 suggesting a 20–44% reduction in mortality. The relative risk was significant in all studies. Notably the risk of mortality from any type of cancer was less than one in all studies and significantly decreased in three studies (50,52,53). However, it is arguable that such results represent the selection of healthier women for ERT therapy. Ultimately, only a randomized clinical trial will provide a clear answer to questions about overall morbidity and mortality for ERT users. The first definitive publications of the Woman's Health Initiative are expected in the year 2005.

Another approach to ERT policy is to use a decision analysis taking into consideration an individual woman's risk factors for breast cancer, heart disease, or osteoporosis. A recent analysis *(54)* suggested that high blood pressure, diabetes, cholesterol profile, and hip fracture risk may be factors that would favor ERT prescription. Family history of breast cancer, was considered a relative contraindication to ERT. However, our review of the breast cancer data suggests there is no basis for the proposition that women with a family history of breast cancer face a greater risk for breast cancer associated with ERT use. Obviously, it is reasonable to individualize the decision about ERT use, but foundations for the decisions must have a firm basis.

CONCLUSION

Fear of cancer may be the principal reason that many women choose not to use ERT. The most convincing association between ERT and cancer relates to endometrial cancer and unopposed ERT, but this is an association that is eliminated by the use of opposed regimens (either continuous use of a progestagen or use of one for at least 10 days per month). The data continues to be conflicting for breast cancer and ERT with recent case-control studies negative and cohort studies positive. Breast cancer arising in the setting of ERT use appears to have a more favorable prognosis, which lessens the impact of any association between breast cancer and ERT on overall mortality. The association between ovarian cancer and ERT must still be clarified. It seems unlikely that opposed regimens particularly those with a continuous progestagen would be associated with increased risk for ovarian cancer because oral contraceptive use has been consistently found to be protective. An emerging association of potentially great importance is a protective effect of ERT use on risk for colon cancer. Perhaps most importantly, studies demonstrate that overall mortality is lower for ERT users compared to nonusers and that includes a significantly lower risk of death from all types of cancer. The woman whose only impediment to ERT use is fear of cancer should be convinced by an objective presentation of the evidence that risk for cancer from ERT use is outweighed by the benefits of its use.

REFERENCES

1. Kaufman DW, Palmer JR, de Mouzon J, Rosenberg L, Stolley PD, Warshauer ME, Zauber AG, Shapiro S. Estrogen replacement therapy and the risk of breast cancer: results from the case-control surveillance study. Am J Epidemiol 1991;134:1375–1385.
2. Palmer JR, Rosenberg L, Clarke EA, Miller DR, Shapiro S. Breast cancer risk after estrogen replacement therapy: results from the Toronto breast cancer study. Am J Epidemiol 1991;134:1386–1395.
3. La Vecchia C, Negri E, Franceschi S, Favero A, Nanni O, Filiberti R, Conti E, Montella M, Veronesi A, Ferraroni M, Decarli A. Hormone replacement treatment and breast cancer risk: a cooperative Italian study. Br J Cancer 1995;72:144–148.
4. Newcomb PA, Longnecker MP, Storer BE, Mittendorf R, Baron J, Clap RW, Bogdan G, Willett WC. Long-term hormone replacement therapy and risk of breast cancer in postmenopausal women. Am J Epidemiol 1995;142:788–795.
5. Stanford JL, Weiss NS, Voigt LF, Daling JR, Habel LA, Rossing MA. Combined estrogen and progestin hormone replacement therapy in relation to risk of breast cancer in middle-aged women. JAMA 1995;274:137–142.
6. Bergkvist L, Adami HO, Persson I, Hoover R, Schairer C. The risk of breast cancer after estrogen and estrogen-progestin replacement. N Engl J Med 1989;321:293–297.

7. Mills PK, Beeson L, Phillips RL, Fraser GE. Prospective study of exogenous hormone use and breast cancer in Seventh-day Adventists. Cancer 1989;64:591–597.

8. Risch HA, Howe GR. Menopausal hormone usage and breast cancer in Saskatchewan: a record-linkage cohort study. Am J Epidemiol 1994;139:670–683.

9. Colditz GA, Hankinson SE, Hunter DJ, Willett WC, Manson JE, Stampfer MJ, Hennekens C, Rosner B, Speizer FE. The use of estrogens and progestins and the risk of breast cancer in postmenopausal women. N Engl J Med 1995;332:1589–1593.

10. Buring JE, Hennekins CH, Lipnick RJ, Willett W, Stampfer MJ, Rosner B, Peto R, Speizer FE. A prospective cohort study of postmenopausal hormone use and risk of breast cancer in US women. Am J Epidemiol 1987;125:939–947.

11. Dupont WD, Page DL, Rogers LW, Parl FF. Influence of exogenous estrogens, proliferative breast disease, and other variables on breast cancer risk. Cancer 1989;63:948–957.

12. Armstrong BK. Oestrogen therapy after the menopause — boon or bane? Med J Australia 1988;148:213,214.

13. Dupont WD, Page DL. Menopausal estrogen replacement therapy and breast cancer. Arch Intern Med 1991;151:67–72.

14. Steinberg KK, Thacker SB, Smith J, Stroup DF, Zack MM, Flanders D, Berkelman RL. A meta-analysis of the effect of estrogen replacement therapy on the risk of breast cancer. JAMA 1991;265:1985–1990.

15. Sillero-Arenas M, Delgado-Rodriguez M, Rodigues-Canteras R, Bueno-Cavanillas A, Galvez-Vargas R. Menopausal hormone replacement therapy and breast cancer: a meta-analysis. Obstet Gynecol 1992;79:286–294.

16. Colditz GA, Egan KM, Stampfer MJ. Hormone replacement therapy and risk of breast cancer: results from epidemiologic studies. Am J Obstet Gynecol 1993;168:1472–1480.

17. Hunt K, Vessey M, McPherson K, Coleman M. Long-term surveillance of mortality and cancer incidence in women receiving hormone replacement therapy. Br J Obstet Gynecol 1987;94:620–635.

18. Bergkvist L, Adami HO, Persson I, Bergstrom R, Krusemo UB. Prognosis after breast cancer diagnosis in women exposed to estrogen and estrogen-progestogen replacement therapy. Am J Epidemiol 1989;130:221–228.

19. Grady D, Gebretsadik T, Kerlikowske K, Ernster V, Petitti D. Hormone replacement therapy and endometrial cancer risk: a meta-analysis. Obstet Gynecol 1995;85:304–313.

20. Horwitz R, Feinstein A. Alternative analytic methods for case-control studies of estrogens and endometrial cancer. N Engl J Med 1978;299:1089–94.

21. Persson I, Adami HO, Bergkvist L, Lindgren A, Pettersson B, Hoover R, Schairer C. Risk of endometrial cancer after treatment with oestrogens alone or in conjunction with progestogens: results of a prospective study. Br Med J 1989;298:147–151.

22. Voigt LF, Weiss NS, Chu J, Daling JR, McKnight B, Van Belle G. Progestagen supplementation of exogenous oestrogens and risk of endometrial cancer. Lancet 1991;338:274–277.

23. Brinton LA, Hoover RN, and The Endometrial Cancer Collaborative Group. Estrogen replacement therapy and endometrial cancer risk: unresolved issues. Obstet Gynecol 1993;81:265–271.

24. Jick SS, Walker AM, Jick H. Estrogens, progesterone, and endometrial cancer. Epidemiology 1993;4:20–24.

25. Beresford SAA, Weiss NS, Voigt LF, McKnight B. Risk of endometrial cancer in relation to use of oestrogen combined with cyclic progestagen therapy in postmenopausal women. Lancet 1997;349:458–461.

26. Whitehead MI, Townsend PT, Pryse-Davis J, et al. Effects of estrogens and progestagen on the biochemistry and morphology of the postmenopausal endometrium. N Engl J Med 1981;305:1599–1605.

27. The Writing Group for the PEPI Trial. Effects of hormone replacement therapy on endometrial histology in postmenopausal women. JAMA 1996;275:370–375.

28. Weiss NS, Lyon JL, Krishnamurthy S, Dietert SE, Liff JM, Daling JR. Noncontraceptive estrogen use and the occurrence of ovarian cancer. JNCI 1982;68:95–98.

29. Cramer DW, Hutchison GB, Welch WR, Scully RE, Ryan KJ. Determinants of ovarian cancer risk. I. Reproductive experiences and family history. JNCI 1983;71:711–716.

30. Tzonou A, Day NE, Trichopoulos D, Walker A, Saliaraki M, Papapostolou M, Polychronopoulou A. The epidemiology of ovarian cancer in Greece: a case-control study. Eur J Cancer Clin Oncol 1984;20:1045–1052.

31. Booth M, Beral V, Smith P. Risk factors for ovarian cancer: a case-control study. Br J Cancer 1989;60:592–598.

32. Kaufman DW, Kelly JP, Welch WR, Rosenberg L, Stolley PD, Warshauer ME, Lewis J, Woodruff J, Shapiro S. Noncontraceptive estrogen use and epithelial ovarian cancer. Am J Epidemiol 1989;130:1142–1151.

33. Whittemore AS, Harris R, Itnyre J, and the Collaborative Ovarian Cancer Group. Characteristics relating to ovarian cancer risk; Collaborative analysis of 12 US case-control studies. II. Invasive epithelial ovarian cancers in white women. Am J Epidemiol 1992;136:1184–1203.

34. Parazzini F, LaVecchia C, Negri E, Vitta A. Estrogen replacement therapy and ovarian cancer risk. Int J Cancer 1994;7:135–136.
35. Rodriguez C, Calle EE, Coates RJ, Miracle-McMahill HL, Thun MJ, Heath CW. Estrogen replacement therapy and fatal ovarian cancer. Am J Epidemiol 1995;141:828–835.
36. Purdie D, Green A, Bain C, Siskind V, Ward B, Hacker N, Quinn M. Estrogen replacement therapy and risk of epithelial ovarian cancer. Am J Epidemiol 1996;143:S43.
37. Risch HA. Estrogen replacement therapy and risk of epithelial ovarian cancer. Gynecol Oncol 1996;63:254–257.
38. Cramer DW, Devesa SS, Welch WR. Trends in the incidence of endometrioid and clear cell cancers of the ovary in the United States. Am J Epidemiol 1981;114:201–208.
39. Jacobs EJ, White E, Weiss NS. Exogenous hormones, reproductive history, and colon cancer. Cancer Causes Contr 1994;5:359–366.
40. Callee EE, Miracle-McMahill HL, Thun MJ, Heath CW, Jr. Estrogen replacement therapy and risk of fatal colon cancer in a prospective cohort of postmenopausal women. J Natl Cancer Inst 1995;87:517–523.
41. Newcomb PA, Storer BE. Post menopausal hormone use and risk of large-bowel cancer. J Natl Cancer Inst 1995;87:1067–1071.
42. Cobleigh MA, Berris RF, Bush T, Davidson NE, Robert NJ, Sparano JA, Tormey DC, Wood WC. Estrogen replacement therapy in breast cancer survivors. JAMA 1994;272:540–545.
43. Matthews PN, Millis RR, Hayward JL. Breast cancer in women who have taken contraceptive steroids. BMJ 1981;282:774–6.
44. Stoll BA. Effect of Lyndiol, an oral contraceptive on breast cancer. BMJ 1967;1:150–153.
45. Stoll BA. Hormone replacement therapy in women treated for breast cancer. Eur J Cancer Clin Oncol 1989;25:1909.
46. Wile AG, Optell DA, Margileth DA, Hoda AC. Hormone replacement therapy does not affect breast cancer outcome. Proc Am Soc Clin Oncol 1991;10:58.
47. DiSaia PJ, Grosen EA, Kurosaki T, Gildea M, Cowan B, Anton-Culver H. Hormone replacement therapy in breast cancer survivors: a cohort study. Am J Obstet Gynecol 1996;174:1494–1498.
48. Eeles RA, Tan S, Wiltshaw E, Fryatt I, A'Hern RP, Shepherd JH, Harmer CL, Blake PR, Chilvers CED. Hormone replacement therapy and survival after surgery for ovarian cancer. BMJ 1991;302:259–262.
49. Criqui MH, Suarez L, Barrett-Connor E, McPhillips J, Wingard DL, Garland C. Postmenopausal estrogen use and mortality. Am J Epidemiol 1988;128:606–614.
50. Hunt K, Vessey M, McPherson K. Mortality in a cohort of long-term users of hormone replacement therapy: an updated analysis. Br J Obstet Gynecol 1990;97:1080–1086.
51. Henderson BE, Paganini-Hill A, Ross RK. Decreased mortality in users of estrogen replacement therapy. Arch Intern Med 1991;151:75–78.
52. Grodstein F, Stampfer MJ, Colditz GA, Willett WC, Manson JE, Joffe M, Rosner B, Fuchs C, Hankinson SE, Hunter DJ, Hennekins CH, Speizer FE. Postmenopausal hormone therapy and mortality. N Engl J Med 1997;336:1769–1775.
53. Schairer C, Adami HO, Hoover R, Persson I. Cause-specific mortality in women receiving hormone replacement therapy. Epidemiology 1997;8:59–65.
54. Col NF, Eckman MH, Karas RH, Pauker SG, Goldberg RJ, Ross Em, Orr RK, Wong JB. Patient-specific decisions about hormone replacement therapy in postmenopausal women. JAMA 1997;277:1140–1147.

11
Nonestrogen Alternatives for Menopause

Ian H. Thorneycroft, PhD, MD

Contents

INTRODUCTION

Before considering estrogen alternatives, the relative and absolute contraindications to estrogen therapy should be considered. The scientific basis for them is limited and in many cases is nonexistent or there is evidence to the contrary.

RELATIVE AND ABSOLUTE CONTRAINDICATIONS TO ESTROGEN THERAPY

Estrogens are generally contraindicated in any of the following conditions.

Known or Suspected Cancer of the Breast, Except in the Appropriately Selected Patients Treated for Metastatic Disease

This is purely theoretical. There are no studies reporting an increase in recurrence or deaths in women with a history of breast cancer, who were subsequently given estrogen replacement therapy (ERT). Estrogens could only stimulate an existing metastasis to grow more rapidly and therefore become clinically apparent earlier, even this has not

From: *Contemporary Endocrinology: Menopause: Endocrinology and Management*
Edited by: D. B. Seifer and E. A. Kennard © Humana Press Inc., Totowa, NJ

been demonstrated. High-dose estrogens prevent recurrence as effectively as tamoxifen, but had more side effects than tamoxifen *(1)*. Furthermore, premenopausal patients with breast cancer are not routinely ovariectomized and patients who conceive after breast cancer are not at higher risk for recurrence than those who do not conceive *(2,3)*.

Eden et al. reported that when compared to patients who were not treated with hormone replacement therapy (HRT), there was a decreased recurrence rate in breast cancer patients treated with either Premarin 0.625 mg or Ogen 1.25 mg per d combined with an average dose of 50 mg of Provera per d *(4)*.

Breast cancer patients should not automatically be denied ERT, particularly in the early stage of the disease. Selected patients, particularly those with severe symptoms and at high risk for cardiac disease and osteoporosis, can be considered for estrogen after appropriate informed consent.

Women with Known or Suspected Estrogen Dependent Neoplasia

This is a theoretical concern. ERT/HRT has been given to patients with endometrial carcinoma. Women with stage I grade 1 endometrial carcinoma given ERT/HRT had fewer recurrences and survived longer than those not treated with estrogens *(3,5)*. Patients with stage I grade 1 disease can probably be treated with estrogens immediately, with appropriate informed consent *(6)*. A small study with stages I and II endometrial cancer was unable to show any difference in recurrences or survival between those given ERT/HRT *(7)*. Endometrial cancer, at stage II or greater, should probably be followed for two to three years. If the course proves to be disease-free, then with proper informed consent, and for severe symptoms, ERT could be initiated.

Known or Suspected Pregnancy

Impossible in a menopausal patient.

Undiagnosed Abnormal Genital Bleeding

Any bleeding in a menopausal patient who does not take estrogens is cancer until proven otherwise and an endometrial biopsy or dilation and curettage and hysteroscopy should be performed before the initiation of ERT.

Active Thrombophlebitis or Thromboembolic Disorders

Medicolegally, it makes no sense during an active thrombotic episode to give estrogen, although if the patient is anticoagulated, estrogen could not cause a thrombosis.

A Past History of Thrombophlebitis, Thrombosis or Thromboembolic Disorders Associated with Previous Estrogen Use

All patients with a previous history of thrombosis are usually eliminated from studies. The risk of ERT in this group is therefore, unknown. Until 1996, all of the literature indicated that ERT was not thrombotic *(8–11)*. Studies have been published since 1996, demonstrating an increased risk with both oral and transdermal ERT *(12–15)*. Patients with Factor V Leiden, antithrombin III deficiency, protein C, or protein S deficiency are at increased risk of thrombosis with oral contraceptives *(16,17)*. The effect of the thrombophilias on ERT is unknown. Tamoxifen increases thrombosis, and in one study, all those with thrombosis had Factor V Leiden *(18)*. Ovariectomy is not recommended for patients with either a thrombophilia or past history of a thrombosis. Most physicians would not give these patients estrogens, Tamoxifen, or Raloxifene.

REASONS FOR ESTROGEN REFUSAL

Many patients refuse estrogens because of the fear of breast cancer and bleeding problems on HRT. Before a decision is made to not prescribe estrogens, patients need to be counseled on the benefits of estrogens, and the risks of not taking estrogens. Lower than usual doses of estrogens (e.g., 0.3 mg Premarin/Estratab or 0.025 mg patch) are probably better than the alternatives to be discussed below. The lower-dose estrogen regimens have fewer estrogen side effects.

MANAGEMENT OF MENOPAUSE WHEN ESTROGEN IS CONTRAINDICATED

An exhaustive discussion of all therapeutic options is not the intent of this chapter. Only agents for preventive therapy that are safe will be discussed. For example, patients with known cardiac disease benefit from estrogen, however, an exhaustive discussion of cardiovascular drugs will not be addressed in this chapter. In addition, only those agents currently available or soon to be available in the United States will be reviewed.

Management of menopausal symptoms poses a significant problem in patients who refuse or have a contraindication to ERT. A number of agents are available that are equivalent to estrogen for relief of vasomotor symptoms and osteoporosis prevention, but no single agent treats both. Alternative therapies for other benefits of estrogen are not as effective or safe as estrogens.

TREATMENT OF VAGINAL ATROPHY AND DRYNESS

It is very difficult to replace estrogens. Lubricants such as Replens will help with lubrication. Estring, a recently introduced product, has no significant peripheral estradiol levels after 48 h and may therefore be the best choice here for all patients.

TREATMENT OF VASOMOTOR SYMPTOMS

A number of both steroid and nonsteroidal agents are available to treat vasomotor symptoms. Common problems encountered when reviewing the data include a prominent placebo effect and interstudy variability. Trials without placebo are not useful. Of the alternative agents, the most commonly employed is medroxyprogesterone acetate (MPA). Clonidine, methyldopa, danazol, naloxone, Bellergal, and Bellergal S have been used with varying success and not always with placebo controls.

Progestins

In two double-blind placebo-controlled crossover studies, oral-MPA and depo-MPA appeared to be equally effective. In the first study, MPA acetate 20 mg po qd relieved vasomotor flushes in 90% of subjects *(19)*. In the second study, Depo Provera at doses of 50, 100, and 150 mg im q 3 mo relieved vasomotor symptoms. The 150-mg dose was the most effective *(20)*. Hot flushes decreased 45% after 12 wk of therapy. Depo MPA acetate 150 mg po qd was as effective as 0.625 mg of Premarin in relieving hot flushes *(21)*. Megace, 20 mg po bid, prevented hot flushes in 70–85% of menopausal women and hypogonadal males *(22,23)*. Side effects including irregular uterine bleeding (43%), depression (10%), headache (7%), and vaginal atrophy limit the usefulness of these agents in some patients *(24)*.

In a small randomized, double-blinded study of eight patients who received 100 mg of Danazol a d, three patients noted 98.5, 80, and 34.7% fewer hot flushes *(25)*. These results need to be confirmed in a larger group of patients before Danazol can be routinely recommended as an alternative to estrogen. Side effects of Danazol also severely limit its usefulness.

Clonidine and Methyldopa

Clonidine relieves hot flushes by diminishing peripheral vascular responsiveness to vasodilator and vasoconstrictor stimuli. Success with clonidine has been variable. A minimum daily dose of 0.1 mg is required, however, most patients require a higher dose of up to 0.4 mg a d *(26)*. Up to a 60% improvement in vasomotor symptoms has been reported *(27)*. Side effects with higher doses can be significant and include dry mouth, insomnia, and hypotension. There is also a rebound hypertension after discontinuing the drug.

Methyldopa 250–500 mg po qd has been used to treat vasomotor symptoms with good results. Women noted a 50–60% improvement in hot flushes and a 77% improvement in well-being in a placebo-controlled study *(28)*. Fatigue (50%) and dry mouth (30%) limit methyldopa's usefulness.

Patients who are hypertensive and not taking the above-mentioned drugs can be switched to these drugs with the hope that both their hypertension and hot flushes can be controlled with the same drug. Nonhypertensive patients can certainly also be tried on them.

Bellergal

Bellergal-S, a combination drug consisting of atropine, ergotamine, and phenobarbital is not useful in treating vasomotor symptoms in placebo-controlled trials *(29)*. It is, however, worthwhile to give a trial when all other agents have failed or are contraindicated. The phenobarbital allows the patient to sleep at night through the hot flushes. The usual regimen is two at night and possibly one in the morning.

In summary, the best nonestrogen alternative for hot flushes is MPA or Megace. As will be discussed below, there is some evidence that Depo Provera may also protect the menopausal patient from bone loss also.

TREATMENT OF OSTEOPOROSIS

A number of agents can be used including MPA, exercise, calcium supplements, fluoride, vitamin D, calcitonin, and the bisphosphonates.

Bisphosphonates

Bisphosphonates exert their effects on bone by inhibiting osteoclast-mediated bone resorption. They are also incorporated into bone, making osteoclastic adsorption more difficult.

Alendronate (Fosamax), 10 mg po qd, when given to patients with existing osteoporosis prevented bone loss and fractures at all skeletal sites. The most pronounced protection was in patients with previous fractures. A lower dose of 5 mg per d has been shown in menopausal patients to prevent osteoporosis. A complication of Fosamax is esophagitis, particularly when the drug is not taken correctly. This is a rare complication. Clearly,

Fosamax is the drug of choice, second to estrogen and is as effective as estrogen in precluding osteoporosis (30–32).

Intermittent cyclic phosphate and etidronate therapy increased bone mass and decreased rates of new vertebral fractures (33). Patients receive 1.0 gm of phosphate twice daily for 3 d, and 400 mg of etidronate for the next 14 d, followed by 500 mg of calcium daily for the next 74 d. This cycle is repeated every 91 d. Also the most pronounced decrease in new fracture rates was seen in patients with diminished vertebral bone mineral density prior to therapy similar to that seen with Fosamax. Long-term fracture data for all skeletal sites is not available.

Progestins

There is little data published regarding progestins when used alone. Women treated with either 0.625 mg Premarin or 150 mg depo MPA had a similar decline in calcium/creatinine and hydroxyproline/creatinine ratios. Bone density was not studied and hydroxyproline is not a very specific marker for bone collagen breakdown (21). With the limited information on progestins, other agents such as bisphosphonates should be used as estrogen substitutes.

SERMs

SERMs are selective estrogen receptor modulators. Examples are tamoxifen, droloxiphene, and raloxifene. In some tissues, they are antiestrogenic and in others estrogenic. In the breast, they are antiestrogens, and in bone, estrogen agonist. The perfect SERM would have all the positive effects of estrogens and be antagonistic in the breast, uterus, and coagulation system. Such an agent is yet to be developed. Low-dose estrogens (e.g., 0.3 mg of Premarin or Estratab) are probably better at the present time.

Breast cancer patients treated with 20 mg per d of Tamoxifen have been noted in several studies to maintain their bone density (30,34). Raloxifene also protects against bone loss in menopausal patients (35).

Exercise

There is little evidence that exercise alone can be beneficial to bone. Walking or dynamic bone-loading exercises seem to be the best (36–38). Exercise is good for a patient's general health so it cannot be harmful to recommend, if all agents are refused.

Calcium

Adult women in the United States have an average daily calcium intake of 500 mg, which is well below the minimum daily requirement of 1000 mg for premenopausal women and 1500 mg for postmenopausal women not receiving estrogen. Calcium appears to be only effective in patients with extremely low calcium intakes of below 200–300 mg per d (39,40). Women receiving 1500 mg of calcium per d continue to lose bone at a rate similar to placebo controls (41,42). A recent Swedish study concluded that only women in the upper-third percentile had protection against osteoporosis (43). Calcium should be used in conjunction with other therapies to maximize their beneficial effects. However, when patients refuse all other effective therapy, calcium supplementation to 1500 mg per d is reasonable.

Fluoride

Sodium fluoride (75 mg daily) is a potent stimulator of bone formation. Increases in trabecular bone density have been observed with this therapy, however, cortical bone density decreases. The new bone formed may be structurally abnormal. Vertebral fractures were the same in study and control groups and nonvertebral fractures were higher in the treatment group *(44)*. Prominent side effects, particularly gastrointestinal, limit its use. Intermittent slow-release fluoride (25 mg bid) and calcium supplementation (1500 mg daily) produce structurally normal bone and a decrease in vertebral fractures *(45,46)*. Side effects are also dramatically reduced. The slow-release fluoride therapy is before the FDA for approval at present and, when approved, will be a good alternative to estrogen. Fluoride should not be used until this particular preparation is available.

Vitamin D

Vitamin D deficiency is rare in the United States and is only seen in patients with a genetic resistance or those who are bedridden and do not get outdoors. Supplementation with 400 U per d is not harmful and would seem reasonable in those patients who do not receive a lot of sunlight.

Calcitonin

Salmon calcitonin has been approved by the Food and Drug Administration (FDA) for the treatment of postmenopausal osteoporosis. It is available as both injectable and intranasal preparations. Long-acting depo preparations are available outside the United States. Calcitonin binds to high affinity receptors on osteoclasts and inhibits their activity. Long-term studies (2 yr) using 50–100 IU 3 times a wk demonstrated a reduction in bone loss comparable to that seen with estradiol *(46)*. Side effects are usually mild (dizziness, flushing, GI upset, nausea) and can be minimized by starting with a low dose (10–25 IU). Intranasal calcitonin has been also demonstrated to decrease bone loss. There are no long-term fracture data and resistance develops with long term use.

SUMMARY OF OSTEOPOROSIS

Agents are available that are as effective as estrogen to reduce bone loss and fractures. These agents do not have the other benefits of estrogen (i.e., prevention of vasomotor symptoms, cardioprotective effects, avoiding urogenital atrophy, etc.) and are therefore only indicated when estrogen is refused or contraindicated. Fosamax or raloxifene are clearly the drugs of choice when estrogen cannot be used or is refused. Breast cancer patients taking tamoxifen are protected. They would have to be switched to Fosamax 5 mg or ralixifene 60 mg after tamoxifen is discontinued. Etidronate, although less expensive, has not been shown in long-term studies to reduce fractures. Similarly, the long-term results with calcitonin are not as efficacious as bisphophonates.

CARDIOVASCULAR BENEFITS

Exercise

Exercise and a low-cholesterol and low-saturated fatty acid diet should be encouraged for all and particularly those menopausal patients at risk for cardiac disease by virtue of family history and other risk factors. Exercise can decrease total and LDL cholesterol and triglycerides *(47)*.

Selective Estrogen Receptor Modulators (SERMs)

Tamoxifen lowers LDL cholesterol and is an antioxidant *(48–51)*. Myocardial infarctions were lower in breast cancer patients taking tamoxifen than those in the pla-

Table 1
Comparison of Estrogen with Nonestrogen Alternatives for Menopause

	Estrogens	Estrogen/ progestin	Tamoxifen	Raloxifene	Fosamax	Provera	Megace	Lubricants	Vasomotor drugs
Beneficial effects									
Osteoporosis	Protect	Protect	Protect	Protect	Protect	Protect	Unknown	No effect	No effect
Hot flushes	Protect	Protect	Aggravate	Aggravate	No effect	Protect	Protect	No effect	Protect
Cardiovascular	Protect	Protect	Possibly	Unknown	No effect	No effect	Unknown	No effect	No effect
Lipids	Improve	Improve	Improve	Improve	No effect	Adverse	Adverse	No effect	No effect
Urological	Protect	Protect	Aggravate	Prob aggravate	No effect	No effect	No effect	No effect	No effect
Vaginal	Protect	Protect	Aggravate	Prob aggravate	No effect	No effect	No effect	Helpful	No effect
Alzheimer's	Prob protect	Unknown	Unknown	Unknown	No effect	Unknown	Unknown	No effect	No effect
Adverse effects									
Breast Cancer	Slight effect	No effect	Prob protect	Prob protect	No effect	No effect	No effect	No effect	No effect
DVT	Increase	Increase	Increase	Increase	No effect	No effect	No effect	No effect	No effect
Endometrial cancer	Increase	Protect	Increase	Prob protect	No effect	Protect	Protect	No effect	No effect

cebo group. Only the Scottish Adjuvant trial was significant *(52,53)*. The US NSABBP Trial reported a nonsignificant reduced risk of 0.85 (95% CI 0.46–1.58) *(54)*. There appears to be a trend to a lower rate of MI with tamoxifen. Raloxifene has similar lipid changes to tamoxifen *(35)*, however, in monkeys the equivalent of 60 mg per d had the same amount of atherosclerosis as placebo and a dose equivalent to 120 mg increased atherosclerosis over placebo *(55)*.

The major benefit of ERT is the decrease in myocardial infarctions. No equivalent nonestrogen alternative exists except for therapeutic cardiac drugs, which are not the subject of the chapter. Patients at risk for cardiac disease are most likely to benefit from ERT and should be encouraged to take estrogen *(56)*.

Alzheimer's Disease

Vitamin E and NSAIDS have been shown to decrease the incidence of Alzheimer's disease *(57,58)*. With the hepatic toxicity and bleeding complications of NSAIDS, it is difficult to recommend them for routine prophylaxis except in patients at high risk. Drugs such as Tacrin and Aricept, which ameliorate the symptoms of Alzheimer's, are not for prevention and Tacrin is associated with liver toxicity. If ERT is truly effective in the prevention of Alzheimer's, there does not appear to be a nonestrogen alternative at the present time except for vitamin E.

Tamoxifen antagonized the beneficial effects on rat neurons *(59)*. Current SERMs have yet to be studied regarding their possible protection against Alzheimer's.

CONCLUSION

There is no single substitute for estrogen. The alternatives for osteoporosis are the only ones that are equivalent to estrogen. With combinations of drugs, many but not all the benefits of ERT can be achieved. Table 1 summarizes the benefits and risks for estrogen and nonestrogen substitutes.

REFERENCES

1. Beex L, Pieters G, Smals A, Koenders A, Benraad T, Kloppenborg P. Tamoxifen versus ethinyl estradiol in the treatment of postmenopausal women with advanced breast cancer. Cancer Treatment Rep 1981;65:179–185.
2. Creasman W. Estrogen replacement therapy: is previously treated cancer a contraindication? Obstet Gynecol 1991;77:308–312.
3. DiSaia P. Hormone-replacement therapy in patients with breast cancer: a reappraisal. Cancer Suppl 1993;71:1490–1500.
4. Eden J, Bush T, Nand S, Wren B. A case-control study of combined continuous estrogen-progestin replacement therapy among women with a personal history of breast cancer. Menopause: JNAMS 1995;2:(2)67–72.
5. Lee R, Burke T, Park R. Estrogen replacement therapy following treatment for stage I endometrial carcinoma. Gynecol Oncol 1990;36:189–191.
6. American College of Obstetricians and Gynecologists. Estrogen replacement therapy and endometrial cancer. Committe opinion: committee on gynecologic practice 1995;126.
7. Chapman JA, DiSaia PJ, Osann K, Roth PD, Gillotte DL, Berman ML. Estrogen replacement in surgical stage I and II endometrial cancer survisors. Am J Obstet Gynecol 1996;1195–1200.
8. Devor M, Barrett-Connor E, Renvall M, Feigal D, Ramsdell J. Estrogen replacement therapy and the risk of venous thrombosis. Am J Med 1992;92:275–282.
9. The Boston Collaborative Drug Surveillance Program. Surgically confirmed gallbladder disease, venous thromboembolism, and breast tumors in relation to postmenopausal estrogen therapy. N Engl J Med 1974;290:15–19.

10. Nachtigall L, Nachtigall R, Nachtigall R, Beckman E. Estrogen replacement therapy II: a prospective study in the relationship to carcinoma and cardiovascular and metabolic problems. Obstet Gynecol 1979;54:74–79.

11. Petitti DB, Wingerd J, Pellegrin F, Ramcharan S. Risk of vascular disease in women: smoking, oral contraceptives, noncontraceptive estrogens, and other factors. JAMA 1979;242:1150–1154.

12. Jick H, Derby L, Myers M, Vasilakis C, Newton K. Risk of hospital admission for idiopathic venous thromboembolism among users of postmenopausal oestrogens. Lancet 1996;348:981–983.

13. Daly E, Vessey M, Hawkins M, Carson J, Gough P, Marsh S. Risk of venous thromboembolism in users of hormone replacement therapy. Lancet 1996;348:977–980.

14. Grodstein F, Stampfer MJ, Goldhaber SZ, Manson JE, Colditz GA, Speizer FE, et al. Prospective study of exogenous hormones and risk of pulmonary embolism in women. Lancet 1996;348:983–987.

15. Gutthann SP, Rodriguez LA, Castellsague J, Oliart AD. Hormone replacement therapy and risk of venous thromboembolis: population based case-control study. BMJ 1997;314:796–800.

16. Pabinger, I, Schneider B. Thrombotic risk of women with hereditary antithrombin III protein C- and protein s-deficiency taking oral contraceptive medication. The GTH Study Group on Natural Inhibitors. Thromb Haemostas 1994;71:548-552.

17. Rintelen C, Mannhalter C, Ireland H, Lane D, Knobl P, Lechner K, et al. Oral contraceptives enhance the risk of clinical manifestation of venous thrombosis at a young age in females homozygous for factor V Leiden. Br J Haematol 1996;93:487–490.

18. Weitz I, Isreal V, Liebman H. Tamoxifen-associated venous thrombosis and activated protein C resistance due to factor V Leiden. Cancer 1997;79:2024–2027.

19. Albrecht B, Schiff I, Tulinchinsky D, Ryan K. Objective evidence that placebo and oral medroxyprogesterone acetate therapy diminish menopausal vasomotor flushes. Am J Obstet Gynecol 1981;136:361.

20. Morrison J, Martin D, Blair R, Anderson G. The use of medroxyprogesterone acetate for relief of climacteric symptoms. Am J Obstet Gynecol 1980;138:99.

21. Lobo R, McCormic W, Singer F, Roy S. Depomedroxyprogesterone acetate compared with conjugated estrogens for the treatment of postmenopausal women. Obstet Gynecol 1984;63:1.

22. Smith JA. A prospective comparison of treatments for symptomatic hot flushes following endocrine therapy for carcinoma of the prostate. J Urol 1994;152:132–134.

23. Loprinzi CL, Michalak JC, Quella SK, O'Fallon JR, Hatfield AK, Nelimark RA, et al. Megestrol acetate for the prevention of hot flashes. N Engl J Med 1994;331:347–352.

24. Gambrell R. Clinical use of progestins in the menopausal patient. J Reprod Med 1983;27:531.

25. Foster G, Zacur H, Rock J Hot flushes in postmenopausal women ameliorated by danazol. Fertil Steril 1985;43:401.

26. Laufer L, Erlik Y, Meldrum D, Judd H. Effect of clonidine on hot flashes in postmenopausal women. Obstet Gynecol 1982;60:583.

27. Nagamani M, Kelver M, Smith E. Treatment of menopausal hot flashes with transdermal administration of clonidine. Am J Obstet Gynecol 1987;156:561.

28. Nesheim B, Saetre T. Reduction of menopausal hot flushes by methyldopa. Eur J Clin Pharmacol 1981;20:413.

29. Bergmans M, Merkins J, Corbey R, Schellekens L. Effect of Bellergal Retard on climacteric complaints: a double-blind, placebo-controlled study. Maturitas 1987;9:227–234.

30. Black DM, Cummings SR, Karpf DB, Cauley JA, Thompson DE, Nevitt MC, et al. Randomised trial of effect of alendronate on risk of fracture in women with existing vertebral fractures. Lancet 1996;348:1535–1541.

31. Hosking D, McConnell M, Ravn P, Wasnich D, Thompson M, Daley M, et al. Alendronate in the prevention of osteoporosis: EPIC study two-year results. Am Soc Bone Mineral Res 1996;1996 Ann Meet.

32. Rimmer DE, Rawls DE. Improper alendronate administration and a case of pill esophagitis [Letter]. Am J Gastroenterol 1996;91:2648–2649.

33. Watts N, Harris S, Genant H, Wasnich R. Intermittent cyclical etidronate treatment of postmenopausal osteoporosis. N Engl J Med 1990;323:7379.

34. Fornander T, Rutqvist L, Wilking N, Carlstrom K, von Schoultz B. Oestrogenic effects of adjuvant tamoxifen in postmenopausal breast cancer. Eur J Cancer 1993;29A:(4)497–500.

35. Draper M, Flowers D, Huster W, Neild J, Harper K, Arnaud C. A controlled trial of rolaxifene (LY139481) HC1: impact on bone turnover and serum lipid profile in healthy postmenopausal women. J Bone Mineral Res 1996;11:835–842.

36. Ayalon J, Simkin A, Leichter, I, Raifmann S. Dynamic bone loading exercises for postmenopausal women: effect on the density of the distal radius. Arch Phys Med Rehab 1987;68:280.

37. White M, Martin R, Yeater R. The effects of exercise on the bones of postmenopausal women. Int Orthoped 1984;7:209.

38. Krolner B, Toft B, Nielsen S, Tondevold E. Physical exercise as prophylaxis against involutional vertebral bone loss: a controlled trial. Clin Sci 1983;64:541.

39. Stevenson J, Whitehead M, Padwick M, Endacott J, Sutton C, Banks L, et al. Dietary intake of calcium and postmenopausal bone loss. BMJ 1988;297:15–17.

40. Dawson-Hughes B. Calcium supplementation and bone loss: a review of controlled clinical trials. Am J Clin Nutr 1991;51:274S–280S.

41. Ettinger B, Genant HK, Cann CE. Postmenopausal bone loss is prevented by treatment with low-dosage estrogen with calcium. Ann Intern Med 1987;106:40–45.

42. Riis B, Thomsen K, Christiansen C. Does calcium supplementation prevent postmenopausal bone loss? N Engl J Med 1987;316:173.

43. Michaelsson R, Bergstron R, Holmberg L, Mallmin H, Wolk A, Ljunghall S. A high dietary calcium intake is needed for a positive effect on bone density in Swedish postmenopausal women. Osteopor Internat 1997;7:155–161.

44. Riggs B, Hodgson S, O'Fallon W, Chao E. Effect of fluoride treatment of the fracture rate in postmenopausal women with osteoporosis. N Engl J Med 1990;322:802.

45. Pak C, Sakhaee K, Adams-Huet B, Piziak, V, Peterson R, Poindexter J. Treatment of postmenopausal osteoporosis with slow-release sodium fluoride — final report of a randomized controlled trial. Ann Intern Med 1995;123:401–408.

46. MacIntyre, I, Whitehead M, Banks L, Stevenson J. Calcitonin for prevention of postmenopausal bone loss. Lancet 1988;900.

47. Lindheim S, Notelovitz M, Feldman E, Larsen S, Kahn F, Lobo R. The independent effects of exercise and estrogen on lipids and lipoproteins in postmenopausal women. Obstet Gynecol 1994;83:167–172.

48. Wiseman H, Cannon M, Arnstein HR, Barlow DJ. The structural minicry of membrane sterols by tamoxifen: evidence from cholesterol coefficients and molecular-modelling for its action as a membrane anti-oxidant and an anti-cancer agent. Biochim Biophys Acta 1992;1138:197–202.

49. McDonald CC, Alexander FE, Whyte BW, Forrest AP, Stewart HJ. Cardiac and vascular morbidity in women receiving adjuvant tamosifen for breast cancer in a randomised trial. The Scottish Cancer Trials Breast Gourp. BMJ 1995;311:977–980.

50. Elisaf M, Bairaktari E, Nicolaides C, Fountzilas G, Tzallas C, Siamopoulos K, et al. The beneficial effect of tamoxifen on serum lipoprotein-A levels: an additional anti-atherogenic property. Anticancer Res 1996;16:2725–2728.

51. Sherwin B. Estrogen and/or androgen replacement therapy and cognitive functioning in surgically menopausal women. Pschoneuroendocrinol 1988;13:345–357.

52. McDonald C, Stewart H. Fatal myocardial infarction in the Scottish adjuvant tamoxifen trial. BMJ 1991;303:435–437.

53. Rutqvist LE, Mattsson A. Cardiac and thromboembolic morbidity among postmenopausal women with early stage breast cancer in a randomized trial of adjuvant tamoxifen. J Nat Cancer Inst 1993;85:1398–1406.

54. Costantino J, Kuller L, Ives D, Fisher B, Dignam J. Coronary heart disease mortality and adjavant tamoxifen therapy. J Nat Cancer Inst 1997;89:776-782.

55. Clarkson TB, Anthony MS, Jerome CP. Lack of effect of raloxifene on coronary artery atherosclerosis of postmenopausal monkeys. J Clin Endo Metab 1988;83(3):721–726.

56. Sullivan J, Zwaag R, Hughes J, Maddock, V, Kroetz F, Ramanathan K, et al. Estrogen replacement therapy and coronary artery disease: effect on survival in postmenopausal women. Arch Intern Med 1990;150:2557–2562.

57. Sano M, Ernesto C, Thomas R, Klauber M, Schafer K, Grundman M, et al. A controlled trial of Selegiline, Alpha-Tocopherol, or both as treatment for Alzheier's disease. N Engl J Med 1997;336:1216–1222.

58. Rich J, Rasmusson D, Folstein M, Carson K, Kawas C, Brandt J. Nonsteroidal anti-inflammatory drugs in Alzheimer's disease. Neurology 1995;45:51–55.

59. Chowen J, Torres-Aleman, I, Garcia-Segura L. Trophic effects of estradiol on fetal rat hypothalamic neurons. Neuroendocrinology 1992;56:895–901.

12

The Use of Antiestrogens in the Postmenopausal Woman

Mark P. Leondires, MD, James H. Segars, MD, and Brian W. Walsh, MD

CONTENTS

INTRODUCTION
REVIEW OF ESTROGEN ACTION
CLINICAL USE OF SERMs AND FINDINGS
CONCLUSIONS
REFERENCES

INTRODUCTION

As women enter the menopause, endogenous estrogen levels fall and this state of estrogen deficiency contributes to several age-related health problems in women. Postmenopausal estrogen replacement therapy (ERT) is designed to take advantage of the positive health benefits of estrogen action in women, which include osteoporosis protection, reduction of cardiovascular risk, urogenital health, improved mood, and possibly, a reduction in Alzheimer's disease risk *(1–3)*. Acceptance of ERT for postmenopausal women by both patients and practitioners has been limited by multiple concerns, including an increased risk of endometrial cancer for those on unopposed ERT; a possible, albeit small, increased risk of breast cancer, discontent with concomitant progestin therapy, and the undesired resumption of vaginal bleeding associated with cyclical therapy. Since the introduction of tamoxifen in 1978 and appreciation of its tissue-specific estrogenic and antiestrogenic actions (*see* the next section), many compounds have been designed to mimic or ablate the estrogenic signal in a tissue-specific fashion. Distinct tissue responsivity to estrogenic compounds is mediated by at least two distinct receptors, as well as, associated nuclear receptor binding proteins, binding to other receptors, and likely additional undefined factors. Because there have been many recent developments in the mechanisms of estrogen and antiestrogen action, this chapter is organized in three parts: the mechanisms of estrogen/antiestrogen action, the pharmacology and design of antiestrogens, and a description of antiestrogens in clinical use for postmenopausal women.

From: *Contemporary Endocrinology: Menopause: Endocrinology and Management*
Edited by: D. B. Seifer and E. A. Kennard © Humana Press Inc., Totowa, NJ

Antiestrogens represent a structurally and functionally diverse group of compounds. They are subclassified into two groups: pure antiestrogens and mixed estrogen agonist/ antagonists. A pure antiestrogen has no estrogenic activity and is based structurally on the steroid ring structure of estrogen. The pure antiestrogens are designed to provide both adjuvant and primary treatment options for patients with breast cancer and are currently in clinical trials. The mixed estrogen agonist/antagonists are agents that either stimulate or inhibit estrogen action depending on the particular tissue and endocrine milieu in which they are used. Of the agents currently used in clinical practice (tamoxifen, toremifene, clomiphene, and raloxifene) none are pure antiestrogens and should be considered selective estrogen receptor modulators (SERMs). These compounds are structurally based on triphenylethylene or benzothiophene rings that are distinct from the steroid ring structure of estrogen. The SERM tamoxifen has proven to be an effective adjuvant in the treatment of breast cancer since its approval in 1978, although its agonistic effect on uterine endometrial tissue has proven troublesome (4). After 20 years of usage tamoxifen has been found not only to improve breast cancer survival, but also to provide protection against osteoporosis and cardiovascular disease exemplifying its mixed estrogen agonist/antagonist activity (4–6). With tamoxifen as a template, SERMs have been designed to take advantage of the positive effects of estrogen while avoiding the unwanted stimulation at breast and endometrial tissues. With further advances SERMs may provide women with more options for hormone replacement therapy to be used with estrogen or alone for the prevention of osteoporosis and protection against cardiovascular disease. Therefore the design of selective estrogen receptor modulators (SERMs) and pure antagonists will lead to therapeutic improvements in breast cancer treatment, hormone replacement therapy (HRT), osteoporosis, hypercholesterolemia, endometriosis, and other yet to be defined areas in the future.

REVIEW OF ESTROGEN ACTION

Classical Understanding of Estrogen Receptor Action

Estrogen receptors are intracellular single chain polypeptides that belong to a superfamily of hormone binding proteins called nuclear hormone receptors. There are two distinct estrogen receptors: ERα and ERβ (see later in the text). This superfamily of proteins is activated by a specific interaction with ligands that are typically small lipophilic molecules and are believed to diffuse into intracellular compartments where the receptors exist in an inactive state. Recent advances in molecular biology have led to cloning and isolation of over 60 members of this superfamily that are related to the estrogen receptor including the thyroid hormone receptor, glucocorticoid receptor, retinoic acid receptor, retinoid X receptor, vitamin D receptor, mineralocorticoid receptor, androgen receptor, and peroxisome proliferator-activated receptor (for review, see refs. 2–4, and references therein [7–9]).

Similar to the other members of this superfamily the polypeptide chain of the estrogen receptor is composed of distinct domains. The three principal regions are characterized by 1) a divergent amino terminus involved in activation of RNA transcription, 2) a more conserved DNA-binding region composed of two zinc-finger motifs, the C domain, and 3) a less well-conserved complex carboxyl region composed of the DEF regions which includes the ligand-binding region, protein:protein interaction regions, the D "hinge region," and a receptor dimerization interface (Fig. 1). Crystallization studies of related

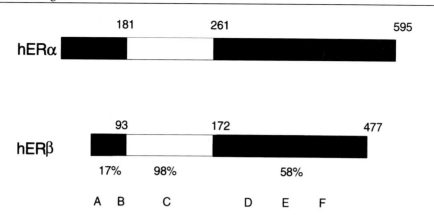

Fig. 1. Schematic of the human estrogen receptors demonstrating the structural domains and comparing the percent homology between hERα and hERβ.

family members as well as other approaches have shown that binding of ligand to the carboxyl region of the nuclear receptors involves noncovalent interactions and the close association with specific peptides in a hydrophobic pocket within the receptor *(10,11)*.

The mechanism by which estrogen gains access to the intracellular compartment containing the estrogen receptor(s) is believed to be by diffusion. Binding of estrogen to the receptor results in a conformational change within the carboxyl region of the receptor, perhaps exposing regions of the protein capable of associating with transcriptionally active proteins (*see* later in the text) *(12–14)*. Additionally, ligand binding to the receptor is accompanied with the release of inhibitory molecules heat-shock protein 90, heat shock protein 70, and other associated molecules *(15,16)*. Thus, ligand binding accomplishes two functions: the release of inhibitory molecules and a conformational change, which is understood to expose specific regions of the receptor that may then participate in signal transduction.

The principal mechanism by which the estrogen receptor alters cellular responses is through binding to specific DNA sequences in the promoter region of hormone responsive genes, resulting in transcription of specific RNA species *(9,17,18)*. The DNA sequences to which the zinc fingers of the ER associate with are called "estrogen response DNA elements" (EREs) and have been described for a number of estrogen-responsive genes. A consensus ERE may be defined as a palindromic sequence of AGGTCA-nnn-TGACCT, with a variable three-base pair spacer region denoted by "n," however, in most promoters the actual sequence may differ widely from the consensus sequence *(19,20)*. Although many genes are regulated by hormone response elements located from 100 to 300 base pairs upstream (5') to the start of transcription, hormone response elements have been described downstream (3') to the gene, within other promoter regions, as well as within the gene itself. Association of the activated (ligand-bound) estrogen receptor with the hormone response element occurs when two separate polypeptide chains dimerize to form a high-affinity DNA-binding interface, which then leads to assembly of a functional preinitiation complex (*see* Fig. 2), recruitment of RNA polymerase II, and generation of specific RNA transcripts (reviewed in ref. *17) (21)*. Unfortunately, association of the receptor with DNA is often more complex than the model presented (Fig. 2), because there is not strict fidelity between the ER and an ERE. Furthermore, other nuclear receptor family members do show affinity for estrogen responsive DNA elements and several groups have described "crosstalk" between nuclear receptors, transcription factors, and

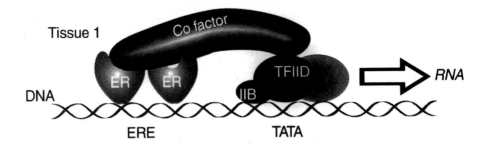

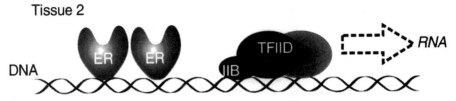

Fig. 2. General mechanism of steroid hormone action. The abbreviations used are E, estrogen; ER, estrogen receptor; ERE, estrogen response element; IIb, transcription factors IIb; IId, transcription factors IId; PolII, RNA polymerase II. See text for details.

estrogen response elements. because "crosstalk" between nuclear receptors, transcription factors, and estrogen response elements *(19,22–24)*.

Interaction of the estrogen receptor with DNA leads to assembly of a functional preinitiation complex. Formation of this complex is facilitated by interaction of the receptor with proteins that comprise essential components of the RNA transcription machinery, for instance, the transcription factor IIB (TFIIB). TFIIB is believed to be a rate-limiting step in the assembly of an active RNA transcription complex *(25–27)*. In addition, receptors have been shown to interact with other proteins in the transcription complex called "TAFs" *(28)*. The number of proteins to which the activated ER may bind includes a greater number than previously realized and include proteins of 120, 125, 140, 160, 168, and 270 kDa molecular mass *(29–35)*. Association of the ER with these auxiliary or receptor cofactors is believed to have physiologic importance, since these proteins not only may facilitate assembly of an active transcription complex, but may also contribute to tissue-specific responses in estrogen action *(36,37)*. As a group, the proteins have been designated "receptor cofactors." Based on their ability to affect receptor function, the receptor cofactors capable of influencing estrogen action may be further classified as "coactivators" if augmenting receptor action; "corepressors" if principally inhibitory in nature; or "integrators" if serving to coordinate the action of other proteins with the estrogen receptor *(36,37)*. The ability of cofactors to influence estrogen receptor may also explain some tissue-specific effects of antiestrogen action and is relevant to the focus of this chapter. Estrogen receptor cofactors that function as integrators include high molecular weight proteins such as Creb binding protein (CBP) (and the related protein, p300) that reside in the nucleus and may bind to several factors including the nuclear receptor binding protein p160, TFIIB, and *jun/fos (38)*. These high molecular weight proteins are believed to coordinate the response of a specific tissue to estrogen with those of other signaling systems (e.g., *fos* and *jun*). Following association of the receptor with the DNA, the receptor complex is recycled, or degraded through processes that are poorly defined. These pathways are summarized in Fig. 3.

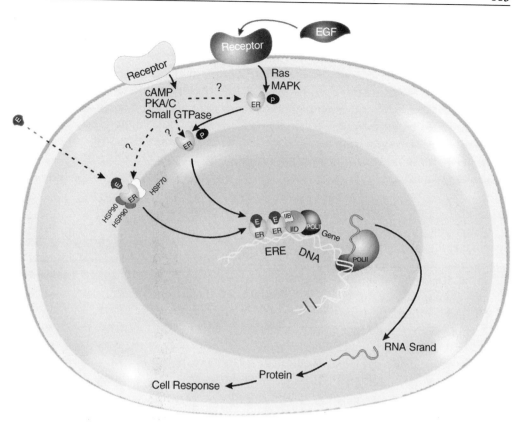

Fig. 3. A schematic model of a cofactor and facilitating the initiation of RNA transcription. See text for details.

In addition to the general mechanism of action, it was recently recognized that the human estrogen receptor exists as a polypeptide chain of two distinct forms, an alpha form (ERα) of 595 amino acids and a more recently isolated beta form (ERβ) of 477 amino acids (Fig. 1). *(39)* Cloning of human ERβ followed isolation of ERβ from the rat *(40)*. The presence of two distinct ER isoforms (α and β) significantly impacts our understanding of estrogen action in reproductive tissues due to differences between ERα and ERβ with regards to their distinct structural features, tissue distribution, ligand affinity, and heterodimerization (reviewed in ref. *38) (41)*. Given the recent identification of the ERβ isoform, it may be helpful to elucidate some of the differences between the ERα and ERβ isoforms. Most significantly, the human ERβ shows 96% amino acid homology with ERα in the DNA-binding region, but only 58% homology in the carboxyl region, suggesting that ERβ may interact with a different set of coactivator proteins than ERα, although this remains to be determined *(39)*. With the exception of the phosphorylation site surrounding serine 118 in ERα, the A/B domain of ERβ is wholly divergent from ERα *(39)*. Likewise, there is little amino acid similarity in the D domain (hinge region) and F domain between the two receptor isoforms. Messenger RNA transcripts for the two receptor isoforms appear to be differently expressed in rat tissues: message for ERα is observed in pituitary, uterus, kidney, adrenal, epidydimus, and testis; whereas ERβ mRNA is found in brain, prostate, ovary, lung, bladder, and testis *(40)*. It is anticipated that protein expression will mirror mRNA expression, but confirmation of this assumption awaits publication of studies with antibodies directed against ERβ. Of particular interest, the two isoforms display different binding affinities for ligands (*see* later) including antiestrogens, no doubt as a result of the structural differences between the two receptors. Finally, in some tissues ERα and ERβ are both expressed, and it has been proposed that heterodimeric combinations of the receptors could alter tissue responses to estrogens based on the differential affinity for ligands and data support this assumption *(41)*. It is clear, however, from the ERα knockout (ERKO) mice that proper function of the alpha isoform of the estrogen receptor is requisite for proper fertility in female and male mice *(42,43)*.

Additional Pathways of Estrogen Action

In addition to RNA transcription, steroid receptors may also alter cellular responses by other mechanisms, which may not be dependent upon RNA transcription. In general, this second pathway of estrogen receptor action is less well characterized, but may be quite important physiologically (reviewed in ref. *41) (44)*. This second pathway has been shown in some cases to involve phosphorylation of the estrogen receptor in response to extracellular stimulation by growth factors. For example, response of the estrogen receptor is influenced by epidermal growth factor (EGF), dopamine, TGFα, insulin-like growth factor-I (IGF-1), cAMP, and heregulin *(45–54)*. This second pathway may result in ligand-independent receptor activation *(47,48)*. Interestingly IGF-1, cholera toxin/3-isobutyl-1-methylxanthine (CT/IBMX), and 8-bromo-cyclic-AMP (8-Br-cAMP) elicited an in vitro response equal to that of estradiol *(51)*. Conversely, activation of the estrogen receptor by protein kinase A (PKA) and protein kinase C (PKC) was ligand-dependent and could be abolished by the addition of the pure antiestrogen ICI-164,384 *(55)*. EGF causes phosphorylation of serine 118 in the amino-terminus of ER through a Ras—Raf—mitogen activated protein kinase (MAPK) signaling pathway, suggesting that small GTPases are also able to influence ER signaling *(45,47,56)*. Furthermore, EGF was capable of inducing nuclear translocation of the ER in the absence of estradiol, emphasizing the importance of these cytoplasmic signaling pathways upon estrogen action *(47)*. At present, while several cytoplasmic signaling pathways have clearly shown the ability to influence either estrogen-dependent or estrogen-independent receptor activation the precise mechanism of how these pathways interrelate with estrogen receptor signaling remain somewhat unclear. These signaling pathways may contribute to tissue-specific estrogen action and thus are assumed to be important to a thorough understanding of estrogen action in women.

Antiestrogen Action

The term antiestrogen covers a spectrum of compounds that range from pure antiestrogens to mixed estrogen receptor agonist/antagonists. The mechanism by which antiestrogens interact with the estrogen receptor and display differential responses when compared to the prototypical estradiol is incompletely understood. It is known that estrogen action is mediated by several factors including goodness of fit, conformational changes, and association with cofactors that implies multiple active pathways which mediate estrogen action. The understanding of these interrelationships is how the complex estrogen/antiestrogen signaling pathways will be further unraveled through a greater understanding of the molecular pharmacology of antiestrogen action. Through this understanding of steroid receptor activation and function, development of a wide array of therapies based on modulation of the steroid receptor is likely in the future.

Antagonists or partial agonists of estrogen action may interfere with receptor action at any point in the pathway of estrogen action. Research into the mechanism of antiestrogen action has suggested that the receptor may have a second binding site for tamoxifen (57,58). Such a site could explain the differential affinities for the receptors to ligand (59). In addition, antiestrogens may cause the receptor to "freeze" in conformational forms that feature partial activity (60). Thus, differential association with the hydrophobic pocket in the receptor, and the resulting altered conformational shape may alter the ability of the antiestrogen bound receptor to function.

Another possible explanation of the tissue-specificity of the SERMs can be explained by the appreciation of two distinct estrogen receptors. There are multiple possibilities how two distinct receptors could explain the tissue-specificity of these compounds. As noted above ERα and ERβ are expressed uniquely in specific tissues, this fact coupled with the amino acid differences in the ligand-binding domains of ERα and ERβ may explain some of the unique aspects of antiestrogen action which remain to be defined. Furthermore, as noted above, ERα and ERβ display different affinities for estrogens and antiestrogens. For the stilbene estrogens, ERα showed the following competition order: diethylstilbesterol > hexestrol > dienestrol > estradiol. In comparison, competition of ERβ for the same compounds showed dienestrol > diethylstilbesterol > hexestrol > estradiol (61). This observation suggests that sequence differences in amino acid in the carboxyl regions of ERα and ERβ may affect binding of ligand to the hydrophobic pocket. For triphenylethylene compounds, both ERα and ERβ showed the following similar affinities: 4OH-tamoxifen >> nafoxidine > clomiphene > tamoxifen (61). Likewise, both ERα and ERβ showed avid binding to pure antiestrogen ICI 164,384. Phytoestrogens are used by many postmenopausal women and it is therefore worth noting that coumestrol and genistein showed a higher affinity for ERβ in comparison with ERα, in keeping with the known effects of these compounds on the prostate, which expresses high levels of ERβ (61,62). Therefore, whereas incompletely understood, the mechanisms of antiestrogen action and tissue-specificity possibly include a unique antiestrogen binding site, unique associations with cofactors and differential actions on ERα and ERβ.

Aims of Drug Development

There are multiple drug design goals for the modulation of estrogen action and the downstream effects of the estrogen receptor. A goal of drug design for postmenopausal HRT is to design a compound that is not mitogenic at the level of the breast or endometrium, but is estrogenic at the CNS, blood vessel wall, liver, bone, and urogenitial region. Such a drug would not only increase the number of women who start HRT and realize its positive health benefits, but might also effect continuation rates. An agents posessing antiestrogenic specificity for endometrial tissues, but without associated estrogenic activity might be used to treat women with endometriosis, endometrial hyperplasia, or possibly endometrial cancer. Furthermore, an endometrial-specific antiestrogen may have contraceptive applications. Agents specifically designed to be antiestrogenic at the level of the breast could provide primary prevention for women deemed at high risk for breast cancer. Such a compound could be used in tamoxifen resistant breast cancer and in all stages of breast cancer treatment. Currently, the design of agents suitable for all of these applications is a focus of research and development.

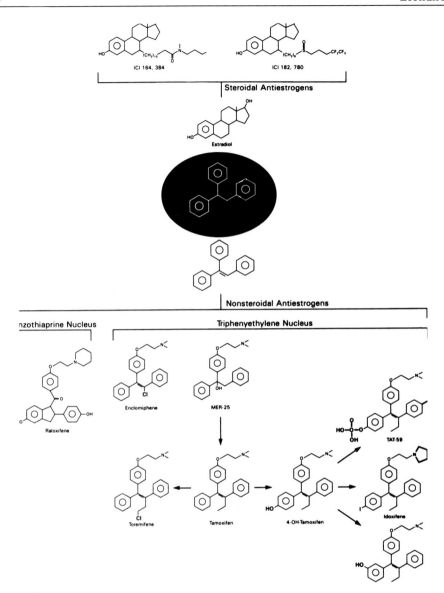

Fig. 4. The chemical structure of the pure antiestrogens, estradiol, and selected SERMs. The steroidal antiestrogens are represented by the top two figures with their structural derivative, estradiol directly below. The structure highlighted in the center of the figure represents the similarity between the triphenylethylene ring structure and the estradiol ring structure. The nonsteroidal antiestrogens are represented in the lower two-thirds of this figure. All of but one, Raloxifene, are based on the triphenylethylene molecule. Of those based on a triphenylethylene ring structure, with tamoxifen as the prototype, the regions distinct from the tamoxifen molecule are highlighted in bold type.

There are two major classifications of antiestrogens: pure antiestrogens and SERMs. The pure antiestrogens belong to the steroidal group as shown in the top section of Fig. 4 are based on substitution at the 7-α position of 17β-estradiol. In contrast, the SERMS belong to the heterogeneous nonsteroidal antiestrogen group as shown in the bottom section of Fig. 4 and exhibit a wide array of actions in a tissue-specific fashion. This group of compounds is under intense investigation not only for breast cancer prevention and treatment applications, but also for general gynecologic and nongynecologic applications such as HRT, endometriosis, endometrial hyperplasia, osteoporosis prevention and treatment, hypercholesterolemia, and Alzheimer's disease risk reduction. This group represents a burgeoning class of pharmaceuticals that will be intensely studied into the next millenium.

Pure Steroidal Antiestrogens

The development of this class of drugs has been driven by the need for treatment of advanced breast cancer after the failure of tamoxifen therapy. The structure of the pure steroidal antiestrogens is based upon estradiol with the addition of a long alkyl side chain at the 7-α position of the B ring (see Fig. 4). ICI 164,384 was shown to be a potent antiestrogen, however, secondary to its hydrophobicity it had reduced bioavailability. ICI 164,384 induces the secretion of TGF-β in fetal fibroblasts devoid of ER receptor as do the nonsteroidal antiestrogens (63). TGF-β is a potent inhibitor of epithelial cell proliferation and is one of the putative mechanism of non-ER-mediated inhibition of tumor growth (64,65). Because of the hydrophobicity of ICI 164,384, ICI 182,780 was developed, which involved the addition of sulfur and fluorine atoms (see Fig. 4). This new compound has affinity for the ER equivalent to that of estradiol and is more bioavailable than ICI 164,384 (66,67).

ICI 182,780 is a pure antiestrogen that not only blocks estrogen binding to the ER but causes destruction of the ER (66,68,69). ICI 182,780 inhibits MCF-7 cell proliferation at low concentrations and is more potent than tamoxifen (66). Importantly several investigators have found ICI 182,780 to inhibit the growth of tamoxifen resistant human breast cancer cell lines (70–72), although, resistance to ICI 182,780 has been reported in vitro (73,74). In the immature rat uterine assay ICI 182,780 blocked estradiol stimulated hypertrophy in a dose dependent fashion and was a complete antiestrogen when administered alone (66). In nude mice, a single dose of ICI 182,780 was as effective of as four weeks of daily tamoxifen therapy in inhibiting the growth of transplanted, estradiol supported MCF-7 human breast cancer cells (66). In premenopausal women ICI 182,780 (12 mg/d IM) treatment for seven ds led to significantly lower ER levels in myometrial cells whereas having no effect on progesterone receptor levels (75).

Currently, there are limited published reports concerning the metabolism of ICI 182,780 in humans, but at a dose of 18 mg/d blood levels of 25 ng/mL are seen after one week of treatment. Additionally, this compound has no effect on luteinizing hormone (LH), follicle stimulating hormone (FSH), lipids, or sex hormone-binding globulin (SHBG) (76,77) concentration. Howell et al. reported on the treatment 19 women with advanced breast cancer resistant to tamoxifen with ICI 182,780. There was a 69% response rate after progression on tamoxifen and there were no apparent negative effects on the liver, brain, or genital tract. Peak levels were achieved in 8–9 d at dosages of either 100 mg or 250 mg administered in a depot form. After six months of multiple dosings some drug accumulation was noted. ICI 182,780 has a very favorable side effect profile in that it did not alter the frequency of hot flushes, night sweats, and none of the patients reported vaginal dryness or decreased libido. Serial endometrial ultrasound evaluations documented in five patients showed no change in endometrial thickness (77). Further studies are required on this compound to confirm its response and to determine the long-term effects of treatment with ICI 182780 and to further define its side effect profile.

Nonsteroidal Antiestrogens

The first nonsteroidal estrogen antagonist was described in 1958 by Lerner et al. *(78)* This compound ethamoxytriphetol (MER 25) is a triphenol ring-based analog and was found to be an antiestrogen in all species tested and importantly inhibited implantation in rats and mice. In human trials MER 25 was found to be an antiestrogen at multiple sites, but this drug exhibited an unacceptable toxicity profile because of central nervous system side effects *(79–81)*. Nonetheless, MER 25 served as a template for many of the nonsteroidal antiestrogens in trials today. Variations on its structural theme which includes three aromatic rings with a basic side chain is the basis for the triphenylethylene family of antiestrogens that includes enclomiphene, tamoxifen, and droloxifene. Raloxifene, another SERM also contains three aromatic rings, but has a benzothiophene nucleus instead of the triphenylethylene of the other SERMs (Fig. 4).

Triphenylethylenes

Tamoxifen

Tamoxifen was first used in the early 1970s for the treatment of advanced breast cancer in postmenopausal woman and has gained wide clinical acceptance, for both metastatic breast cancer and adjuvant therapy. Currently, tamoxifen is being studied for the chemoprevention of breast cancer in healthy women at high risk for the disease *(82)*. The use of tamoxifen has expanded over the years because of its efficacy in prolonging overall and disease free survival as well as reducing the incidence of contralateral breast cancer *(83)*. Tamoxifen is a mixed estrogen agonist/antagonist or SERM which is estrogenic on bone, uterus, liver, and the cardiovascular system whereas acting as an antiestrogen at the level of the breast at least in part because of its inhibition of breast cancer cell mitogenesis *(4–6)*.

Tamoxifen is easily absorbed and metabolized through the cytochrome P450 system to the potent antiestrogen, 4-hydroxytamoxifen, and to the relatively inactive compound α-hydroxytamoxifen. 4-hydroxytamoxifen (4-OH-TAM) binds with a higher affinity to the estrogen receptor than tamoxifen itself and inhibits vaginal cornification at doses approx 25 times lower than tamoxifen *(84–89)*. The metabolism of tamoxifen does lead to glucuronide metabolites which are primarily excreted in the urine and feces with very low levels of α-hydroxytamoxifen found in the serum *(90)*. The half life of tamoxifen is 9–12 h after the initial dose, and 7 d with chronic dosage *(91)*. Tamoxifen also seems to influence several growth factors. Tamoxifen therapy suppresses the levels of IGF-1 in plasma and downregulates TGF-α expression in ER positive cells *(92,93)*. Additionally Knabbe et al. found that tamoxifen induced the secretion of TGF-β, a potent inhibitor of epithelial cell growth, from ER positive MCF-7 breast cancer cells *(94)*. Because of the paradoxical finding that ER negative tumors often respond to tamoxifen therapy *(95,96)*, Colletta et al. investigated the role of antiestrogens in inducing TGF-β production. Tamoxifen was found to induce TGF-β production in ER negative human fetal fibroblasts *(63)*. These observations provided a putative nonER mediated action of tamoxifen inhibition of breast cancer cell mitogenesis via stromal cell production of TGF-β. These findings support additional roles of antiestrogens and their actions independent of the estrogen receptor, although one must interpret this data carefully considering the discovery of ERβ.

Tamoxifen exerts a proliferative effect on human endometrium and is associated with a two to threefold increase in the risk of endometrial carcinoma and endometrial polyp formation *(4)*. Therefore, whereas being an antiestrogen for breast tissue it acts as a partial estrogen at the endometrium. The increase in polyp formation, vaginal bleeding, and endometrial carcinoma presents a problem for patients and practitioners alike. Vaginal bleeding on tamoxifen is not uncommon and must be evaluated via biopsy and treated as appropriate. Endometrial carcinomas in these patients are likely to be detected at an early stage and therefore more likely to be successfully treated. The uterotropic activity of tamoxifen presents as an undesirable side effect of tamoxifen therapy and exemplifies the mixed agonist/antagonist activity of the compound and underlines the need for development of additional compounds with better side effect profiles.

Tamoxifen acts as an estrogen favorably in other human organ systems. The cardiovascular system is positively effected as shown by the induction of lower LDL-cholesterol levels, fibrinogen levels, and a reduction in the incidence of myocardial infarction *(6,97,98)*. Tamoxifen acts as an estrogen on bone metabolism and has been found to increase bone density *(99)*. Tamoxifen does decrease LH levels in postmenopausal women it increases the incidence of hot flushes, therefore tissue-specific actions on the central nervous system and passage across the blood-brain-barrier are unclear *(100)*. Association with Alzheimer's disease protection is not known at this time for tamoxifen.

In humans tamoxifen increases sex hormone binding globulin and decreases LDL-cholesterol and therefore functions as an estrogen agonist in the liver *(101)*. Interestingly, tamoxifen exhibits unique effects in different species. In rats tamoxifen induces nodular hyperplasia in the liver, hepatocellular adenoma, and is a potent hepatic carcinogen *(102–105)*. This finding has led to concern for liver carcinogenisis in humans and stimulated efforts to design a SERM without this property. Theories concerning the mutagenic action of tamoxifen in rats involve the mitogenic effect of estrogenic compounds, a possible role as a tumor promoter, and most likely a direct genotoxic action. In the rat the metabolism of tamoxifen leads to the generation of DNA adducts which are hypothesized to be responsible for the hepatocarcinogenesis *(103)*. Although DNA adducts are readily identified in mouse and rat hepatocytes, they are not detected in human hepatocytes *(106)*. Synthetic estrogens are known promoters of hepatocellular carcinoma as evidenced by the 10-fold increase in risks in women taking oral contraceptives. In the rat model, not only are there DNA adducts formed at a 300-fold higher level in the rat than the human, but in rat studies the animals receive 20 times more tamoxifen from 6 wk of age and develop liver tumors at 2 yr of age. With comparison to the human system this would be equivalent to a 14-yr-old girl taking 20 times the normal dose for 40 yr *(107)*. The direct relevance of rat pharmaco-physiology to the human system is difficult to ascertain, but these data are nevertheless concerning. Concerns about the promotion of endometrial cancer and possibly hepatocarcinogenesis have led to the design and development of other SERMs that are not uterotropic or associated with hepatocarcinogenicity while retaining their positive estrogen agonist and antagonist actions.

Toremifene

Toremifene or chlorotamoxifen is the result of chlorination of the ethyl side chain of tamoxifen *(see* Fig. 4*)*. Toremifene's actions are similar to tamoxifen in most respects, but unlike tamoxifen it does not produce DNA adducts in the rat liver. *(108)* Like tamoxifen, toremifene has an antagonistic effect on the growth of ER positive MCF-7 cells at concentrations from 10^{-7} to 10^{-6} mol/L and is oncolytic at higher concentrations *(109,110)*. Toremifene is effective in inhibiting the growth of MCF-7 (ER positive) cell lines in athymic mice but is not inhibitory for MDA-MB-231 (ER negative) breast cancer cells *(111)*. Toremifene like tamoxifen increases the production of TGF-β production from human fetal fibroblasts (63). In addition, like tamoxifen, resistance to inhibition is reported with long-term therapy in athymic mice with MCF-7 cell tumors (87).

Toremifene is easily absorbed and extensively metabolized in humans (110,112). The elimination half-lives for toremifene and its major metabolite N-desmethyltoremifene were long at 6.2 and 21 ds, respectively. These long half-lives may be a result of extensive tissue-specific metabolism, enterohepatic circulation, and plasma protein binding. Toremifene shows estrogenicity in the postmenopausal patient with slight increase in SHBG, and a slight decrease in the gonadotropins (FSH, LH) (113). Like tamoxifen, toremifene is estrogenic on the histology of the postmenopausal endometrium (114).

Toremifene is FDA approved for the treatment of metastatic breast cancer. In clinical trails versus tamoxifen, toremifene has shown similar efficacy (115–117). Patients who are resistant to tamoxifen also appear to be resistant to toremifene (118,119). Toremifene does not produce DNA adducts in rat liver and has a reduced ability to induce rat liver tumors in comparison to tamoxifen (108,120). Therefore, if concerns about the hepatocarcinogenicity of tamoxifen are founded toremifene may be an appropriate replacement for tamoxifen in breast cancer treatment (121).

Droloxifene

Droloxifene or 3-hydroxytamoxifen was developed by modifying the tamoxifen metabolite 3,4-hydroxytamoxifen leaving it hydroxlyated in the 3 position (see Fig. 4). Unlike its derivative, 3,4-hydroxytamoxifen, it has a high-binding affinity for the estrogen receptor. In fact in comparison to tamoxifen, droloxifene has a 10-fold higher binding affinity to the estrogen receptor (122,123).

Droloxifene is more effective in inhibiting the growth of ER positive breast cancer cells than tamoxifen (123,124). In addition, droloxifene induces TGF-β production in greater proportion than either tamoxifen or toremifene (123). Droloxifene has demonstrated antitumor activity in several animal models including NMU-induced tumors and in ER-positive breast tumors implanted into athymic mice (125,126). Droloxifene is a weaker estrogen and a more potent antiestrogen in the rat immature uterine weight test when compared to tamoxifen (85,124). Studies by Ke et al. have demonstrated that not only does droloxifene maintain bone density in the ovarectomized rat model, but that there was no significant increase in uterine size or epithelial thickness associated with treatment (127).

Droloxifene is rapidly excreted and does not accumulate like tamoxifen and toremifene and has a half life of only 27 h at a dose of 100 mg daily. There are several metabolites of droloxifene and all are present in serum as both free and glucuronide conjugates. This is different from both tamoxifen and toremifene which do not have appreciable levels of serum glucuronide metabolites (128,129). Therefore, although a potent analog at the estrogen receptor, secondary to its short half life, five times the daily dose of tamoxifen is currently in clinical trials (100 mg daily). At this dose, SHBG increases while the levels of the gonadotropins decrease (122,130). There have been several clinical trials involving droloxifene in patients with metastatic breast carcinoma with varying results (131–133). In rats droloxifene does not produce DNA adducts or induce hepatocellular carcinoma (123). In addition, droloxifene is inactive in the ability to transform Syrian hamster embryo cells in vitro, whereas tamoxifen and its metabolite 4-hydroxytamoxifen produce a significant level of transformation further supporting droloxifene's potential as a nontumorogenic compound (134).

Idoxifene

Idoxifene was designed to take advantage of the antiestrogenicity of tamoxifen whereas reducing potential carcinogenicity thought to be secondary to tamoxifen metabolites. Therefore, idoxifene is the result of modification of tamoxifen's most antiestrogenic metabolite 4-hydroxytamoxifen. An iodine was placed at the "4" position to prevent rapid glucuronidation, urinary excretion and to prolong tissue-specific half-life. Furthermore in order to avoid liver carcinogenicity thought to be associated with the alkylaminoethoxy side chain of tamoxifen and formaldehyde production a pyrrolidine ring was substituted for the dimethylamino group of tamoxifen (*see* Fig. 4) *(135)*.

Idoxifene has a binding affinity for the ER that is about 2.5- to fivefold that of tamoxifen *(135)*. Therefore, idoxifene is slightly more effective in the inhibition of ER positive MCF-7 breast cancer cell growth *(136)*. Idoxifene demonstrates antitumor properties in the N-nitrosomethylurea (NMU)-induced rat mammary carcinoma model *(136)*. Idoxifene is less potent antiestrogen in the immature uterine rat assay when compared to tamoxifen conversely, it is less uterotropic when administered alone.

Idoxifene was designed to circumvent the toxicity problems associated with liver carcinogenicity associated with tamoxifen while having affinity for the ER and being metabolically stable *(86,137)*. Preliminary studies with radioiodine 125 and 131 demonstrated no metabolism up to 48 h after administration, but further metabolic studies have not been reported *(138,139)*. Idoxifene in phase I trials had an initial half-life of 15 h with a mean terminal half-life of 23.3 d. Pace et al. have reported 100 times less DNA liver adduct formation associated with idoxifene treatment as compared to tamoxifen *(140)*. There have been no published evaluations concerning idoxifene and rat liver carcinogenisis.

TAT-59

TAT-59 is a derivative of the most antiestrogenic tamoxifen metabolite, 4-hydroxytamoxifen (Fig. 4). 4-Hydroxytamoxifen (4-OH-TAM) is a potent antiestrogen in vitro, while in vivo high doses are required to produce equivalent effects secondary to its rapid phase II metabolism *(141,142)*. TAT-59 drug was designed to take advantage of the potent antiestrogenicity of the tamoxifen metabolite, 4-hydroxytamoxifen (4-OH-TAM) whereas protecting it from phase II metabolism. Therefore, TAT-59 is phosphorylated at the 4-hydroxy position.

TAT-59 shows similar binding affinity to the ER as does it metabolite 4-OH-TAT-59. 4-OH-TAT-59 and 4-OH-TAM were found to be equivalent in binding to the rat uterine ER *(143,144)*. In ER positive MCF-7 cells 4-OH-TAT-59 was more effective in inhibiting growth than 4-OH-TAM *(145)*. In a comparison with other SERMs TAT-59 was more effective than droloxifene, toremifene, and tamoxifen in MCF-7 cell growth inhibition *(146)*. Compared to tamoxifen, TAT-59 was 10 times more effective against dimethylbenzanthracene (DMBA)-induced mammary tumors in rats *(147)*. Toko et al. reported higher levels of TGF-β in conditioned media from ER positive MCF-7 cells treated with 4-OH-TAT-59 compared to those treated with 4-OH-TAM. Additionally, this conditioned media was able to inhibit growth in ER-negative cell lines. There have been no published human trials of this drug currently under investigation primarily in Japan.

Benzothiophenes

Raloxifene

Raloxifene is a compound derived from a benzothiophene family of antiestrogens with a high affinity for the ER that is antiestrogenic in the rat uterus while being estrogenic at the level of rat bone and lipids (Fig. 4) *(148,149)*. Raloxifene binds the ER with slightly higher affinity than that of estradiol and is unique in its a lack of uterotropic effect in ovariectomized rats *(148,150)*.

Raloxifene inhibits the growth of MCF-7 cells and ZR-75-1 cells in culture *(150,151)*. In addition, it inhibits the growth of both NMU and DMBA induced tumors in mice *(152,153)*. Raloxifene was shown to reduce cholesterol and maintain bone density in the ovariectomized rat *(154–156)*. Raloxifene exhibits an extremely low degree of estrogenicity, in the immature rat uterine weight test. A unique feature of raloxifene in the uterotrophic assay is that as the dose of the compound increases, the modest increase in uterine weight seen at lower doses decreases *(124,148,156)*.

Raloxifene is rapidly absorbed and cleared from the circulation with the serum half-life of 12 h associated with a 200-mg oral dose *(157,158)*. Raloxifene is subject to conjugation with glucuronide acid and/or sulfate and primarily excreted in the feces *(159,160)*. No rat liver hepatocarcinogenicity studies have been published, although rats given dosages of 25 mg/kg per d did not develop hepatocellular carcinomas *(161)*. Raloxifene was not genotoxic, with or without metabolic activation in any of the in vitro or in vivo test systems used including: Ames assay, unscheduled DNA repair synthesis test, mouse lymphoma assay, sister chromatid exchange test, mouse micronucleus test, and the chromosome aberration assay *(162)*.

CLINICAL USE OF SERMS AND FINDINGS
Raloxifene

Clinical Studies

Raloxifene was first studied in humans in a limited fashion in 1982 as a possible treatment for metastatic breast cancer. Large-scale clinical trials were not initiated until 1994, primarily to assess its efficacy in the prevention and treatment of osteoporosis in otherwise healthy postmenopausal women. To date, more than 14,000 women worldwide have been enrolled in raloxifene studies, of whom 8000 women were assigned treatment with raloxifene. Although most of these studies are ongoing, interim and short-term results have been published.

Effect on Bone

Raloxifene has been found to preserve bone density in postmenopausal women. Treatment with 60 mg daily for 2 yr was found to increase bone density (compared to calcium-supplemented placebo groups) of the lumbar spine by 2.4 ± 0.4 percent, the total hip by 2.4 ± 0.4 percent (Fig. 5), the femoral neck by 2.5 ± 0.4 percent, and the total body by 2.0 ± 0.4 percent. All of these changes were statistically significant. This study also evaluated the 30 mg and 150 mg daily doses of raloxifene, which had essentially the same effects on bone density as the 60 mg dose *(163)*. A second study evaluated women who had previously undergone hysterectomy, and were randomly assigned to treatment with conjugated equine estrogen 0.625 mg daily, raloxifene 60 mg daily, or to calcium-supple-

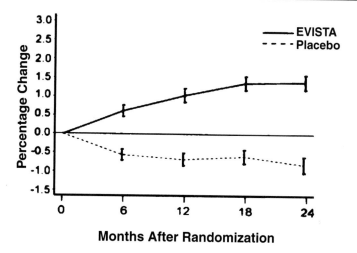

Fig. 5. Mean percent change in bone mineral density of the total hip in postmenopausal women given Raloxifene 60 mg daily (solid lines) or placebo (dotted lines) for 2 yr. The bars show the standard errors for the median changes.

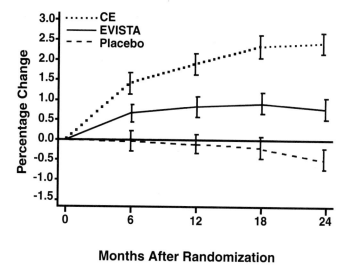

Fig. 6. Mean percent change in bone mineral density of the total hip in hysterectomized postmenopausal women given conjugated estrogens 0.625 mg daily (dotted lines), Raloxifene 60 mg daily (solid lines), or placebo (dashed lines) for 2 yr. The bars show the standard errors for the median changes.

mented placebo. Compared to the placebo group, treatment with estrogen for 2 yr was found to increase bone density of the total hip by 3.0%, which was double the 1.5% change seen with raloxifene 60 mg daily (Fig. 6) *(162)*. Based on these data, the Food and Drug Administration granted approval in December 1997 for the use of raloxifene, 60 mg daily, for the *prevention* of osteoporosis. The effect of raloxifene on the incidence of osteoporotic fractures is expected to be reported in the latter part of 1998. It is anticipated, however, that raloxifene will reduce the incidence of fractures because histomorphic evaluation of iliac crest bone biopsies in 10 women treated with raloxifene for 6 mo were normal. There was no evidence of mineralization defects, woven bone, marrow fibrosis,

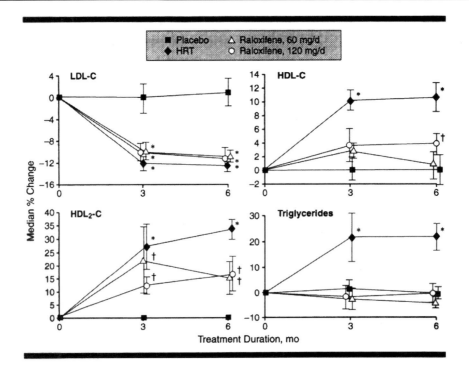

Fig. 7. Median percentage changes in LDL-C, HDL-C, HDL$_2$-C, and triglyceride levels in healthy postmenopausal women during six months' treatment with raloxifene 60 mg/d, raloxifene 120 mg/d, hormone replacement therapy (conjugated equine estrogen 0.625 mg/d and medroxyprogesterone acetate 2.5 mg/d), or placebo. The bars show the standard errors for the median changes.

osteomalacia, or osteocyte damage *(162)*. Bone formation rate per unit bone volume as well as activation frequency were decreased to a lesser extent with raloxifene compared to estrogen treatment *(162)*.

Effects on Markers of Cardiovascular Risk

Raloxifene favorably alters several markers of cardiovascular risk in healthy post-menopausal women, by lowering the levels of LDL-cholesterol, fibrinogen, and lipoprotein(a); and by not raising triglyceride levels. However, in contrast to HRT, raloxifene has no effect on HDL-C and PAI-1 levels and a lesser effect on HDL$_2$-C and lipoprotein(a) levels. This was shown in a clinical trial *(164)* (Figs. 7 and 8) of 390 healthy postmenopausal women who received one of four possible treatments for 6 mo: raloxifene 60 mg/d, raloxifene 120 mg/d, HRT (conjugated equine estrogen 0.625 mg/d and medroxyprogesterone acetate 2.5 mg/d), or placebo. Compared with placebo, both doses of raloxifene significantly lowered LDL-C by 12% ($p < 0.001$), similar to the 14% reduction seen with HRT ($p < 0.001$). Both doses of raloxifene significantly lowered lipoprotein(a) by 7–8% ($p < 0.001$), which was less than the 19% decrease observed with HRT ($p < 0.001$). Raloxifene increased HDL$_2$-C by 15%-17% ($p < 0.005$), which was less than the 33% elevation seen with HRT (p < 0.001). Raloxifene did not significantly change HDL-C, triglycerides, and PAI-1; whereas HRT increased HDL-C by 10% and triglycerides by 20%, and decreased PAI-1 by 19% (for all, $p < 0.001$). Raloxifene significantly lowered fibrinogen by 10–12% ($p < 0.001$), unlike HRT which had no

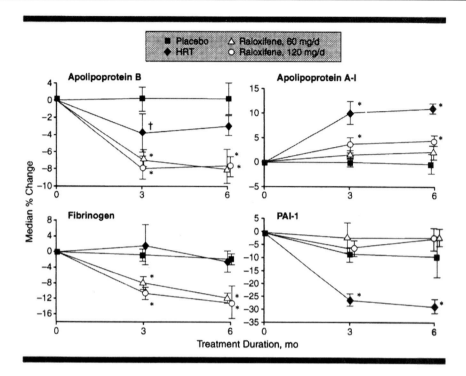

Fig. 8. Median percentage changes in apolipoproteins A-I and B, fibrinogen, and PAI-1 levels in healthy postmenopausal women during 6 months' treatment with raloxifene 60 mg/d, raloxifene 120 mg/d, hormone replacement therapy (conjugated equine estrogen 0.625 mg/d and medroxyprogesterone acetate 2.5 mg/d), or placebo. The bars show the standard errors for the median changes.

effect. Neither treatment changed index of coagulation activation, fibrinopeptideA, or prothrombin fragment. For all these effects, there were no significant differences between the two doses tested.

The decrease in LDL-cholesterol induced by raloxifene would be expected to reduce the risk of coronary artery disease. Epidemiological studies have found that the levels of LDL-C are related to risk of coronary artery disease among both men and women. Moreover, clinical trials that lowered LDL-cholesterol levels in women have been found to reduce the incidence of a second cardiac event. One such trial of a lipid-lowering agent found that a 30% reduction in LDL-cholesterol levels in women was associated with a 46% reduction in cardiovascular events *(165)*. This suggests that the 12% reduction in LDL levels observed in this study, if sustained over time, might lower the incidence of heart disease by as much as 18%. The 7% reduction in lipoprotein(a) levels may reduce this risk even more.

The decline in fibrinogen levels induced by raloxifene treatment may also serve to lower cardiovascular risk. Fibrinogen levels have been found to be an independent risk factor for heart disease, with a reduction of 0.5% for every 0.01 g/L decrease in fibrinogen levels *(166)*. We may hypothesize that the 0.42 g/L reduction in fibrinogen induced by raloxifene in this study could, therefore, translate into an additional 21% reduction in cardiovascular events. This is speculative, because there is no evidence to date from a clinical trial that shows that lowering the fibrinogen level of an individual will reduce her cardiovascular risk.

Table 1
Comparison of the effects of Raloxifene, Tamoxifen, and HRT on Markers
of Cardiovascular Risk in Healthy Postmenopausal Women.
Percentage Change Compared to Placebo Treatment

Cardiovascular Risk Marker	Tamoxifen 20 mg/d	Raloxifene 60 mg/d	HRT
LDL-Cholesterol	**−16***	**−12**	**−14**
HDL-Cholesterol	+2* 0	**+10**	
HDL$_2$-Cholesterol	**+2***	**+15**	**+33**
Triglycerides	0*	−4	**+20**
Apolipoprotein A1	**+7***	+3	**+12**
Apolipoprotein B	−7[†]	**−9**	−3
Lipoprotein(a)	**−32**[†]	−7	**−19**
Fibrinogen	**−24***	**−10**	−1
Plasminogen activator inhibitor-1	−15[‡]	+8	**−19**
Prothrombin fragment 1 and 2	+1[‡]	+5	**+19**
Fibrinopeptide A	+11[‡]	−4	+3

Data on raloxifene and HRT (hormone replacement therapy with conjugated equine
estrogen 0.625 mg/d and medroxyprogesterone acetate 2.5 mg/d) are from the current
study. Data on tamoxifen are from references *97,169,* and *170,* which reported the effect
from 3–6 mo treatment. Statistically significant changes are shown in boldface type.

Although there are similarities between the effects of raloxifene and estrogen on lipid
and coagulation factors, there are differences as well. This indicates that the serum levels
of these factors are controlled by processes which operate by independent mechanisms.
Some of these processes appear to be alterable by estrogen only, some by raloxifene only,
and some by both. This independence of mechanisms is consistent with the observation
that the magnitudes of the changes in LDL, HDL, and triglyceride levels induced by
estrogen treatment are not significantly correlated within individual subjects. *(167)* One
noteworthy difference between estrogen and raloxifene is in their effect on HDL-choles-
terol, HDL$_2$-cholesterol, and apolipoprotein A1 levels, which were only marginally
increased by raloxifene. Raloxifene, therefore, does not appear to have full agonist activity
against the target(s) that estrogen modulates to increase HDL. In contrast, LDL-cholesterol lowering represents an estrogen-agonist effect of raloxifene and is similar in magnitude to the estrogen effect. This is consistent with the in vitro observation that raloxifene
lowers LDL-C by binding to the estrogen receptor *(168)*.

In contrast, the effect of raloxifene on markers of cardiovascular risk bore a greater
resemblance to the pattern previously reported for tamoxifen (Table 1) *(97,169,170)*.
Because these data are not derived from the same clinical trial, the percent changes seen
may not be directly comparable among the different treatment groups. However, these
trials were all performed in similar groups of healthy postmenopausal women, and illustrate that the raloxifene and tamoxifen effect on HDL-C, HDL$_2$-C and apolipoprotein A1
are both distinctly smaller than estrogen's effect. The overall similarity of the effects of
raloxifene and tamoxifen is noteworthy, since the changes induced by tamoxifen on
cardiovascular risk markers could be responsible for its apparent cardioprotective effect.

This cardioprotective effect is supported by the observation that postmenopausal women with breast cancer who received tamoxifen in a randomized, controlled clinical trial were found to have a significantly lower incidence of fatal myocardial infarction (odds ratio, 0.37; 95% confidence 0.18 to 0.77) (6). In another such controlled clinical trial (98), women randomized to tamoxifen treatment had fewer hospital admissions due to cardiac disease (relative risk, 0.68; 95% confidence interval, 0.48–0.97). A third such trial (171) found a trend toward fewer cardiovascular deaths in women given tamoxifen, but this did not reach statistical significance (relative risk, 0.85; 95% confidence interval, 0.47–1.58). The Tamoxifen Breast Cancer Prevention Trial showed no difference in myocardial infarction rates between the tamoxifen and placebo groups, which could be due to the young age and premenopausal status of the participants and limited duration of treatment.

In summary, raloxifene favorably alters a number of lipid and coagulation markers of cardiovascular risk. For the most part, the direction of the response parallels that of HRT, although not necessarily of the same magnitude. The pattern of response bears a greater similarity to tamoxifen than HRT. Because of these beneficial effects on biochemical markers of cardiovascular risk, it can be speculated that raloxifene might reduce the risk of heart disease in postmenopausal women. Conclusive proof would require a clinical trial with cardiovascular events as the definitive endpoint. Such a study is currently underway.

Effect on Venous Thromboembolic Disease (VTE)

To date, there have been 51 episodes of VTE experienced by women enrolled in raloxifene trials: 19 had pulmonary emboli and 32 had deep vein thrombosis (172). The relative risk of VTE with raloxifene treatment is 3.4 (95% confidence interval, 1.5–8.0), which is similar to that reported for postmenopausal estrogen treatment (173–175). The greatest risk for VTE appeared during the first 4 mo of treatment. Many of these cases occurred in women who had a prior history of thrombophlebitis. For this reason, a past history of VTE is one of the few contraindications to raloxifene treatment (the others are hepatic dysfunction and premenopausal use). Because of this risk, patients should be advised to discontinue raloxifene at least 72 h prior to prolonged immobilization (e.g., for elective surgery) and to resume it only when fully ambulatory.

Effect on the Uterus

Raloxifene does not appear to stimulate the endometrium. The incidence of vaginal bleeding over the course of 2 yr was 3.0% with the 60 mg dose, and 2.2% with placebo (163). In a 6 month study with an estrogen/progestin treatment arm, the rates of bleeding in women with intact uteri was 6% for both 60 mg of raloxifene and for placebo. This was considerably lower than the 64% incidence with hormone treatment. (167) Thus, episodes of vaginal bleeding, which occur during raloxifene treatment, warrant clinical evaluation.

A 12-mo study found no histopathologic changes in endometrial biopsies obtained in 43 raloxifene-treated women. In contrast, 13 of 37 women treated with estrogen-developed proliferative changes (162). Endometrial thickness was also assessed in a 2-yr study of 831 women who underwent transvaginal ultrasound every 6 mo. Endometrial thickness was indistinguishable between the raloxifene and placebo-treated groups (163). To date, there have been 12 new cases of endometrial cancer in women enrolled in raloxifene studies. The relative risk of endometrial cancer for raloxifene users was not increased at 0.84 (95% confidence interval: 0.25–2.87) (172).

Effect on the Breast

Raloxifene does not appear to cause breast tenderness. The incidence of breast tenderness over the course of 2 yr was 3.3% with the 60 mg dose, and 2.0% with placebo *(163)*. In a 6 mo study with an estrogen/progestin treatment arm, the rate of breast tenderness was 4% for 60 mg of raloxifene and 6% for placebo, which was much lower than the 38% incidence with hormone treatment *(164)*. To date, there have been 45 new cases of breast cancer in women enrolled in raloxifene studies. The relative risk of breast cancer for raloxifene users was significantly lower at 0.33 (95% confidence interval: 0.19–0.52). Of those 45 women, 25 were diagnosed after taking study drug for more than 18 mo. For this subgroup, the relative risk of breast cancer among raloxifene users was even lower at 0.23 (95% confidence interval 0.10–0.49). The apparent protective effect of raloxifene appeared to be limited to estrogen receptor positive tumors. Inclusion and exclusion of the small number of cases of ductal carcinoma *in situ* did not alter the results *(176)*.

Effect on the Central Nervous System

Raloxifene appears to increase the incidence of hot flashes. The difference in the incidence of hot flashes between raloxifene and placebo-treated groups is 5–6% in prior studies *(163,164)*. Moreover, raloxifene is not an appropriate treatment for women who seek relief from menopausal symptoms. The effect of raloxifene on cognitive functioning and on the incidence of Alzheimer's disease is unknown.

Tamoxifen

Clinical Studies

Tamoxifen has been used for the treatment of advanced breast cancer in the United States since 1978. Tamoxifen has been found to prolong survival for women with both node-positive and node-negative breast cancer, and to prevent the occurrence of contralateral breast cancer *(177,178)*. Initially, there were concerns that tamoxifen, acting as an estrogen-antagonist, would predispose women to osteoporosis and heart disease. On the contrary, tamoxifen was actually found to increase bone density *(99)*, lower LDL-cholesterol and fibrinogen levels *(97)*, and to reduce the incidence of myocardial infarction *(6,98)*. Tamoxifen was found to increase the incidence of endometrial cancer *(4)*. Thus, it appears that for most organs (except most notably for breast), tamoxifen acts like an estrogen.

Because tamoxifen has been found to prevent contralateral breast cancer, it could play a role in the prevention of breast cancer in high-risk women. To answer that question, a multicenter study enrolled 13,000 women into a placebo-controlled clinical trial. Subjects were required to be older than 35 yr, and to be at increased risk of breast cancer, equal to that of the average 60-year-old woman. A large number of subjects were premenopausal: 40% were younger than age 49. The study was terminated 14 mo early because a clear treatment benefit for the reduction of breast cancer was observed. The mean duration of treatment was 4 yr. The relative risks (95% confidence intervals) of breast cancer with tamoxifen treatment was reduced in all age groups: for ages 49 and under: 0.65 (0.43–0.98); for ages 50–59: 0.52 (0.32–0.85); and for ages 60 and over: 0.47 (0.29–0.77) *(179)*. The reduction in risk was observed for both invasive breast cancer as well as for ductal carcinoma *in situ* (Table 2). Of interest is that tamoxifen treatment was also found to increase endometrial cancer (relative risk, 2.4) and to decrease bone fractures

Table 2
Tamoxifen Breast Cancer Prevention Trial: Clinical Outcomes

Outcome	Placebo group	Tamoxifen group	Relative risk
Malignancies (total)	256	203	0.79
Breast, invasive	154	85	0.55
Endometrial	14	33	2.36
Other	88	85	0.97
Breast, ductal cancer in situ	59	31	0.52
Thromboembolic events			
Pulmonary emboli	6	17	2.8
Deep vein thrombosis	19	30	1.6
Cardiovascular events			
Myocardial infarction	28	27	0.96
Anginal surgery	12	12	1.00
Stroke	24	34	1.41
Fractures (total)	71	47	0.66
Hip	20	9	0.45
Colles'	12	7	0.58
Spine	39	31	0.79

Table 3
The Effects of Estradiol and Selected Antiestrogens on Physiologic Systems

	Estradiol	ICI 182,780	Tamoxifen	Toremifene	Raloxifene	Droloxifene	Idoxifene
Breast tissue	↑	↓	↓	↓	↓	↓	↓
Bone	↑	—	↑	↑	↑	↑	—
HDL-c	↑	NC	NC	↑	NC	NC	—
LDL-c	↓	NC	↓	↓	↓	↓	—
SHBG	↑	NC	↑	↑	↑	↑	NC
Endometrium	↑	NC	↑	↑	↓	—	—
Vasomotor instability	↓	NC	↑	↑	↑	↑	—
FSH/LH	↓	NC	↓	↓	↓	↓	↓

NC = No significant change; — = No data available.

(relative risk, 0.66). There was no difference in myocardial infarction rates between the tamoxifen and placebo groups, which could be due to the young age and premenopausal status of many of the participants as well as the limited duration of treatment.

CONCLUSIONS

The development of tamoxifen has created multiple opportunities for drug design with applications throughout medicine. This review has described the properties of several agents being tested and has discussed the multiple therapeutic options for these agents that modulate estrogen signaling. Evaluations of these new compounds have led to a greater understanding, not only of antiestrogens, but also of the mechanisms of estrogen signaling in general. All of the drugs discussed in this article require further evaluation to define their effects on the endometrium, bone mineral density, and lipid profiles, as well as to evaluate their potential negative side effects as compared to estrogen. Table 3 illustrates the principal differences of selected compounds discussed in this review.

Antiestrogens were used first as regulators of ovulation, and later as a treatment for breast cancer. Currently, compounds such as clomiphene, tamoxifen, toremifene, and raloxifene are in clinical use and other compounds are in clinical trials, while pure antiestrogens are in clinical trials for women with tamoxifen-resistant breast cancers. All of these compounds are designed to take advantage of our understanding of estrogen action on reproductive tissues as well as cardiovascular systems, bone metabolism, and neural function. Only after the collection of more data will an optimal regimen for postmenopausal HRT be defined. This will not only address the long-term health maintenance needs of postmenopausal women, but will overcome some of the current limitations of ERT. This regimen may be a single compound or involve a combination with estrogen. Further research into the role of estrogen signaling throughout the body will lead to the development of new compounds with many possible therapeutic applications. These lines of investigation create an exciting atmosphere for understanding of steroid hormone action and will clearly improve our treatment options for women in both the postreproductive and reproductive years.

REFERENCES

1. Kiel D, Felson D, Anderson J, Wilson P, Moskowitz M. Hip fracture and the use of estrogen in post menopausal women: the Framingham study. N Engl J Med 1987;317:1169–1174.
2. Colditz G, Willitt W, Stampfer M, Rosner B, Speizer F, Hennekens C. Menopause and the risk of heart disease in women. N Engl J Med 1987;316:1105–1110.
3. Paganini-Hill A, Henderson V. Estrogen deficiency and risk of Alzheimer's disease in women. Am J Epidemiol 1994;140:256–261.
4. van Leeuwen FE, Benraadt J, Coebergh JW, Kiemeney LA, Gimbrere CH, Otter R, Schouten LJ, Damhuis RA, Bontenbal M, Diepenhorst FW, van den Belt-Dousebout A, van Tinteren H. Risk of endometrial cancer after tamoxifen treatment of breast cancer. Lancet 1994;343(8895):448–452.
5. Ward R, Morgan G, Dalley D, Kelly P. Tamoxifen reduces bone turnover and prevents lumbar spine and proximal femoral bone loss in early postmenopausal women. Bone and Mineral 1993;22:87–94.
6. McDonald C, Stewart H. Fatal myocardial infarction in the Scottish adjuvant tamoxifen trial. The Scottish Breast Cancer Committee. BMJ 1991;303:435–437.
7. Kastner P, Mark M, Chambon P. Nonsteroid nuclear receptors: what are genetic studies telling us about their role in real life? Cell 1995;83(6):859–869.
8. Mangelsdorf DJ, Evans RM. The RXR heterodimers and orphan receptors. Cell 1995;83(6):841–850.
9. Tsai MJ, O'Malley BW. Molecular mechanisms of action of steroid/thyroid receptor superfamily members. Annu Rev Biochem 1994;63:451–486.
10. Parker M, Arbuckle N, Daubois S, et al. Structure and function of the estrogen receptor. Ann NY Acad Sci 1993;684:119–126.
11. Bourguet W, Ruff M, Chambon P, Gronemeyer H, Moras D. Crystal structure of the ligand-binding domain of the human nuclear receptor RXR-alpha. Nature 1995;375(6530):377–382.
12. Fritsch M, Leary CM, Furlow JD, Ahrens H, Schuh TJ, Mueller GC, Gorski J. A ligand-induced conformational change in the estrogen receptor is localized in the steroid binding domain. Biochemistry 1992;31(23):5303–5311.
13. Beekman JM, Allan GF, Tsai SY, Tsai MJ, O'Malley BW. Transcriptional activation by the estrogen receptor requires a conformational change in the ligand binding domain. Mol Endocrinol 1993;7(10):1266–1274.
14. Zhuang Y, Katzenellenbogen BS, Shapiro DJ. Estrogen receptor mutants which do not bind 17 beta-estradiol dimerize and bind to the estrogen response element in vivo. Mol Endocrinol 1995;9(4):457–466.

15. Murdoch FE, Gorski J. The role of ligand in estrogen receptor regulation of gene expression. Mol Cell Endocrinol 1991;78(3):103–108.
16. Pratt W, Welsh M. Chaperone functions of the heat shock proteins associated with steroid receptors. Semin Cell Biol 1994;5:83–93.
17. Klein-Hitpass L, Schorpp M, Wagner U, Ryffel GU. An estrogen-responsive element derived from the 5' flanking region of the Xenopus vitellogenin A2 gene functions in transfected human cells. Cell 1986;46(7):1053–1061.
18. Seiler-Tuyns A, Walker P, Martinez E, Merillat AM, Givel F, Wahli W. Identification of estrogen-responsive DNA sequences by transient expression experiments in a human breast cancer cell line. Nucleic Acids Res 1986;14(22):8755–8770.
19. Burbach JP, Lopes da Silva S, Cox JJ, Adan RA, Cooney AJ, Tsai MJ, Tsai SY. Repression of estrogen-dependent stimulation of the oxytocin gene by chicken ovalbumin upstream promoter transcription factor I. J Biol Chem 1994;269(21):15,046–15,053.
20. Evans RM. The steroid and thyroid hormone receptor superfamily. Science 1988;240(4854):889–895.
21. Beato M, Sanchez-Pacheco A. Interaction of steroid hormone receptors with the transcription initiation complex. Endocr Rev 1996;17(6):587–609.
22. Glass CK, Holloway JM, Devary OV, Rosenfeld MG. The thyroid hormone receptor binds with opposite transcriptional effects to a common sequence motif in thyroid hormone and estrogen response elements. Cell 1988;54(3):313–323.
23. Segars JH, Marks MS, Hirschfeld S, Driggers PH, Martinez E, Grippo JF, Brown M, Wahli W, Ozato K. Inhibition of estrogen-responsive gene activation by the retinoid X receptor beta: evidence for multiple inhibitory pathways [published erratum appears in Mol Cell Biol 1993 Jun;13(6):3840]. Mol Cell Biol 1993;13(4):2258–2268.
24. Ambrosino C, Cicatiello L, Cobellis G, Addeo R, Sica V, Bresciani F, Weisz A. Functional antagonism between the estrogen receptor and Fos in the regulation of c-fos protooncogene transcription. Mol Endocrinol 1993;7(11):1472–1483.
25. Zawel L, Reinberg D. Common themes in assembly and function of eukaryotic transcription complexes. Annu Rev Biochem 1995;64:533–561.
26. Ha I, Roberts S, Maldonado E, Sun X, Kim LU, Green M, Reinberg D. Multiple functional domains of human transcription factor IIB: distinct interactions with two general transcription factors and RNA polymerase II. Genes Dev 1993;7(6):1021–1032.
27. Hisatake K, Roeder RG, Horikoshi M. Functional dissection of TFIIB domains required for TFIIB-TFIID-promoter complex formation and basal transcription activity. Nature 1993;363(6431):744–747.
28. Jacq X, Brou C, Lutz Y, Davidson I, Chambon P, Tora L. Human TAFII30 is present in a distinct TFIID complex and is required for transcriptional activation by the estrogen receptor. Cell 1994;79(1):107–117.
29. LeDouarin B, Zechel C, Garnier JM, Lutz Y, Tora L, Pierrat P, Heery D, Gronemeyer H, Chambon P, Losson R. The N-terminal part of TIF1, a putative mediator of the ligand- dependent activation function (AF-2) of nuclear receptors, is fused to B-raf in the oncogenic protein T18. Embo J 1995;14(9):2020–2033.
30. Onate SA, Tsai SY, Tsai MJ, O'Malley BW. Sequence and characterization of a coactivator for the steroid hormone receptor superfamily. Science 1995;270(5240):1354–1357.
31. Cavailles V, Dauvois S, F LH, Lopez G, Hoare S, Kushner PJ, Parker MG. Nuclear factor RIP140 modulates transcriptional activation by the estrogen receptor. Embo J 1995;14(15):3741–3751.
32. Cavailles V, Dauvois S, Danielian PS, Parker MG. Interaction of proteins with transcriptionally active estrogen receptors. Proc Natl Acad Sci USA 1994;91(21):10,009–10,013.
33. Halachmi S, Marden E, Martin G, MacKay H, Abbondanza C, Brown M. Estrogen receptor-associated proteins: possible mediators of hormone-induced transcription. Science 1994;264(5164):1455–1458.
34. Chen JD, Evans RM. A transcriptional co-repressor that interacts with nuclear hormone receptors. Nature 1995;377(6548):454–457.
35. Horlein AJ, Naar AM, Heinzel T, Torchia J, Gloss B, Kurokawa R, Ryan A, Kamei Y, Soderstrom M, Glass CK, et al. Ligand-independent repression by the thyroid hormone receptor mediated by a nuclear receptor co-repressor. Nature 1995;377(6548):397–404.
36. Katzenellenbogen JA, O'Malley BW, Katzenellenbogen BS. Tripartite steroid hormone receptor pharmacology: interaction with multiple effector sites as a basis for the cell- and promoter-specific action of these hormones. Mol Endocrinol 1996;10(2):119–131.
37. Horwitz KB, Jackson TA, Bain DL, Richer JK, Takimoto GS, Tung L. Nuclear receptor coactivators and corepressors. Mol Endocrinol 1996;10(10):1167–1177.

38. Kamei Y, Xu L, Heinzel T, Torchia J, Kurokawa R, Gloss B, Lin SC, Heyman RA, Rose DW, Glass CK, Rosenfeld MG. A CBP integrator complex mediates transcriptional activation and AP-1 inhibition by nuclear receptors. Cell 1996;85(3):403–414.

39. Mosselman S, Polman J, Dijkema R. ER beta: identification and characterization of a novel human estrogen receptor. FEBS Lett 1996;392(1):49–53.

40. Kuiper GG, Enmark E, Pelto-Huikko M, Nilsson S, Gustafsson JA. Cloning of a novel receptor expressed in rat prostate and ovary. Proc Natl Acad Sci U S A 1996;93(12):5925–5930.

41. Kuiper GG, Gustafsson JA. The novel estrogen receptor-beta subtype: potential role in the cell- and promoter-specific actions of estrogens and anti-estrogens. FEBS Lett 1997;410(1):87–90.

42. Hess RA, Bunick D, Lee KH, Bahr J, Taylor JA, Korach KS, Lubahn DB. A role for oestrogens in the male reproductive system. Nature 1997;390(6659):509–512.

43. Korach KS. Insights from the study of animals lacking functional estrogen receptor. Science 1994;266(5190):1524–1527.

44. O'Malley B, Schrader WT, Mani S, Smith C, Weigel NL, Conneely OM, Clark JH. An alternative ligand-independent pathway for activation of steroid receptors. Recent Prog Horm Res 1995;50:333–347.

45. Kato S, Endoh H, Masuhiro Y, Kitamoto T, Uchiyama S, Sasaki H, Masushige S, Gotoh Y, Nishida E, Kawashima H, Metzger D, Chambon P. Activation of the estrogen receptor through phosphorylation by mitogen- activated protein kinase. Science 1995;270(5241):1491–1494.

46. Katzenellenbogen BS, Fang H, Ince BA, Pakdel F, Reese JC, Wooge CH, Wrenn CK, William L. McGuire Memorial Symposium. Estrogen receptors: ligand discrimination and antiestrogen action. Breast Cancer Res Treat 1993;27(1–2):17–26.

47. Bunone G, Briand PA, Miksicek RJ, Picard D. Activation of the unliganded estrogen receptor by EGF involves the MAP kinase pathway and direct phosphorylation. Embo J 1996;15(9):2174–2183.

48. Ignar-Trowbridge DM, Teng CT, Ross KA, Parker MG, Korach KS, McLachlan JA. Peptide growth factors elicit estrogen receptor-dependent transcriptional activation of an estrogen-responsive element. Mol Endocrinol 1993;7(8):992–998.

49. Power RF, Mani SK, Codina J, Conneely OM, O'Malley BW. Dopaminergic and ligand-independent activation of steroid hormone receptors. Science 1991;254(5038):1636–1639.

50. Smith C, Conneely O, O'Malley B. Modulation of the ligand-independent activation of the human estrogen receptor by hormone and antihormone. Proc Natl Acad Sci U S A 1993;90(13):6120–6124.

51. Aronica SM, Katzenellenbogen BS. Stimulation of estrogen receptor-mediated transcription and alteration in the phosphorylation state of the rat uterine estrogen receptor by estrogen, cyclic adenosine monophosphate, and insulin-like growth factor-I. Mol Endocrinol 1993;7(6):743–752.

52. Ma ZQ, Santagati S, Patrone C, Pollio G, Vegeto E, Maggi A. Insulin-like growth factors activate estrogen receptor to control the growth and differentiation of the human neuroblastoma cell line SK-ER3. Mol Endocrinol 1994;8(7):910–918.

53. Denner LA, Weigel NL, Maxwell BL, Schrader WT, O'Malley BW. Regulation of progesterone receptor-mediated transcription by phosphorylation. Science 1990;250(4988):1740–1743.

54. Pietras RJ, Arboleda J, Reese DM, Wongvipat N, Pegram MD, Ramos L, Gorman CM, Parker MG, Sliwkowski MX, Slamon DJ. HER-2 tyrosine kinase pathway targets estrogen receptor and promotes hormone-independent growth in human breast cancer cells. Oncogene 1995;10(12):2435–2446.

55. Cho H, Katzenellenbogen BS. Synergistic activation of estrogen receptor-mediated transcription by estradiol and protein kinase activators. Mol Endocrinol 1993;7(3):441–452.

56. Rubino D, Driggers P, Arbit D, Kemp L, Miller B, Coso O, Pagliai K, Gray K, Gutkind S, Segars J. Characterization of Brx, a novel Dbl family member that modulates estrogen receptor action. Oncogene 1998;16(19):2513–2526.

57. Jensen E. Steroid Hormone Antagonist. Summary and future challenges. Ann N Y Acad Sci 1995;761:1–4.

58. Hedden A, Muller V, Jensen EV. A new interpretation of antiestrogen action. Ann N Y Acad Sci 1995;761:109–120.

59. Berthois Y, Pons M, Dussert C, Crastes de Paulet A, Martin PM. Agonist-antagonist activity of anti-estrogens in the human breast cancer cell line MCF-7: an hypothesis for the interaction with a site distinct from the estrogen binding site. Mol Cell Endocrinol 1994;99(2):259–268.

60. McDonnell DP, Clemm DL, Hermann T, Goldman ME, Pike JW. Analysis of estrogen receptor function in vitro reveals three distinct classes of antiestrogens. Mol Endocrinol 1995;9(6):659–669.

61. Kuiper GG, Carlsson B, Grandien K, Enmark E, Haggblad J, Nilsson S, Gustafsson JA. Comparison of the ligand binding specificity and transcript tissue distribution of estrogen receptors alpha and beta. Endocrinology 1997;138(3):863–870.

62. Adlercreutz H, Markkanen H, Watanabe S. Plasma concentrations of phyto-oestrogens in Japanese men. Lancet 1993;342(8881):1209–1210.

63. Colletta A, Wakefield L, Howell F, vanRoozendaal K, Danielpour D, Ebbs S, Sporn M, Baum M. Antiestrogens induce the secretion of active transforming growth factor beta from human fetal fibroblast. Br J Cancer 1990;62:405–409.

64. Wakefield L, Kim S-J, Glick A, Winokur T, Colletta A, Sporn M. Regulation of transforming growth factor-β subtypes by members of the steroid hormone superfamily. J Cell Sci Suppl 1990;13:139–148.

65. Wakefield LM, Sporn MB. Suppression of carcinogenesis: a role for TGF-βeta and related molecules in prevention of cancer. Immunol Ser 1990;51:217–243.

66. Wakeling A, Dukes M, Bowler J. A potent specific pure antiestrogen with clinical potential. Cancer Res 1991;51:3867–3873.

67. Wakeling A, Bowler J. Novel antiestrogens without partial agonist activity. J Steroid Biochem 1988;31:645–653.

68. Dauvois S, White R, Parker M. The antiestrogen ICI 182,780 disrupts estrogen receptor nucleocytoplasmic shuttling. J Cell Sci 1993;106:1377–1388.

69. Gibson M, Nemmas L, Beckman W, et al. The mechanism of ICI 164,384 antiestrogenicity involves rapid loss of estrogen receptor in uterine tissue. Endocrinology 1991;129:2000–2010.

70. Coopman P, Garcia M, Brunner N, et al. Antiproliferative and anti-estrogenic effects of ICI 164,384 and ICI 183,780 in 4–OH-tamoxifen resistant human breast cancer cells. Int J Cancer 1994;56:295–300.

71. Lykkesfeldt A, Madsen M, Briand P. Altered expression of estrogen-regulated genes in a tamoxifen-resistant and ICI 164,384 and ICI 182,780 in sensitive human breset cancer cell line, MCF-7/TAM[R]-1. Cancer Res 1994;54:1587–1595.

72. Brunner N, Frandsen TL, Holst-Hansen C, Bei M, Thompson EW, Wakeling AE, Lippman ME, Clarke R. MCF7/LCC2: a 4-hydroxytamoxifen resistant human breast cancer variant that retains sensitivity to the steroidal antiestrogen ICI 182,780. Cancer Res 1993;53(14):3229–3232.

73. Larsen SS, Madsen MW, Jensen BL, Lykkesfeldt AE. Resistance of human breast-cancer cells to the pure steroidal anti- estrogen ICI 182,780 is not associated with a general loss of estrogen- receptor expression or lack of estrogen responsiveness [In Process Citation]. Int J Cancer 1997;72(6):1129–1136.

74. Brunner N, Boysen B, Jirus S, Skaar TC, Holst-Hansen C, Lippman J, Frandsen T, Spang-Thomsen M, Fuqua SA, Clarke R. MCF7/LCC9: an antiestrogen-resistant MCF-7 variant in which acquired resistance to the steroidal antiestrogen ICI 182,780 confers an early cross-resistance to the nonsteroidal antiestrogen tamoxifen. Cancer Res 1997;57(16):3486–3493.

75. Dowsett M, Howell R, Salter J, et al. Effects of the pure anti-oestrogen ICI 182780 on oestrogen receptors, progesterone receptros and Ki67 antigen in human endometrium in vivo. Human Reprod 1995;10:262–267.

76. DeFriend D, Howell A, Nicholson R, et al. Investigation of a pure antiestrogen (ICI 182780) in women with primary breast cancer. Cancer Res 1994;54:408–414.

77. Howell A, DeFriend D, Robertson J, Blamey R, Anderson L, Anderson E, Sutcliffe F, Walton P. Pharmacokinetics, pharmacological and anti-tumour effects of the specific anti-oestrogen ICI 182780 in women with advanced breast cancer. Br J Cancer 1996;74(2):300–308.

78. Lerner L, Holthaus F, Thompson C. A non-steroidal estrogen antagonist 1-(p-diethylamino-ethoxyphenyl) 1-phenyl-2-p-methoxyphenyl ethanol Endocrinology 1958;63:295–318.

79. Lerner L. The first non-steroidal antioestogen—MER-25. In: Sutherland R, Jordan V, eds. Non-Steroidal Antioestroen: Molecular Pharmacclogy and Antitumour Activity. Academic, Sydney, 1986, pp. 1–16.

80. Kistner R, Smith O. Observations on the use of a non-steroidal estrogen antagonist: MER 25. Surg Forum 1960;10:725–729.

81. Kistner R, Smith O. Observations on the use of a non-steroidal estrogen antagonist MER 25 II. Effects in endometrial hyperplasia and Stein-Leventhal syndrome. Fertil Steril 1961;12:121–141.

82. Jordan V. A current view of tamoxifen for the treatment and prevention of breast cancer. Br J Pharmacol 1993;110:507–517.

83. Jordan V, ed. Long-Term Tamoxifen Treatment for Breast Cancer. University of Wisconsin Press, Madison, WI, 1994, pp. 1–289.

84. Katzenellenbogen BS, Montano MM, Le Goff P, Schodin DJ, Kraus WL, Bhardwaj B, Fujimoto N. Antiestrogens: mechanisms and actions in target cells. J Steroid Biochem Mol Biol 1995;53(1–6):387–393.

85. Loser R, Seibel K, Roos W, et al. In vivo and in vitro antiestrogenic action of 3-hydroxy-tamoxifen, tamoxifen, and 4-hydroxy-tamoxifen. Eur J Cancer Clin Oncol 1985;21:985–990.

86. McCague R, LeClercq G, Legros N, et al. Derivatives of tamoxifen. dependency of estrogenicity on the 4 substituent. J Med Chem 1989;32:2527–2533.

87. Osborne C, Jarman M, McCague R, et al. The importance of tamoxifen metabolism in tamoxifen-stimulated breast tumor growth. Cancer Chemother Pharmacol 1994;34:89–95.

88. Coezy E, Borgna JL, Rochefort H. Tamoxifen and metabolites in MCF7 cells: correlation between binding to estrogen receptor and inhibition of cell growth. Cancer Res 1982;42(1):317–323.

89. Allen K, Clark E, Jordan V. Evidence for the metabolic activation of non-steroidal anti-oestrogens: A study of structure-activity relationships. Br J Pharmacol 1980;71:83–89.

90. Poon G, Walter B, Lonning P, Horton M, McCague R. Identification of tamoxifen metabolites in human HEP G2 cell line, human liver homogenate adn patients on long tem therapy for breast cancer. Drug Metab Dispos 1995;23:377–382.

91. Fabian C, Sternson L, El-Serafi M, Cain L, Hearne E. Clinical pharmacology of tamoxifen in patients with breast cancer: correlation with clinical data. Cancer 1981;48(4):876–882.

92. Jordan V, Murphy C. Endocrine pharmacology of antiestrogens as antitumour agents. Endocrine Rev 1990;11:578–610.

93. Nogochi S, Matomura K, Inaji H, et al. down regulation of transforming growth- factor- alpha by tamoxifen in human breast cancer. Cancer 1993;72:131–136.

94. Knabbe C, Lippman M, Wakefield L, Flanders K, Kasid A, Derynck R, Dickson R. Evidence that transforming growth factor beta is a hormonally regulated negative growth factor in human breast cancer cells. Cell 1987;48:417–428.

95. "Nolvadex" Adjuvant Trial Organisation. Controlled trial of tamoxifen as a single adjuvant agent in the management of early breast cancer. Br J Cancer 1988;57(6):608–611.

96. Adjuvant tamoxifen in the management of operable breast cancer: the Scottish Trial. Report from the Breast Cancer Trials Committee, Scottish Cancer Trials Office (MRC), Edinburgh. Lancet 1987;2(8552):171–175.

97. Grey AB, Stapleton JP, Evans MC, Reid IR. The effect of the anti-estrogen tamoxifen on cardiovascular risk factors in normal postmenopausal women. J Clin Endocrinol Metab 1995;80(11):3191–3195.

98. Rutqvist LE, Mattsson A. Cardiac and thromboembolic morbidity among postmenopausal women with early-stage breast cancer in a randomized trial of adjuvant tamoxifen. The Stockholm Breast Cancer Study Group. J Natl Cancer Inst 1993;85(17):1398–1406.

99. Love RR, Mazess RB, Barden HS, Epstein S, Newcomb PA, Jordan VC, Carbone PP, DeMets DL. Effects of tamoxifen on bone mineral density in postmenopausal women with breast cancer. N Engl J Med 1992;326(13):852–856.

100. Luciani L, Oriana S, Spatti G, et al. Hormonal and receptor status in postmenopausal women with endometrial cancer before and after treatment with tamoxifen. Tumori 1984;1984:189–192.

101. Jordan V, Fritz N, Langan-Fahey S, Thompson M, Tormey M. Alternation of endocrine parameters in premenopausal women with breast cancer during long-term adjuvant therapy with tamoxifen as a single agent. J Natl Cancer Inst 1991;83:1488–1491.

102. Hirsimaki P, Hirisimaki Y, Nieminen L. The Effects of tamoxifen citrate and toremifene citrate on the ultrastructure of the rat liver. Inst Phys Conf Ser 1988;6:643–658.

103. Williams G, Iatropoulos M, Djordjevic M, Kaltenberg O. The triphenylethylene drug tamoxifen is a strong liver carcinogen in the rat. Carcinogenisis 1993;14:315–317.

104. Carthew P, Martin E, White I, et al. Tamoxifen induces short term cumulative DNA damage and liver tumours in rats: promotion by phenobarbital. Cancer Res 1995;55(3):544–547.

105. Greaves P, Goonetilleke R, Nunn G, Topham J, et al. Two-year carcinogenicity study of tamoxifen in Alderly Park Wistar derived-rats. Cancer Res 1993;53:3919–3924.

106. Phillips D, Carmichael P, Hewer A, et al. Activation of tamoxifen and its metabolite α-hydroxytamoxifen to DNA-binding products: comparisons between human, rat, and mouse hepatocytes. Carcinogenesis 1996;17:89–94.

107. Jordan V, Piette M, Cisneros A. Metabolism of Antiestrogens. In: Lindsay R, Dempster D, Jordan V, eds. Estrogens and Antiestrogens: Basic and Clinical Aspects. Lippincott-Raven, Philiadelphia, PA, 1998, pp. 29–39.

108. Hard G, Iatropoulos M, Jordan K, Radi L, Kaltenberg O, Imordi A, Williams G. Major differences in hepatocarcinogenicity and DNA adduct forming ability between toremifene and tamoxifen in female Crl:CD (BR) rats. Cancer Res 1993;53:4534–4541.

109. Grenman R, Laine K, Klemi P, et al. effect of the antiestrogen toremifene on growth of the human mammary carcinoma cell line MCF-7. J Cancer Res Clin Oncol 1991;117:223–226.

110. Kangas L. Review of the pharmacological properties of toremifene. J Steroid Biochem 1990;36:191–195.

111. Robinson S, Jordan V. Antiestrogen action of toremifene on hormone dependent , independent and heterogenious breast tumor growth in the athymic mouse. Cancer Res 1989;49:1758–1762.

112. Anttila M, Valavaara R, Kivinen S, Maenpaa J. Pharmacokinetics of toremifene. J Steroid Biochem 1990;36:249–252.

113. Kivinen S, Maenpaa J. Effect of toremifene on clinical hematological and hormonal parameters at different dose levels in healthy postmenopausal volunteers: phase I study. J Steroid Biochem 1990;36:217–220.

114. Tomas E, Kauppila A, Blanco G, Apaja-Sarkkinen M, Laatikainen T. Comparison between the effects of tamoxifen and toremifene on the uterus in postmenopausal breast cancer patients. Gynecol Oncol 1995;59:261–266.

115. Ebbs S, Roberts J, Baum M. Response to toremifene (Fc-1157a) therapy in tamoxifen failed patients with breast cancer. Preliminary communication. J Steroid Biochem 1990;36(3):239.

116. Stenbygaard L, Herrstedt J, Thomsen J, Svendsen K, Engelholm S, Dombernowsky P. Tormeifene and tamoxifen in advanced breast cancer- a double blind crossover trial. Breast Cancer Res Treat 1993;25:57–63.

117. Hayes D, Van Zyl J, Hacking A, et al. Randomized comparison of tamoxifen and two separate doses of toremifene in post-menopausal patients with metastatic breast cancer. J Clin Oncol 1995;113:2556–2566.

118. Pyrhonen S, Valavaara R, Vuorinen J, Hajba A. High dose troemifene in advanced breast cancer resistant to or relapsed during tamoxifen treatment. Breast Cancer Res Treat 1994;29:223–228.

119. Vogel C, Shemano I, Schoenfelder J, et al. Multicenter phase II efficacy trial of toremifene in tamoxifen refractory patients with advanced breast cancer. J Clin Oncol 1993;11:345–350.

120. Dragan Y, Vaughn J, Jordan V, Pitot H. Comparison of tamoxifen and toremifene on liver and kidney tumor promotion in female rats. Carcinogenesis 1995;16(11):2733–2741.

121. Prentice R. Epidemiologic data on exogenous hormones and hepatocellualr carcinoma and selected other cancers. Prev Med 1991;20:38–46.

122. Kvinnsland S. Droloxifene: a new antiestrogen. Am J Clin Oncol [Suppl 2] 1991;14: S45–S51.

123. Hasman M, Rattel B, Loser R. Preclinical data for droloxifene. Cancer Lett 1994;84:101–116.

124. Eppenberger U, Wosikowski K, Kung W. Pharmacologic and biological properties of droloxifene, a new antiestrogen. Am J Clin Oncol [suppl 2] 1991;14: S5–S14.

125. Winterfeld G, Hauff P, Gorlich M, Arnold W, Fichtner I, Staab H. Investigations of droloxifene and other hormonal manipulations on N-nitrosomethyl-urea-induced rat mammary tumours. J Cancer Res Oncol 1992;119:91–96.

126. Kawamura I, Mizota T, Lacey E, Tanaka Y, Manda T, Shimomura K, Kohsaka M. Pharmacologic and biologic properties of droloxifene, a new antiestrogen. Jpn J Pharmacol 1993;63:27–34.

127. Ke H, Simmons H, Pirie C, Crawford D, Thompson D. Droloxifene, a new estrogen antagonist/agonist, prevents bone loss in ovariectomized rats. Endocrinology 1995;136:2435–2441.

128. Grill H, Pollow K. Pharmacokinetics of droloxifene and its metabolites in breast cancer patients. Am J Clin Oncol 1991;14 (supp 2): S30–S35.

129. Lein E, Ander G, Lonning P, et al. Determination of droloxifene and two metabolites in serum by high pressure liquid chromatography. Ther Drug Monit 1995;17:259–265.

130. Geisler J, Ekse D, Hosch S, et al. Influence of droloxifene (3–hydroxytamoxifen) 40 mg daily on plasma gonadotrophins, sex hormone binding globulin and estrogen levels in postmenopausal breast cancer patients. J Steroid Biochem Mol Biol 1995;55:193–195.

131. Buzdar A, Kau S, Hortobagyi G, et al. Phase I trial of droloxifene in patients with metastatic breast cancer. Cancer Chemother Pharmacol 1994;33:313–316.

132. Bellmunt J, Sole L. European early phase II dose finding study of droloxifene in advanced breast cancer. Am J Clin Oncol 1991;14:536–539.

133. Rausching W, Pritchard K. Droloxifene, a new antiestrogen: Its role in metastatic breast cancer. Breast Cancer Res Treat 1994;31:83–94.

134. Metzler M, Schiffmann D. Structural requirments for the in vitro transformation of Syrain hamster embryo cells by stilbene estrogens and triphenylthylene-type antiestrogens. Am J Clin Oncol 1991;14 (suppl 2): S30–S35.

135. Coombes RC, Haynes BP, Dowsett M, Quigley M, English J, Judson IR, Griggs LJ, Potter GA, McCague R, Jarman M. Idoxifene: report of a phase I study in patients with metastatic breast cancer. Cancer Res 1995;55(5):1070–1074.

136. Chander S, McCague R, Luqmani Y, Newton C, Dowsett M, Jarman M, Coombes R. Pyrrolidino-4-iodotamoxifen and 4-iodotamoxifen, new analogues of the antiestrogen tamoxifen for the treatment of breast cancer. Cancer Res 1991;51:5851–5858.

137. McCague R, Parr I, Haynes B. Metabolism of the 4 iodo derivative of tamoxifen by isolated rat hepatocytes. demonstration that the iodine atom reduces metabolic conversion and identification of four metabolites. Biochem Pharmacol 1990;40:2277–2283.

138. Carnochan P, Trivedi M, Young H, Eccles S, Potter G, Haynes B, Ott R. Biodistribution and kinetics of radiolabelled pyrrolidino-4-iodo-tamoxifen: prospects for pharmacokinetic studies using PET. J Nucl Biol Med 1994;38(4 Suppl 1):96–98.

139. Young H, Carnochan P, Trivedi M, Potter GA, Eccles SA, Haynes BP, Jarman M, Ott RJ. Pharmaco-kinetics and biodistribution of radiolabelled idoxifene: prospects for the use of PET in the evaluation of a novel antioestrogen for cancer therapy. Nucl Med Biol 1995;22(4):405–411.

140. Pace P, Jarman M, Phillips D, Hewer A, Bliss J, Coombes RC. Idoxifene is equipotent to tamoxifen in inhibiting mammary carcinogenesis but forms lower levels of hepatic DNA adducts. Br J Cancer 1997;76(6):700–704.

141. Jordan VC, Allen KE. Evaluation of the antitumour activity of the non-steroidal antioestrogen monohydroxytamoxifen in the DMBA-induced rat mammary carcinoma model. Eur J Cancer 1980;16(2):239–251.

142. Gottardis MM, Robinson SP, Jordan VC. Estradiol-stimulated growth of MCF-7 tumors implanted in athymic mice: a model to study the tumoristatic action of tamoxifen. J Steroid Biochem 1988;30(1–6):311–314.

143. Toko T, Matsuo K, Shibata J, Wierzba K, Nukatsuka M, Takeda S, Yamada Y, Asao T, Hirose T, Sato B. Interaction of DP-TAT-59, an active metabolite of new triphenylethylene- derivative (TAT-59), with estrogen receptors. J Steroid Biochem Mol Biol 1992;43(6):507–514.

144. Toko T, Sugimoto Y, Matsuo K, Yamasaki R, Takeda S, Wierzba K, Asao T, Yamada Y. TAT-59, a new triphenylethylene derivative with antitumor activity against hormone-dependent tumors. Eur J Cancer 1990;26(3):397–404.

145. Toko T, Shibata J, Nukatsuka M, Yamada Y. Antiestrogenic activity of DP-TAT-59, an active metabo-lite of TAT-59 against human breast cancer. Cancer Chemother Pharmacol 1997;39(5):390–398.

146. Tominaga T, Yoshida Y, Matsumoto A, Hayashi K, Kosaki G. Effects of tamoxifen and the derivative (TAT) on cell cycle of MCF-7 in vitro. Anticancer Res 1993;13(3):661–665.

147. Toko T, Shibata J, Sugimoto Y, Yamaya H, Yoshida M, Ogawa K, Matsushima E. Comparative pharmacodynamic analysis of TAT-59 and tamoxifen in rats bearing DMBA-induced mammary carcinoma. Cancer Chemother Pharmacol 1995;37(1–2):7–13.

148. Black L, Jones C, Falcone J. Antagonism of estrogen action with a new benzothiophene derived antiestrogen. Life Sci 1983;32:1031–1036.

149. Sato M, Rippy M, Bryant H. Raloxifene, tamoxifen, nafoxidine or estrogen effect on reproductive and nonreproductive tissues in ovariectomized rats. FASEB J 1996;10:905–912.

150. Fuchs-Young R, Magee D, Cole H, Short L, Glasebrook A, Rippy M, Termine J, Bryant H. Raloxifene is a tissue specific anti-estrogen that blocks tamoxifen or estrogen stimulated uterotropic effects. Endocrinology 1995;136(suppl): S57.

151. Poulin R, Merand Y, Poirier D, et al. Antiestrogenic properties of keoxifene, trans 4-hydroxy tamoxifen, and ICI 164,384, a new steroidal antiestrogen in ZR-75-1 human breast cancer cells. Breast Cancer Res Treat 1989;14:655–667.

152. Gottardis MM, Jordan VC. Antitumor actrions of keoxifene and tamoxifen in the N-nitrosomethylurea-induced rat mammary carcinoma model. Cancer Res 1987;47:367–369.

153. Clemens J, Bennet D, Black L, et al. Effects of a new antiestrgen keoxifene (LY15678) on growth of carcinogen induced mammary tumors and on LH and prolactin levels. Life Sci 1983;32:2869–2875.

154. Sato M, Kim J, short L, et al. Longitudinal and crosssectional analysis of raloxifene effects on tibiae from ovariectomized rats. J Pharmocal Exp Ther 1995;272:1252–1259.

155. Evans G, Bryant H, Magee D, et al. The effects of raloxifene on tibia histomorphometry in ovariec-tomized rats. Endocrinology 1994;134:2283–2288.

156. Black L, Sato M, Rowley E, et al. Raloxifene (LY139481 HCL) prevents bone loss and reduces serum sholesterol without causing uterine hypotrophy in ovariectomized rats. J Clin Invest 1994;93:63–69.

157. Balfour JA, Goa KL. Raloxifene. Drugs Aging 1998;12(4):335–41;discussion 342.

158. Dodge JA, Lugar CW, Cho S, Short LL, Sato M, Yang NN, Spangle LA, Martin MJ, Phillips DL, Glasebrook AL, Osborne JJ, Frolik CA, Bryant HU. Evaluation of the major metabolites of raloxifene as modulators of tissue selectivity. J Steroid Biochem Mol Biol 1997;61(1–2):97–106.

159. Ni L, Allerheiligen S, Basson R, et al. Pharmacokinetics of raloxifene in men and postmenopuasal women. Pharm Res 1996;13:S-430.

160. Forgue S, Rudy A, Knadler M, et al. Raloxifene pharmacokinetics in healthy postmenopausal women. Pharm Res 1996;13:S-429.
161. Liehr JG, Folse DS, Roy D. Lack of effectiveness of antiestrogens RU 39,411 or keoxifene in the prevention of estrogen-induced tumors in Syrian hamsters. Cancer Lett 1992;64(1):23–29.
162. Eli Lilly and Company, Evista® (raloxifene hydrochloride) tablets prescribing information. 1997.
163. Delmas PD, Bjarnason NH, Mitlak BH, Ravoux AC, Shah AS, Huster WJ, Draper M, Christiansen C. Effects of raloxifene on bone mineral density, serum cholesterol concentrations, and uterine endometrium in postmenopausal women. N Engl J Med 1997;337(23):1641–1647.
164. Walsh BW, Kuller LH, Wild RA, Paul S, Farmer M, Lawrence JB, Shah AS, Anderson PW. Effects of raloxifene on serum lipids and coagulation factors in healthy postmenopausal women. Jama 1998;279(18):1445–1451.
165. Sacks FM, Pfeffer MA, Moye LA, Rouleau JL, Rutherford JD, Cole TG, Brown L, Warnica JW, Arnold JM, Wun CC, Davis BR, Braunwald E. The effect of pravastatin on coronary events after myocardial infarction in patients with average cholesterol levels. Cholesterol and Recurrent Events Trial investigators. N Engl J Med 1996;335(14):1001–1009.
166. Kannel WB, Wolf PA, Castelli WP, RB DA. Fibrinogen and risk of cardiovascular disease. The Framingham Study. Jama 1987;258(9):1183–1186.
167. Walsh BW, Schiff I, Rosner B, Greenberg L, Ravnikar V, Sacks FM. Effects of postmenopausal estrogen replacement on the concentrations and metabolism of plasma lipoproteins. N Engl J Med 1991;325(17):1196–1204.
168. Yang NN, Venugopalan M, Hardikar S, Glasebrook A. Identification of an estrogen response element activated by metabolites of 17beta-estradiol and raloxifene [published erratum appears in Science 1997 Feb 28;275(5304):1249]. Science 1996;273(5279):1222–1225.
169. Mannucci PM, Bettega D, Chantarangkul V, Tripodi A, Sacchini V, Veronesi U. Effect of tamoxifen on measurements of hemostasis in healthy women. Arch Intern Med 1996;156(16):1806–1810.
170. Shewmon DA, Stock JL, Rosen CJ, Heiniluoma KM, Hogue MM, Morrison A, Doyle EM, Ukena T, Weale V, Baker S. Tamoxifen and estrogen lower circulating lipoprotein(a) concentrations in healthy postmenopausal women. Arterioscler Thromb 1994;14(10):1586–1593.
171. Costantino JP, Kuller LH, Ives DG, Fisher B, Dignam J. Coronary heart disease mortality and adjuvant tamoxifen therapy. J Natl Cancer Inst 1997;89(11):776–782.
172. Data on file, Lilly Research Laboratories.
173. Grodstein F, Stampfer MJ, Goldhaber SZ, Manson JE, Colditz GA, Speizer FE, Willett WC, Hennekens CH. Prospective study of exogenous hormones and risk of pulmonary embolism in women. Lancet 1996;348(9033):983–987.
174. Daly E, Vessey MP, Hawkins MM, Carson JL, Gough P, Marsh S. Risk of venous thromboembolism in users of hormone replacement therapy. Lancet 1996;348(9033):977–980.
175. Jick H, Derby LE, Myers MW, Vasilakis C, Newton KM. Risk of hospital admission for idiopathic venous thromboembolism among users of postmenopausal oestrogens. Lancet 1996;348(9033):981–983.
176. Jordan V, Glusman J, Eckert S, Lippman M, Powles T, Costa A, Morrow M, Norton L. Incident primary breast cancers are reduced by raloxifene: integrated data from multicenter, double-blind, randomized trials in ~12,000 postmenopausal women. American Society of Clinical Oncology, 1998, Los Angeles, CA, 1998 program/Proceedings of the American Society of Clinical Oncology. Abstract 466 p. 122a.
177. Early Breast Cancer Trialists' Collaborative Group. Systemic treatment of early breast cancer by hormonal, cytotoxic, or immune therapy. 133 randomised trials involving 31,000 recurrences and 24,000 deaths among 75,000 women. Lancet 1992;339(8785):71–85.
178. Early Breast Cancer Trialists' Collaborative Group [see comments]. Systemic treatment of early breast cancer by hormonal, cytotoxic, or immune therapy. 133 randomised trials involving 31,000 recurrences and 24,000 deaths among 75,000 women. Lancet 1992;339(8784):1–115.
179. Smigel K. Breast Cancer Prevention Trial shows major benefit, some risk [news]. J Natl Cancer Inst 1998;90(9):647–648.

13

Androgen Replacement in Postmenopausal Women

Elizabeth S. Ginsburg, MD

CONTENTS

INTRODUCTION

Androgen replacement therapy (ART) in postmenopausal women is controversial, in part because the role androgens play in women is unclear. Are androgens "extra" hormones in women, or are they vital to the maintenance of normal bone metabolism, libido, and sense of well being? If androgen replacement does enhance the sense of well being, sexual interest and sexual function, as well as bone density, then replacement postmenopausally may make medical, as well as biological, sense. This chapter will review the androgen milieu present in premenopausal and postmenopausal women, and will summarize the findings to date on androgen replacement in menopause.

ANDROGENS IN PREMENOPAUSAL WOMEN

The metabolic clearance rates of testosterone and androstenedione are stable from the premenopausal to postmenopausal years, although the aromatization of androstenedione to estrone, but not testosterone to estradiol, increases over time *(1)*. There is some evi-

From: *Contemporary Endocrinology: Menopause: Endocrinology and Management*
Edited by: D. B. Seifer and E. A. Kennard © Humana Press Inc., Totowa, NJ

Table 1
Ovarian Vein and Peripheral Estrogen and Androgen Levels
in Menopause[a]

Steroid	Ovarian vein	Peripheral
Estrone (pg/mL)	105.3 + 54.5	44.4 + 25.6
Estradiol (pg/mL)	143.3 ± 58.2	13.9 + 11.0
Testosterone (ng/mL)	1.11 + 1.06	10.30 + 0.27
androstenedione (ng/mL)	2.30 ± 1.13	10.83 + 2.47
DHEAS (ng/mL)	2.79 + 1.45	12.47 + 0.40

[a]From ref. 3.

dence that diet affects circulating androgen levels. In omnivores serum testosterone, androstenedione, and free testosterone correlate with dietary protein and fat intake. Carbohydrate, grain, total fiber, and grain fiber intakes are inversely correlated to these androgens (2).

ANDROGENS IN POSTMENOPAUSAL WOMEN

The postmenopausal ovary continues to secrete androgens after menopause. Large amounts of testosterone, and moderate amounts of androstenedione, estrone, and dehydroepiandrosterone (DHEA) are secreted into the peripheral and ovarian venous circulation, as documented in a study of 42 postmenopausal women (Table 1) (3). After oophorectomy in postmenopausal women, estradiol levels are unchanged and serum testosterone and androstenedione decrease by 50% (4). There is also evidence that there is reduced 17,20 desmolase enzymatic activity in postmenopausal women. DHEA pulse frequency is the same in postmenopausal women as in premenopausal women, however the pulse amplitude is diminished. In addition, dehydroepiandrosterone sulfate and DHEA response to corticotropin releasing factor, but not cortisol, are diminished. These data indicate that the conversion of 17 hydroxyprogesterone to DHEA and 17 hydroxyprogesterone to androstenedione by 17,20 desmolase are reversed (5).

RELATIONSHIP BETWEEN ANDROGEN LEVELS
AND SEXUAL BEHAVIOR/DESIRE IN PREMENOPAUSAL
AND POSTMENOPAUSAL WOMEN

Up to 50% of postmenopausal women complain of decreased libido on presentation to their physician (6,7). Part of the reason for decreased libido after menopause is due to vaginal atrophy, when narrowing of the vagina and thinning and loss of elasticity of the vaginal mucosa causes dyspareunia. However, the decrease in circulating ovarian androgens that occurs after menopause may contribute to decreased libido.

DHEA, androstenedione, testosterone, and dihydrotestosterone (DHT) were measured in a study of healthy married women. Postmenopausal women were compared to premenopausal women by questionnaire, and responses were correlated with serum androgen levels. Older women reported the same levels of sexual desire and arousal as the younger women, but intercourse frequency and sexual gratification were lower. Androgen levels were correlated with stages of the four-stage sexual response process (8).

Another cohort of 141 women age 40–60 yr was studied with a baseline interview and weekly interviews and blood sampling over the following 4 wk. Multiple parameters including age, menopausal status, body mass index, smoking, ovarian steroids, and adrenal androgens were analyzed using multivariate analysis. None of the hormonal parameters predicted measures of sexuality. The most important predictors of sexual function were sexual attitudes and measures of well being. DHEA was related to well being (9). A small study of 16 perimenopausal women involved questionnaires and blood drawing every 4 mo until 1 yr after the last menstrual period. Not surprisingly, estradiol and testosterone levels declined over time as ovarian function waned. Declining testosterone levels were consistently associated with decreases in coital frequency. Women experienced significant declines in the number of sexual thoughts and fantasies in this transitional period as well, and were less satisfied with their partners as lovers after menopause (10).

However, data do not consistently link decreased androgens to decreased libido or sexual function after menopause. Sixty-nine postmenopausal women who were defined as being coitally active (intercourse >3x/mo) were compared to 29 coitally inactive postmenopausal women studied in a single interview and blood testing. Inactive women rarely had coitus or any sexual activity. No women were on hormone replacement or had had hysterectomy and/or bilateral oophorectomy. Dyspareunia was found to correlate with desire for less coital frequency, and less than ideal coital frequency. No correlation was found between current or ideal sexual frequency and estrone, estradiol, testosterone, or androstenedione levels. Of unclear significance is the fact that LH levels were significantly higher in sexually active women. Testosterone levels were higher, though not significantly so, in the active women (161 ± 57.9 versus 144.7 ± 36.9). One can hypothesize that the elevated luteinizing hormone (LH) levels in the active patients increased testosterone concentrations in these women, and that the small number of women in the study gives it insufficient power to demonstrate significant differences (11).

In a cohort study of 59 healthy postmenopausal women age 60–70 yr, sexual behavior was correlated with hormone levels. In women, higher free-testosterone levels were correlated with increased sexual desire compared to the rest of the cohort (12).

Available data are clearly contradictory concerning the effects of postmenopausal endogenous androgen levels on libido and sexual response. The possible relationship between endogenous androgens and sense of well being is intriguing and warrants further investigation.

REASONS TO CONSIDER ANDROGEN REPLACEMENT IN MENOPAUSE

Decreased Libido

Decreased libido is a common problem for postmenopausal women (12). It is difficult to assess what constitutes a decrease in sexual function. Decreases in desire and difficulty with arousal or orgasm are all reported complaints. There are no standards to help determine what level of activity is abnormal. What is acceptable for one woman may represent significant deficiency to another. It is therefore difficult to look to a particular standard in assessing the patient. It may be best to find out in what ways the woman's sexual life has diminished by taking a careful social and psychiatric history. Alcohol dependence, changes in life situation, fatigue, stress at work, depression, the use of antidepressants, and interpersonal relationship conflict may all contribute to decreased sexual function.

Well-Being Enhancement

Another reason to consider androgen replacement in a postmenopausal women is if she complains of general feelings of loss of energy, without signs or symptoms of depression or mental or interpersonal disorder. In general, such women should be on ERT, as the loss of REM sleep that occurs with estrogen deficiency after menopause can cause fatigue and energy loss as well.

EFFECTS OF ORAL TESTOSTERONE REPLACEMENT ON LIBIDO

A prospective, randomized, crossover study of androgen replacement in 53 surgically menopausal women found that exogenous androgens enhanced the intensity of sexual desire and arousal and frequency of sexual fantasies in hysterectomized and oophorectomize women, but there was no increase in sexual intercourse. Subjects were randomized to two 3-mo blocks of treatment with a placebo month in between as a washout period. Subjects received an androgen–estrogen preparation, estrogen alone, androgen alone, or placebo as one of the 3-mo treatments *(13)*.

In a 10-wk double-blind placebo-controlled study of 40 naturally postmenopausal women, Premarin (0.625 mg), Premarin/Provera (0.625 mg/5 mg), Premarin/methyltestosterone (0.625/5 mg), and placebo were evaluated for effects on mood ratings, sexual behaviors, and arousal. Premarin/methyltestosterone treatment increased reports of pleasure from masturbation compared to the other three groups. However, other aspects of sexual functioning were not affected. This study indicates that high-dose androgen replacement enhances self-stimulatory behavior alone *(14)*.

INTRAMUSCULAR TESTOSTERONE USE

In a study of eight women receiving monthly intramuscular testosterone enanthate and estradiol dienanthate and estradiol benzoate (Climacteron, Merck, Frosst, Montreal, Canada), plasma testosterone levels were approximately twice as high (range 1.8 to 1.19 ng/mL over 42 d) as the upper limit of normal for women (0.6 ng/mL). Sexual desire, fantasies, and arousal varied directly with plasma steroid levels and were highest the first two weeks after injection. Rates of coitus and orgasm were unrelated to steroid hormone levels *(15)*.

TESTOSTERONE IMPLANTS FOR LIBIDO

Seventeen postmenopausal women in a nonrandomized study were treated with a single application of 40 mg estradiol and 100 mg testosterone implants due to insufficient response to estrogen replacement alone. Women with uteri received monthly cyclic medroxyprogesterone-acetate withdrawal. Maximal testosterone levels rose threefold from baseline peaking at 6.7 nmol/L (ng/mL) at 1 mo, with levels falling to 2.5 nmol/L at 5 mo. Libido improved, as did enjoyment of sex and lack of concentration. However, there was no placebo arm, so a placebo effect cannot be ruled out *(16)*.

A randomized study of 40 healthy postmenopausal women with regular sexual partners and complaints of decreased libido, assigned women to either 50 mg estradiol or 50 mg estradiol plus 100 mg testosterone implants. By two months of treatment, libido and sexual responsiveness, as well as psychological, somatic, and vasomotor symptoms, were equally improved over baseline in both treatment groups, with no further improvement at the end of the six-month study *(17)*.

It is interesting that there have been so few randomized, placebo-controlled randomized studies of androgen replacement in postmenopausal women. Essentially, all preparations used in the cited studies used supraphysiologic androgen doses. Even at these high levels, libido was not consistently improved. It is possible that there is a U-shaped curve, above and below which testosterone receptors are not optimally occupied and activated. Clearly, larger studies employing standardized sexual function and psychometric questionnaires would be definitive. The question that would still remain is whether the optimal replacement regimen for postmenopausal women would entail physiologic levels of testosterone or other androgens. This has not yet been studied.

TRANSDERMAL TESTOSTERONE REPLACEMENT

Oral androgens, even if given in combination with estrogen, reduce HDL and increase LDL cholesterol. Long-term effects of these metabolic changes could be to remove the protective effects of female sex and estrogen on cardiovascular risk and lead to atherogenic serum lipoprotein profiles and cardiovascular disease. To avoid first-pass effects of oral replacement and the discomfort of intramuscular or pellet therapy, transdermal testosterone is now under development. Dosages are being formulated to mimic levels in the mid- and upper-normal premenopausal female ranges in an effort to minimize side effects (Theratek Inc., Salt Lake City, UT). Whether such dosages will be effective in improving complaints of decreased libido is not yet known.

DHEA THERAPY

Six obese (30–50% above ideal body weight) postmenopausal women were given 1600 mg/d in 4 divided doses over a 4-wk period. DHEA levels rose rapidly to a peak at 180–240 min of sixfold over baseline, with dehydroepiandrosterone sulfate (DHEAS) and androstenedione rising 12-fold, testosterone 2.5-fold, and DHT 15-fold. Estradiol, estrone, and serum hormone-binding globulin (SHBG) were unchanged. By week 2, all levels were increased still more (DHEA 15-fold, testosterone ninefold, DHEAS 20-fold, androstenedione 20-fold, DHT 20-fold, and estradiol and estrone were twice basal by 4 wk. HDL levels fell 20% within the first week and remained depressed. LDL, VLDL, and triglycerides fell slightly. Peak insulin levels also rose, with no change in fasting glucose levels *(18)*.

EFFECTS OF ANDROGENS ON WELL-BEING

In a study of 43 surgically menopausal women estrogen–androgen (Climacteron), testosterone enanthate 200 mg, estrogen alone, and placebo treatments were randomly assigned to patients after hysterectomy with bilateral salpingo-oophorectomy in a double-blind placebo-controlled crossover study. All medications and placebo were given by intramuscular injection every 28 d during 3 mo treatment arms. Ten women who underwent hysterectomy with ovarian conservation served as controls. Estrogen–androgen combination and androgen alone increased well being, energy level, and appetite as compared to estrogen alone and placebo *(19)*. Androgen levels resulting from replacement were fourfold higher than preoperative levels after androgen–estrogen replacement, and approximately double preoperative baseline after testosterone enanthate alone. The results of the study suggest that supraphysiologic androgen replacement after hysterectomy and bilateral oophorectomy may improve postoperative well being.

EFFECTS OF ANDROGENS ON BONE DENSITY

There is evidence that androgens are important predictors of bone density, with higher androgen levels correlating with greater bone density. In 16 women with an average age of 66 (range 58–75) who were at least 5 yr postmenopausal from spontaneous menopause, lumbar bone density measured by CT scanning was positively correlated with DHEAS and androstenedione levels, but not with estradiol or estrone (20). In another study of 28 postmenopausal women, bone density in the forearm was correlated with the amount of free testosterone, indicating that SHBG levels might modify effects of sex steroids on bone metabolism. The study is significantly flawed, however, by not taking into account circulating estradiol levels, which affect SHBG levels as well as bone density (21). Hip fracture incidence has also been found to be related to levels of estrogens and androgens in postmenopausal women (22). In addition, vertebral bone density has been found to be related to serum DHEAS levels (23).

There is evidence that androgen–estrogen replacement therapy increases bone formation, whereas estrogen alone decreases resorption only as shown in a study comparing bone formation and resorption markers in two groups of postmenopausal women, one on 1.25 mg CEE, and the other on 1.25 mg esterified estrogens plus 2.5 mg MT (24). Androgens are thought to act by increasing osteoblastic activity in bone, as has been demonstrated in vitro (25). In one 2-yr double-blind randomized study of 34 postmenopausal women, those who were treated with androgen–estrogen subdermal implants had higher hip and spinal bone densities than those treated with estrogen alone (26). In another double-blind randomized study, conjugated estrogen–methyltestosterone users had a 3.4% increase in spinal bone density compared to no change in women using estrogens alone (27).

There is evidence from randomized studies that androgen replacement with intramuscular nandrolone deconate may increase peripheral bone density in postmenopausal women with established osteoporosis, where estrogen replacement plus calcium does not. The largest study of 191 women found that women receiving nandrolone had increases in forearm bone density, whereas those receiving estrogen, calcium, and/or calcitrol did not (28,29). The data suggest that estrogen–androgen replacement probably increases bone density by 2–4%, whereas estrogen replacement alone prevents loss (29).

TYPES OF ANDROGENS AVAILABLE FOR REPLACEMENT IN WOMEN

Most studies evaluate estrogen–testosterone replacement rather than testosterone replacement alone. However, there are only three products in the United States that the FDA has approved for use in women, and they are approved solely for the relief of hot flashes (Estratest, Estratest HS, Solvay Pharmaceuticals, Marietta, GA; Premarin with methyltestosterone, Wyeth-Ayerst). Unfortunately, there are a plethora of androgens available that have not been studied at all. DHEA is a weak androgen, but is easily accessible in nearly all pharmacies and health food stores without prescription. As has been previously discussed, it results in significant and concerning decreases in HDL cholesterol *(18)*. Testosterone creams and pellets are made to order by compounding pharmacies with physician prescription. It can be uncomfortable using medications with unknown efficacy or side effects. Patients unhappy with their symptoms may strongly lobby for treatment. One might argue that patients will be safer taking prescribed androgens under physician supervision, than self-treating without monitoring. Injected androgens are formulated for use in men. Testosterone formulations can be measured by standard testosterone assays, and can be dosed to target normal premenopausal female levels, which would be approx 1/8 those of men. The dosing can be adjusted accordingly. Table 2 lists androgen preparations.

RISKS AND SIDE EFFECTS OF ANDROGEN REPLACEMENT

In general, androgens have hepatic effects that antagonize those of estrogens, and lead to increases in LDL cholesterol and decreases in HDL cholesterol. Oral methyltestosterone has a first-pass effect, with 44% of the drug cleared by the liver, indicating that hepatic levels are quite high (*see Physician's Desk Reference*). In oophorectomized postmenopausal women, oral methyltestosterone 2.5 mg in combination with 1.25 mg conjugated equine estrogens lowers HDL by 16.4%, and increases the total cholesterol ratio by approx 10%. These changes potentially represent increases in cardiovascular risk, and in some women could contribute to the occurrence of cardiovascular events. However, if androgens are given parenterally in combination with estrogens, adverse lipid changes may not always occur. In one study of 42 postmenopausal women given androgen and estrogen combination replacement therapy (Climacteron), there was no significant difference in lipoproteins between those women and others using intramuscular estrogen replacement alone (Delestrogen, i.e., estradiol valerate) *(30)*. After implantation of 40 mg estradiol and 100 mg testosterone pellets, total and HDL cholesterol and triglycerides were unchanged *(16)*.

Masculinization

Few reports of androgen replacement in menopause mention androgenic side effects. Part of the reason for this may be that studies are nearly all of short duration, with treatment arms less than six months in most studies. In one study of eight women receiving 100 mg testosterone and 40 mg estradiol implants, one patient experienced hirsutism and another deepening of the voice over a 5-mo period. Circulating testosterone levels were supraphysiologic at double the upper limit of the normal range for women *(16)*. The incidence of 25% masculinizing side effects is concerning, but it is surprising that terminal hair growth would occur so rapidly. With longer term use, the incidence and severity of masculinizing side effects with testosterone doses so high could potentially be severe.

SUMMARY

There are contradictory data concerning the relationship of endogenous androgens to libido in premenopausal and postmenopausal women. Likewise, there is no consistency between data concerning effects of androgen replacement on libido in postmenopausal women. There may be a role for androgen replacement in women following hysterectomy and bilateral oophorectomy. Studies on libido and well being are limited due to the use of unvalidated questionnaires. Data are stronger concerning beneficial effects of androgens on bone density. Larger, well-defined studies using validated psychological and

Table 2
Forms of Androgen Replacement

Name of product/ manufacturer	Type of androgen	Dose	Route of delivery	Comments
Estratest (Solvay Pharmaceuticals, Marietta, GA)	Methyltestosterone (MT)	2.5 mg MT 1.25 mg esterified estrogens: daily	Oral	Methyltestosterone not measured in testosterone assays
Estratest HS (Solvay Pharmaceuticals, Marietta, GA)	Methyltestosterone	1.25 mg MT 0.625 mg esterified estrogens daily	Oral	As above
Premarin with methyltestosterone (Wyeth-Ayerst, Philadelphia, PA)	Methyltestosterone	1.25 mg CEE with 10 mg MT; 0.625 mg CEE with 5 mg MT QD	Oral	As above
Testred capsules (ICN Pharmaceuticals, Costa Mesa, CA)	Methyltestosterone	10 mg MT daily (men)	Oral	For use in men
Android 10 mg capsules (ICN Pharmaceuticals, Costa Mesa, CA)	Methyltestosterone	10 mg MT daily (men)	Oral	For use in men
Delatestryl 200 mg (Bio-technology General Pharmaceuticals, Iselin, NJ)	Testosterone enanthate	Male dosing; 50–400 mg q 2–4 wk; 25–50 mg monthly if given to women	im	Can measure testosterone levels
Androderm 12.2 mg patches (SmithKline Beecham Pharmaceuticals, Philadelphia, PA)	Testosterone	Two 12.2 mg patches daily (men)	Transdermal	Delivers 5 mg testosterone/24 h; for use in men
Testoderm (ALZA Corp, Palo Alto, CA)	Testosterone	6 mg or 4 mg daily (men)	Transdermal to shaved scrotal skin	For use in men
Testopel (Bartor Pharmaceuticals)	Testosterone	10-100 mg implant every 3–6 mo	Skin incision and pellet inserter needed, in upper buttocks or abdominal wall	Must titrate dose to serum testosterone levels; studies use suraphysiologic level minimal data on long-term use and side effects available

(continued)

Table 2 *(continued)*
Forms of Androgen Replacement

Name of product/ manufacturer	Type of androgen	Dose	Route of delivery	Comments
Testosterone powder (Paddock Labs) For testosterone cream formulation by compounding pharmacies	Testosterone	2% nightly	Apply to clitoris	Can monitor blood levels. No studies available
Climacteron (Merck Frosst)	Testosterone enanthate benzilic acid hydrozone estradiol benzoate estradiol dienanthate	Daily	Oral	Unavailable
Valertest (Hyrex Pharmaceuticals)	Testosterone enanthate estradiol valerate	360 mg testosterone enanthate, 16 mg estradiol valerate/2 mL	Single injection im within 1 wk of delivery	For postpartum lactation suppression
Depo-Testosterone 100 mg (Pharmacia & Upjohn, Kalamazoo, MI)	Testosterone cypionate	Approved for use in men, 50–400 mg q 2–4 wk	im	For use in men
Halotestin (Upjohn, Kalamazoo, MI)	Fluoxymesterone	For use in men; 2, 5, 10 mg tablets daily	Oral	For use in men
Virilon IM (Star Pharmaceuticals, Pompano Beach, CA)	Testosterone cypionate	25–50 mg im q month	im	Approved for use in men.
Compounded methyltestosterone	Methyltestosterone	0.5–1.0 mg daily (for women)	Oral	Monitor lipo-proteins if use is long term
Prasterone (Elge)	Dehydroepiandro-sterone	50 mg qd to bid	Oral	FDA unapproved. Monitor lipo-proteins if use is long term. No studies of efficacy available

well being questionnaires that evaluate androgen replacement for at least one year are needed to adequately assess efficacy, safety, and side effects of androgen replacement in menopause. Data are insufficient to document either efficacy or safety of available regimens on psychosexual functioning.

RECOMMENDATIONS

Lack of proof that androgen replacement in postmenopausal women improves psychosexual functioning does not mean that it is necessarily ineffective. In the absence of data confirming long-term safety, it is important for the clinician to be judicious in its use. Estrogen replacement, with its well-documented benefits and risks, should be given before androgen replacement. Screen for lipoprotein abnormalities and take a careful history with attention to signs of depression, which can also cause loss of libido, energy, and sense of well being. It is prudent to monitor lipids once patients begin therapy. Only natural testosterone preparations, i.e., implants or creams can be monitored by serum levels in an effort to avoid levels so supraphysiologic that they are perhaps more likely to cause side effects such as acne and hirsutism. Loss of libido can be very painful for women accustomed to satisfying sexual relationships, and a trial of androgen replacement with judicious monitoring should be offered. With the advent of the bisphosphonates, bone density alone should not be an indication for their use.

REFERENCES

1. Longcope C, Johnston CC. Androgen and estrogen dynamics: stability over a two year interval in perimenopausal women. J Steroid Biochem 1990;35:91–95.
2. Aldercreutz H, Hamalainen E, Gorbach SL, Goldin BR, Woods MN, Dwyer JT. Diet and plasma androgens in postmenopausal vegetarian and omnivorous women and postmenopausal women with breast cancer. Am J Clin Nutr 1989;49:433–442.
3. Ushiroyama T, Sugimoto O. Endocrine function of the peri and postmenopausal ovary. Horm Res 1995;44:64–68.
4. Hughes CL, Wall LL, Creasman WT. Reproductive hormone levels in gynecologic oncology patients undergoing surgical castration after spontaneous menopause. Gynecol Oncol 1991;40:42–45.
5. Liu CH, Laughlin GA, Fischer UG, Yen SS. Marked attenuation of ultradian and circadian rhythms of dehydroepiandrosterone in postmenopausal women: evidence for a reduced 17,20 desmolase enzymatic activity. J Clin Endocrinol Metab 1990;71:900–906.
6. Bachmann GA, Leiblum SR, Sandler B, et al. Correlates of sexual desire in postmenopausal women. Maturitas 1985;7:211–216.
7. Studd JWW, Collins WP, Chakravarti S, et al. Oestradiol and testosterone implants in the treatment of psychosexual problems in the post-menopausal woman. Br J Obstet Gynaecol 1977;84:314,315.
8. Persky H, Dreisback L, Miller WR, et al. The relation of plasma androgen levels to sexual behaviors and attitudes of women. Psyosom Med 1982;44:305–319.
9. Cahwood EH, Bancroft J. Steroid hormones, the menopause, sexuality and well-being of women. Pshychol Med 1996;26:925–936.
10. McCoy NL, Davidson JM. A longitudinal study of the effects of menopause on sexuality. Maturitas 1985;7:203–210.
11. Bachmann GA, Leiblum SR, Kemmann E, Colburn DW, Swartzman L, Shelden R. Sexual expression and its determinants in the post-menopausal woman. Maturitas 1984;6:19–29.
12. Bachman GA, Leiblum SR. Sexuality in sexagenarian women. Maturitas 1991; 13:43–50.
13. Sherwin BB, Gelfand MM, Brender W. Androgen enhances sexual motivation in females: a prospective, crossover study of sex steroid administration in the surgical menopause. Psychosom Med 1985;47:339–351.
14. Myers LS, Dixen J, Morrissette D, Carmichael M, Davidson JM. Effects of estrogen, androgen and progestin on sexual psychophysiology and behavior in postmenopausal women. J Clin Endocrinol Metab 1990;70:1124–1131.
15. Sherwin BB. Changes in sexual behavior as a function of plasma sex steroid levels in postmenopausal women. Maturitas 1985;7:225–233.
16. Burger HD, Hailes J, Menelaus M, Nelson J, Hudson B, Balazs N. The management of persistent menopausal symptoms with oestradiol-testosterone implants: clinical, lipid and hormonal results. Maturitas 1984;6:351–358.
17. Dow MG, Hart DM, Forrest CA. Hormonal treatments of sexual unresponsiveness in postmenopausal women: a comparative study. Br J Obstet Gynecol 1983;90:361–366.

18. Mortola JF, Yen SSC. The effects of oral dehydroepiandrosterone on endocrine-metabolic parameters in postmenopausal women. J Clin Endocrinol Metab 1990;71:696–704.
19. Sherwin BB, Gelfand MM. Differential symptom response to parenteral estrogen and/or androgen administration in the surgical menopause. Am J Obstet Gynecol 1985;151:153–160.
20. Deutsch 5, Benjamin F, Seltzer V. Tafreshi M, Kocheril G, Frank A. The correlation of serum estrogens and androgens with bone density in the late postmenopause. Int J Gynaecol Obstet 1987;25:217–222.
21. Brody S, Carlstrom K, Lagrelius A, Lunell NO, Mollerstrom G, Pousette A. Serum sex hormone binding globulin (SHBG) testosterone/SHBG index, endometrial pathology and bone mineral density in postmenopausal women. Acta Obstet Gynecol Scand 1987;66:357–360.
22. Davidson BJ, Ross RK, Pagnanini-Hill A, et al. Total and free estrogens and androgens in postmenopausal women with hip fractures. J Clin Endocrinol 1982;54:115–120.
23. Nordin BEC, Robertson A, Seamark RE, et al. The relationship between calcium absorption, serum dihydroepiandrosterone and vertebral mineral density in postmenopausal women. J Clin Endocrinol Metab 1985;60:651–657.
24. Raisz LG, Wiita B, Artis A, et al. Comparison of the effects of estrogen alone and estrogen plus androgen on biochemical markers of bone formation and resorption in postmenopausal women. J Clin Endocrinol Metab 1996;81:37–43.
25. Kasperk CH, Wergedal JE, Farley JR, Linkart TA, Twiner RJ, Baylink DJ. Androgens directly stimulate proliferation of bone cells in vitro. Endocrinol 1988;124:1576–1578.
26. Davis SR, McCloud P, Strauss BJG, et al. Testosterone enhances estradiol's effects on postmenopausal bone density and sexuality. Maturitas 1995;21:227–236.
27. Watts NB, Notelovitz M, Timmons MC, et al. Comparison of oral estrogens and estrogens plus androgen on bone mineral density, menopausal symptoms, and lipidlipoprotein profiles in surgical menopausal women. Obstet Gynecol 1995;85:529–537.
28. Need AG, Chaterton BE, Walker CJ, et al. Comparison of calcium, calcitrol ovarian hormones and nandrolone in the treatment of osteoporosis. Maturitas 1986;8:275–280.
29. Rosenberg MJ, King TDN, Timmons MC. Estrogen-androgen for hormone replacement. J Reprod Med 1997;42:394–404.
30. Sherwin BB, Gelfand MM, Schucher R, Gabor J. Postmenopausal estrogen and androgen replacement and lipoprotein lipid concentrations. Am J Obstet Gynecol 1987;156:414–419.

14 Calcium Requirements and Sources in Postmenopausal Women

Brinda N. Kalro, MD and Sarah L. Berga, MD

CONTENTS

CALCIUM HOMEOSTASIS — PHYSIOLOGY AND UTILIZATION

Calcium is an important constituent of bones and teeth and plays a vital role in a number of physiologic and biochemical processes, including the blood coagulation cascade, enzyme activity, release of hormones and neurotransmitters, and regulation of nerve and muscle function. It is also an important mediator of intracellular hormone action where it functions as a second messenger. Cell division and secretion are initiated by the movement of calcium from the extracellular compartment to the cytosol.

The calcium content of the adult human body is about 1100 g (1.5% of body weight), approximately 98% of which is found in the skeleton in its phosphated form known as hydroxyapatite crystals. These provide the inorganic and structural framework of the skeleton. Most of the calcium circulating in the plasma is protein bound and therefore only partly diffusible. There are two types of calcium pools in the bone, a smaller pool that is a readily exchangeable reservoir (2% of bone calcium) and a larger, more stable, pool of calcium that is less readily exchangeable. There are two mechanisms of homeo-

From: *Contemporary Endocrinology: Menopause: Endocrinology and Management*
Edited by: D. B. Seifer and E. A. Kennard © Humana Press Inc., Totowa, NJ

stasis that operate independently of each other. One system maintains plasma levels of calcium utilizing calcium from the smaller, but readily exchangeable, pool. The other system is involved with bone remodeling by a process of bone resorption and deposition that accounts for 95% of bone formation. In the circulating plasma, calcium exists in three forms: bound to plasma proteins (primarily albumin), complexed with organic acids, and free or in an ionized state. About 6% of the total calcium is complexed with citrate, phosphate, and other anions. The remainder is divided almost equally between a protein-bound form and an ionized (unbound form), which is maintained at between 4.45 and 5.26 mg/dL and is the biologically active fraction. Deviations in the ionized calcium fraction can be life threatening and therefore are clinically significant.

Thirty to forty percent of ingested calcium is absorbed from the gastrointestinal tract and the amount absorbed is dependent on the presence of 1,25-dihydroxycholecalciferol (1,25-DHC), the levels of which vary inversely with serum calcium and dietary calcium levels. Calcium absorption is also decreased by substances like phosphates and oxalates that form insoluble salts with calcium and alkalis that form insoluble soaps of calcium. A diet rich in protein increases calcium absorption, but in normal individuals administration of sulfur-containing amino acids increases the acidity of urine and leads to increased urinary loss of calcium (1). There is, however, no evidence to suggest that increased protein intake is associated with a higher risk of fractures (2). Calcium absorption increases in the presence of dietary deficiency and decreases in the presence of excess calcium.

Calcium is filtered by the kidney in significant amounts, but about 98% of this is reabsorbed, mostly in the proximal convoluted tubule. The remainder is reabsorbed in the distal convoluted tubule under the influence of parathyroid hormone (PTH) from the parathyroid gland. There is also an obligatory loss of calcium from the intestines in the form of digestive juices and desquamated epithelial cells (some of which is reabsorbed) and from the skin, both amounting to about 200–250 mg/d. If calcium intake is increased, 10% of the increased fraction is absorbed, 6% excreted in the urine, only 4% being retained, exclusive of dermal loss (3).

Calcium concentration and disposition are regulated by various hormones, particularly, PTH, 1,25-DHC, and calcitonin. PTH increases bone resorption and mobilizes calcium from the bone to the plasma and increases the reabsorption of excreted calcium in the distal tubule of the kidneys. PTH increases the formation of 1,25-DHC in the kidneys, which is the active metabolite of vitamin D.

PTH also increases the permeability of osteoblasts and osteoclasts to calcium and favors the entry of calcium into these cells. Osteoclastic activity is increased by the action of PTH, which also promotes formation of more osteoclasts. Excess PTH causes demineralization of bones characterized by the formation of multiple bone cysts.

Calcitonin is a calcium-lowering hormone and exerts this effect by direct inhibition of bone resorption and increased excretion of calcium by the kidneys. Its secretion is increased during skeletal development in young adults and is believed to have a partial protective effect on the bones of the mother from excessive calcium loss during pregnancy and lactation by inhibiting bone resorption.

The active form of vitamin D is 1,25-DHC (calcitriol or D_3). It is generated in the kidneys from its less active form, 25-hydroxycholecalciferol (calcidiol or 25-hydroxy D_2). 1,25-DHC not only increases calcium absorption from the gut, but it also increases calcium reabsorption in the kidneys. In bone, it increases the number of mature osteoclasts and thus mobilizes calcium and phosphate. Also, it stimulates osteoblasts, but the net effect is mobilization of calcium. Vitamin D is synthesized by the skin in the presence of ultraviolet light of a particular wavelength. An important dietary source of vitamin D is milk, most of which is now fortified with 400 IU of vitamin D per quart. Other dairy products are not normally fortified with vitamin D. Those who avoid milk, live in more extreme latitudes, are vegans, or are lactose intolerant are at an increased risk of developing vitamin D deficiency.

CALCIUM AND THE CENTRAL NERVOUS SYSTEM

Calcium is essential for the fusion of storage granules within neuronal plasma membrane. It has recently been recognized that estrogens have a positive effect on the cognitive function in postmenopausal women. Estrogens facilitate outgrowth of neuronal processes from larger neurons with subsequent formation of synapses essential for memory function only in the presence of calcium. It is therefore very likely that calcium has an extended role to play other than merely increasing bone mass.

OBLIGATORY LOSS OF CALCIUM

An appreciable daily loss of calcium occurs from the skin, intestines, and kidneys and this obligatory loss must be countered by an adequate intake to maintain a positive balance. The exact amount of calcium lost in this manner is difficult to define, but kinetic studies have estimated the daily loss in healthy adults at about 200–250 mg/d, a small proportion of which is reabsorbed. This form of calcium loss has been shown to correlate strongly with bone mass status and to a significant extent with the amount of calcium ingested *(4)*. Loss can increase with age and in diseased states. Calcium supplementation can therefore be beneficial in replacing this fraction of lost calcium, thereby reducing some degree of bone loss.

Dermal loss of calcium occurs in the form of desquamated epithelium and sweat amounting to about 60 mg/d *(5)*. This loss increases with exercise and through loss of nail and hair. Dermal loss also correlates significantly with serum calcium levels and weakly with increased body surface area.

Urinary calcium levels vary greatly and do not correlate well with the amount of calcium absorbed *(6)*. Both absorption and excretion are nonlinearly related to the intake *(3)*. Urinary excretion of calcium, however, increases if there is primary bone loss, such as in patients who have been immobilized for prolonged periods of time.

There is very little, if any, obligatory loss of calcium from the kidneys, which are capable of preserving calcium particularly in patients with a diminished ability to absorb calcium. Urinary calcium loss is determined by sodium and protein intake. Fasting induces very low levels of urinary calcium in some, but not all, women *(7)*. Higher nitrogen intake is associated with increased urinary calcium excretion, but there is no net difference in calcium excretion with varying levels of phosphorus. Caffeine intake increases both urinary excretion and intestinal secretion of calcium *(8)*.

Advancing age and disease processes can increase this obligatory loss. Replacing this lost calcium by increasing intake may be one way of helping to prevent osteoporosis. Ingested calcium in the presence of dietary deficiency suppresses PTH levels and bone resorption, thereby stabilizing bone mass to a certain extent *(9)*. In the presence of estrogen deficiency, bone appears to be more sensitive to the resorbing effects of PTH *(10)*.

Intestinal calcium lost in digestive juices and desquamated epithelia amounts to 140 mg/d and is unrelated to plasma calcium levels. A fraction of this is reabsorbed (11). Intestinal disease can exacerbate this loss and worsen calcium deficiency.

WHY IS CALCIUM IMPORTANT?

Calcium is essential to maintain skeletal integrity. It is estimated that approx 55–60% of postmenopausal women ingest less than the recommended daily allowance of calcium of 1000 mg/d and that 10–15% of these have an intake of < 400 mg/d. A large proportion of younger women have a reduced calcium intake and 5–20% of these go on to have decreased cortical bone mass by age 34 (12). Reduced bone mass weakens the skeleton. Although only 2–6% of falls in elderly women result in fractures, this rate significantly increases in the presence of weaker bones. Soft-tissue mass is also important in reducing fracture rates by absorbing some of the impact of a fall, as is evidenced by the fact that overweight women have a reduced fracture rate by a third. Low bone mass is therefore a critical factor, with as little as 5% difference in bone mass altering the fracture risk by 40% (13).

Peak bone mass is achieved by about age 25 and plateaus between ages 25–35. This is determined by genetic programming under the influence of gonadal and other hormones, mechanical stresses, and an adequate dietary calcium intake. Accumulation of bone mass then begins to gradually decline, with the rate of skeletal loss being close to 5–10% per decade in population studies, until menopause, when estrogenic effects on the bone abruptly cease, leading to a rapid loss of bone mass. Loss of bone mass cannot be prevented altogether or replaced at this stage by merely ensuring adequate or even excess calcium intake. However, calcium deficiency may accelerate the loss, because when calcium needs exceed the amount absorbed, the body compensates by drawing calcium from the bone reserve. If this continues over a length of time and the "borrowed" calcium is not replaced, the skeleton becomes weak and lost bone cannot be replaced regardless of the intake, making the skeletal damage irreversible.

Calcium therefore plays an important role in reducing significant bone loss and helps prevent osteoporosis with time. It achieves this by building up bone mass in the younger years and maintaining this accumulated mass in the later years. A population-based prospective study showed a 60% reduction in hip fracture rates in men and women with high calcium intake (> 765 mg/d) over a prolonged period (14). Another study showed that women whose calcium intake was 1200 g/d, on average, as teenagers had 6% more bone density in their hips as adults. In some individuals "catch-up" mineralization can occur in their thirties secondary to their higher calcium-retention values (15).

BONE LOSS IN MENOPAUSE

The accelerated bone loss related to estrogen withdrawal appears to be intrinsic and is not influenced by nutritional or other extrinsic factors. This is a rapid exponential bone loss during the first 1–3 yr of estrogen deficiency. However, individual variations do exist. Hence, high calcium intake and exercise can only partially correct this rapid loss (16). In a study by Dawson-Hughes (8,17), women were seen not to benefit from increased calcium intake during the first 5 yr of menopause. Calcium supplementation of about 1000 mg elemental calcium/d reduced, but did not cease, bone loss from the radius in these women. However, calcium intake at this time did not have any effect on bone loss from the spine *(18)*. In a more recent case-controlled study by Reid et al., postmenopausal women approx 9 yr after their last menstrual period whose mean daily calcium intake was 750 ± 290 mg/d were shown to benefit from a calcium supplement of 1000 mg/d in both the axial and the appendicular skeleton *(19)*. Bone loss in the placebo group occured at most sites at the rate of 1% per year and this was reduced by a third to a half in the calcium-supplemented group over a period of 2 yr, but the difference tended to decrease with time.

Calcium Intake and Bone Loss

As the time from menopause increases, bone loss slows. Recent studies indicate that calcium supplements modestly slow bone loss, but it is debatable whether calcium intake protects from bone loss due to the new onset of hypoestrogenism that follows immediately after menopause *(17)*. The bone-sparing effects of calcium are primarily mediated through inhibition of PTH secretion. PTH levels rise in response to a deficient calcium intake and increase the extent and activation of bone resorption, thus leading to loss of bone mass. The protective effects of calcium supplements were primarily seen in women who had low dietary calcium intake of less than 400 mg/d. Calcium supplementation in these women blocks bone resorption, but whether this is due to a mechanism other than causing a fall in PTH secretion is unclear. Urine hydroxyproline levels correlate poorly with the extent of bone resorption, but a few clinical trials have demonstrated reduced urinary hydroxyproline levels following calcium supplementation in postmenopausal women with and without osteoporosis *(20–22)*. On the other hand, another group showed that in perimenopausal women, the levels of urinary hydroxyproline decreased in response to estrogens, but not to calcium *(23)*. Postmenopausal women absorb calcium less effectively from their diets and this may be secondary to either decreased levels or activity of calcitriol (1,25 dihydroxycholecalciferol). Urinary calcium excretion in this group of women is greater in early menopause and the net result is negative calcium balance. Calcium supplementation possibly slows the loss of compact bone, but does not alter the rate of loss of trabecular bone as effectively as estrogens *(23)*.

Involutional loss continues at a much slower rate with increasing age and this phase of calcium loss depends on factors such as nutritional status, extent of muscle mass, and reduced exposure to mechanical stress. At this stage, bone mass reaches a new equilibrium. This could be one reason for the difference in calcium requirements of early and late postmenopausal women. Estrogen deficiency decreases calcium absorption by about 7% at the same time, increasing its urinary excretion as evidenced by the calcium:creatinine ratio in the urine over a 24-h period after an overnight fast. Estrogens have a positive effect on tubular absorption of calcium similar to that of sodium *(24)*. Estrogen administration appears to decrease calcium excretion as well as reduce urinary-hydroxyproline values and plasma-alkaline-phosphatase activity (a direct measure of osteoclastic activity). Thus estrogens act at the level of the kidney and the bone to maintain calcium balance and bone mass. Several laboratory studies determined calcium requirements in nonestrogenized states and concluded that it increased by about 50 mg/d in the absence of estrogens *(19,25,26)*. It is estimated that menopause accounts for 38% of bone loss and advancing age (>55 yr) for about 62% until age 70. Even a 1% reduction in bone loss rate per year would significantly affect total postmenopausal bone loss and the fracture risk of this population of women *(24)*.

Approximately 25–50% of women will have reached a bone mass below the theoretical fracture threshold by their early sixties. The question then arises: is increased dietary

Table 1
Revised Recommendations for the Daily Dietary Intake of Calcium

Group (women)	Optimal daily intake (mg of elemental calcium)
25–30 yr	1,000
Over 50 yr (postmenopausal)	
On estrogens	1,000
Not on estrogens	1,500
Over 65 yr	1,500
Pregnant and Nursing	1,200–1,500

calcium or calcium supplementation *per se* of much value in conserving bone mass in postmenopausal women? This appears to be a controversial issue. There is no doubt that estrogen replacement with concurrent calcium intake is of maximum benefit, particularly to the axial skeleton, but the role of increased calcium intake alone is less clear. This is further confused by the fact that individual variations exist with respect to initial bone mass prior to menopause, rates of menopausal bone loss, and concurrent conditions. Other dietary constituents, bioavailability of calcium in the gut, rate of absorption and excretion can further confound the issue. Several studies support the concept that calcium alone reduces the rate of cortical bone loss, but not that of trabecular bone.

SOURCES OF CALCIUM: DIETARY VS SUPPLEMENTATION

Calcium is present in food and can also be consumed as supplements. Recommended daily intake of calcium has been revised recently, as shown in Table 1. Ideally, the best source is dietary and as implied by the name, a supplement should be administered as an adjunct if dietary calcium intake is insufficient and its use as a substitute discouraged unless otherwise indicated. Foods rich in calcium are often good sources of other nutrients too. Apart from calcium and vitamin D, other nutrients essential for normal bone formation are zinc, manganese, copper, ascorbic acid, B vitamins, and proteins. This has been adequately demonstrated by Delmi et al. in a study of elderly patients with femoral neck fractures, where substitution of a protein-enriched supplement improved clinical outcome by improving recovery rates and reducing the rates of complications and deaths (27).

Commercially available calcium supplements include a variety of salts like carbonate, citrate, gluconate, lactate, and phosphate, each of which contain differing amounts of elemental calcium. Carbonate and phosphate salts have the highest concentration of elemental calcium, at about 40%, with smaller amounts of 21%, 13%, and 9% in citrate, lactate, and gluconate, respectively (28). Derivative salts of natural products such as oyster shell and bone are also available, although the dolomite and lead content in these sources were reported to achieve toxic levels (29). Calcium supplements should be selected based on the amount of bioavailable elemental calcium and not the total weight of the calcium product. The bioavailability of calcium from different salts varies in that some deliver a higher amount of calcium on a weight-per-weight basis. In excess, calcium has adverse effects such as constipation, increased risk of renal stone formation, and excessive gas with resultant intestinal bloating. There is some evidence that side effects are more likely when calcium intake is derived from supplements as compared with diary

Table 2
Representative Medications that May Interfere with the Absorption or Disposition of Calcium

Interacting drug	Adverse effect	Mechanism
Tetracycline antibiotics Quinolone antibiotics Iron salts Alendronate	Therapeutic effects of these drugs are reduced	Calcium binds with these drugs in the gut to form insoluble complexes, thereby reducing their absorption. Calcium supplements should therefore be given 3–4 h prior to or after these drugs.
Phosphates Cholestyramine Thiazide diuretics	Reduced absorption of calcium Hypercalcemia and milk-alkali syndrome	Insoluble complexes are formed in the gut. Thiazides decrease calcium excretion by increasing distal tubular reabsorption. Hypercalcemia and metabolic alkalosis may occur if they are combined with high doses of clacium supplements (5 to 10 g/d,chronically)
Calcium channel blockers	Inhibition of activity of calcium channel blockers	Pharmacologic antagonism. Calcium has been used to reverse toxicity associated with calcium channel blockers.

sources. Excess serum levels of calcium, particularly its carbonated salt, can induce milk-alkali syndrome and cause severe renal damage and ectopic calcification. Several drugs may interfere with the absoprtion of calcium and its metabolism (Table 2). Calcium also interferes with the absorption of phosphates and other minerals such as fluoride, iron, manganese, and zinc (30). The extent to which calcium interferes with iron absorption depends on the source of calcium. Deehr et al. demonstrated that calcium in milk or as a citrate-malate salt had a negative influence on the iron absorption, the latter exerting a smaller effect (30).

If calcium citrate-malate is taken with orange juice, the absorption of iron (particularly the nonheme form) is less affected because the citric and ascorbic acids in orange juice enhance absorption of nonheme iron. The exact mechanism of iron-calcium interactions is not clearly understood as yet and appears to be quite complex.

A study by Recker and Heaney looked at the absorption of calcium from milk as compared to no intervention in a small number of healthy postmenopausal women. Their results suggested that calcium in milk and dairy products was effective in suppressing bone remodeling to some extent, that the phosphorus content of the diet did not significantly affect the absorption of calcium, and that reduced dietary protein content enhanced calcium absorption (31).

Calcium-containing antacids can be used as a calcium supplement. Among all the salts, elemental calcium content is greatest (about 40%) in the carbonate and phosphate preparations. With advancing age, less calcium is absorbed.

Most of the calcium is probably absorbed in its ionic form, in the acid environment of the stomach. In the presence of other anions in food such as phosphate and oxalate and in the alkaline medium of the lower bowel, calcium absorption is reduced when encased in solid fecal matter *(32)*. Calcium carbonate is highly soluble in the acid environment of the stomach, its solubility being directly proportional to the amount of gastric acid secreted. In the absence of food, formation of calcium complexes with bicarbonate (in pancreatic secretions) is minimal. Some calcium carbonate may also be absorbed in the mild acid environment of the distal bowel that is free of fecal matter. Calcium phosphate is virtually insoluble in the absence of gastric acid and is highly soluble at peak acid secretion. It tends to precipitate in the duodenum in the presence of bicarbonate from pancreatic juices. The bioavailability from this salt is therefore limited. Calcium citrate (solid and liquid forms) is more soluble than carbonate for a given level of acid secretion as it is a poorer buffer of gastric acid. However, a significant amount forms complexes with bicarbonate and therefore decreases the bioavailability. The liquid form is richer in citrate than the solid form and its solubility is independent of gastric pH. It is neutralized by pancreatic juices, but may be absorbed by the mucosa of the distal bowel free of fecal matter.

In the absence of gastric acid secretion, the availability of ionic calcium from the carbonate and phosphate salts is very limited *(33)*. Calcium citrate (especially the liquid form) is the supplement of choice in the absence of food in patients with achlorhydria, diminished acid secretion, those receiving H_2-receptor antagonists, and in women who prefer to take the supplements without food *(34)*. Calcium carbonate is more efficient as a source of ionic calcium in younger persons with normal gastric acid secretion and especially when it is taken with food. Brennan et al. determined the in vitro dissolution of 27 available commercial calcium supplements and concluded that it is the filler in these preparations that determines the extent of dissolution of the tablets *(35)*. It has been shown that the percentage of calcium absorbed varies inversely with the increase in calcium load and that the daily administered dose of calcium is more effective if taken in divided doses.

Certain types of foods can alter the amount of gastrin or gastric acid secretion and can affect the absorption of calcium by providing an acid or alkaline milieu. The best dietary sources are milk, dairy products, and certain vegetables. Milk and its products have more calcium than other foods on a weight-for-weight basis *(36)*. The calcium content of low- and nonfat milk and dairy foods is equivalent to those with high fat content. Hence, the use of skim milk and other dairy foods with reduced fat content is recommended to protect against the age-related risk of atherosclerosis and cardiovascular disease, particularly in women whose baseline risk of heart disease is increased by declining or minimal estrogen levels. Besides calcium, milk also provides other essential nutrients including vitamins D, A, and B_{12}, and potassium, phosphorus, magnesium, protein, niacin, and riboflavin.

Calcium in milk is readily absorbable due to its presence in a more soluble form and the presence of lactose. Individuals with milder forms of lactose intolerance, which may constitute 25% of the adult United States population, therefore may be unable to absorb calcium efficiently from this source. Lactose intolerance in adults tends to be induced by lack of exposure to dietary sources of lactose. The intestine stops making lactase when it is chronically not needed. As the formation of the enzyme lactase by the epithelial cells of the small intestine is inducible by exposure to lactose-containing foods, it has been recommended that incremental addition of dairy products to a diet that is otherwise

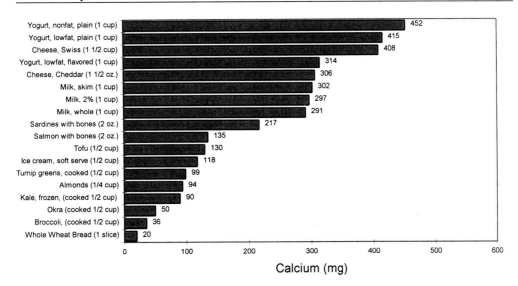

Fig. 1. Calcium contribution of foods. Source: USDA Agriculture Handbook No. 8-1.

devoid of lactose helps overcome this intolerance. In those with genuine lactose intolerance, milk should be ingested with solid food or enzyme supplements in the forms of tablets or drops. These strategies lead to fewer symptoms of lactose malabsorption. These individuals also tolerate milk with added sucrose (chocolate and skim milk) better.

Foods such as steak and other meat favor an acid environment and increase the solubility of calcium salts, but they also contain significant levels of phosphates, which counter the beneficial effects. Despite its high calcium content, spinach forms insoluble calcium oxalate when ingested with calcium carbonate and reduces calcium absorption *(37).* However, this effect of spinach is less with the citrated salt of calcium. Kale, in contrast, contains a more readily absorbable form of calcium. The potential calcium content of several foods is displayed in Fig. 1.

Citrus juices contain significant amounts of citrate, which forms calcium citrate when ingested with calcium carbonate salts and thereby provides a greater amount of ionized calcium for absorption even in the presence of achlorhydria. However, excessive amounts of citrate can complex solubilized calcium and limit its absorption. Phosphates and phytates in bran products also limit calcium availability as does the high dietary fiber content in wheat bran and beans. Soy beans yield better absorption of calcium than do other common beans. Knox et al. demonstrated in their study that calcium absorption in the presence of high fiber was independent of the gastric acidity and that calcium was absorbed just as effectively in achlorhydric individuals as the control group *(38).* Most of the calcium of plant origin is bound to its fiber content and is not available for absorption in the neutral pH of the small intestine where the fiber remains undigested. In the colon, the bacterial flora ferment more than 80% of the fiber and release the bound calcium, thereby making it available for absorption. Despite the reduced capacity of the colon to absorb calcium as opposed to the small intestine, the colon may have some role to play in calcium absorption as the transit time of food is several times greater than the small intestine *(39).*

Long-term calcium deficiency, apart from causing osteopenia and osteoporosis, is also believed to increase the risk of hypertension, a major risk factor for cardiovascular disease and stroke *(40)*. However, one prospective, cross-sectional study cast a shadow of doubt on the beneficial role of calcium on maintenance of blood pressure in the normotensive range, but concluded that calcium supplementation might be of some benefit in those subjects whose intake is extremely low *(40)*.

THE ROLE OF VITAMIN D

When first discovered, vitamin D was classified as a nutrient and grouped with the other fat-soluble vitamins, A, E, and K, as its deficiency led to defective bone mineralization. Since then, the understanding of the structure and function of this compound has improved significantly and it is now regarded as a hormone, synthesized by the kidneys, with a host of possibly unidentified intracellular functions, apart from its most important effect on calcium homeostasis *(41)*. It also suppresses cell proliferation and cell differentiation and may have a place in the treatment of psoriasis.

When the skin is exposed to solar ultraviolet radiation of wavelength 230–313 nm (UV-B radiation), it forms vitamin D_3 (cholecalciferol) from a precursor, 7-dehydrocholesterol. Emission of UV radiation of the wavelength required for vitamin D synthesis occurs only during certain seasons in the year as one moves away from the equator. This beneficial effect is further reduced by clothing and sunscreens, which block UV-B radiation and, to a lesser extent, UV-A radiation *(42)*. Among different kinds of fabrics studied, black wool reduced transmission of UV-B radiation by 98.6%, white cotton by only 47.7%, and polyester in the intermediate range. Regular seasonal street clothing decreases vitamin D formation in the skin, but not nearly as much as heavier garments *(42)*. Vitamin D_3 differs from vitamin D_2 (ergocalciferol), which is formed from a steroid ergosterol by fungi under the influence of the Sun's ultraviolet light.

Vitamin D_1 is the collective name for the combination of vitamin D_2 and other sterols and is no longer used. Vitamin D_3 (commonly referred to as vitamin D) is required in small amounts by the body and plays a key role in the body calcium homeostasis, along with PTH and calcitonin. It is necessary, albeit in small quantities, for the absorption of calcium from the intestines (especially in the presence of deficiency states, low dietary supply, and increased body requirements), bone turnover, and renal excretion of calcium.

Vitamin D produced in skin is by itself inactive. It has to be hydroxylated in two stages to its biologically active form. The first stage is the conversion to 25-hydroxycholecalciferol in the endoplasmic reticulum of the liver cells (a dihydroxylated metabolite). This is then released into the blood stream where it circulates bound to a specific vitamin D binding globulin. In the cells of the proximal convoluted tubule during the second stage, it is converted to its trihydroxylated active form, 1,25-dihydroxycholecalciferol (DHC), which is secreted into the blood to exert the desired effect on the target cells.

Vitamin D and calcium have been implicated in reducing the risk of colonic cancer, the third largest cause of mortality secondary to cancer among men in the United States. It is believed that calcium in the diet forms insoluble calcium soaps in the colonic lumen with secondary bile acids and ionized free-fatty acids, which would otherwise be toxic to the epithelial lining of the colon. Vitamin D in rats has been shown to reduce tumorigenesis and may exert a protective role in humans by possibly influencing the regulation of cell proliferation in the gut *(43)*.

MECHANISM OF ACTION OF 1,25 (OH)$_2$-D (1,25 DIHYDROXYCHOLECALCIFEROL)

Target cells elaborate an intranuclear receptor protein, which serves as a binding site for 1,25(OH)$_2$-D. The combination of the receptor protein and 1,25(OH)$_2$-D then binds to the regulatory sequences on the chromosomal DNA, which induces the transcription of specific messenger RNA that code for proteins responsible for cellular function of vitamin D. Vitamin D receptors have now been identified in osteoblast cell lines, osteoblasts, and osteoprogenitor cells in intact bone, but not in fully differentiated osteoclasts. This mechanism of action is similar to that of steroid hormones and this is why it is now believed that vitamin D is more likely a hormone than a nutrient.

Vitamin D is useful in stimulating bone formation from a low turnover state by promoting differentiation of osteoblasts, but once this is complete prolonged effects of excess vitamin D could have the unwanted effect of inhibiting the final stages of bone formation. Therefore one has to bear in mind not to administer excessive amounts of vitamin D to treat bone loss that is not secondary to vitamin D deficiency. Because of concerns about toxicity, few foods are fortified with vitamin D. An 8-oz glass of milk contains 100 IU and most vitamin tablets contain 400 IU. Up to 800 IU daily of vitamin D is safe and at least 200 IU is needed daily in young adults and children.

IMPACT OF AGE AND ESTROGENS ON VITAMIN D AND CALCIUM METABOLISM

Several studies using radioisotope absorption techniques have shown that intestinal absorption of calcium decreases with age more so in those with osteoporosis. Vitamin D and estrogens appear to correct this age-related defect *(44)*.

Postmenopausal women who showed an increase in the calcium absorption from the intestines in response to both estrogens and 25-hydroxycholecalciferol (the precursor of 1,25 (OH)$_2$_D) had increased levels of 1,25(OH)$_2$_D, whereas those who did not respond did not have increased levels of 1,25(OH)$_2$_D *(45)*. The reason for decreased levels of 1,25(OH)$_2$_D with advancing age is not clear and might be due to decreased production by an aging kidney that is also estrogen deprived. These mechanisms probably account for the fall in the intestinal absorption of calcium with age. It is also possible that the intestine becomes more resistant to the action of vitamin D, thereby reducing the transport of calcium. Vitamin D metabolites and 1,25(OH)$_2$_D levels have been shown to be reduced in elderly subjects over age 65 and may further increase the risk of fractures associated with aging. In a subgroup of the elderly population, despite normal blood levels of these metabolites, there is reduced absorption of calcium suggesting a degree of tissue resistance probably as a consequence of aging or reduced levels of vitamin D receptors. 1,25(OH)$_2$_D production by the kidneys is less efficient in the elderly and those with declining renal function and does not respond to an increase in PTH levels.

How useful then is vitamin D administration in the prevention and treatment of osteoporosis? Several studies have confirmed that supplementation of vitamin D with calcium in the elderly population who were mildly vitamin D and calcium deficient increased femoral and vertebral bone density and decreased the incidence of hip, vertebral, and nonvertebral fractures *(46,47)*. Milk is currently the best source of vitamin D, each glass providing about 100 IU and 300 mg of elemental calcium. Several multivitamin preparations are commercially available with 400 IU of vitamin D. In the absence of vitamin D, calcium absorption from milk is reduced to less than 10% *(48)*.

VITAMIN D TOXICITY

Vitamin D is a fat-soluble vitamin and accumulates in the body when synthetic preparations are administered orally, even in small amounts over a prolonged period of time. Surprisingly, prolonged exposure to sunlight does not produce excess vitamin D in the body despite inducing a sunburn. The toxic action of oral vitamin D can be so potent that its use has extended to being a commercial rodenticide, which kills mice and rats within 24–48 h of ingestion in concentrations of 0.1% of their diet *(49)*. The mechanism of toxicity is believed to lie in its capacity to induce hypercalcemia with metastatic calcification of soft tissues and a generalized disturbance in whole-body calcium homeostasis. The toxic action is probably mediated via 25(OH)-D, the concentration of which rises to greater than 20 times the normal level in hypervitaminosis D despite the level of $1,25(OH)_2$-D remaining unchanged *(50)*.

CLINICAL RECOMMENDATIONS

As clinicians, it is important to reiterate the importance of an adequate calcium and vitamin D intake from a young age and educate the public with regard to simple measures that are vital in preventing the crippling disease of osteoporosis. This can be achieved by counseling women of all ages, beginning at as early an age as possible, particularly in those with known risk factors or a family history of osteoporosis. Maintaining diaries and records with respect to topics discussed and review dates may be beneficial to both patients and clinicians. Prevention at a primary level is less expensive, more effective, and relatively easier to achieve than correcting an established condition.

Fortunately, even after the window of opportunity for bone accretion has passed, lifestyle factors such as adequate calcium intake and exercise still help. In established osteoporosis, calcium intake buttresses the effects of pharmacologic agents such as estrogens, bisphosphonates, and calcitonin. Throughout the life cycle, adequate calcium intake is crucial to bone and overall health. An informed and interested physician can then serve as the guardian of bone health by encouraging healthy behaviors, including sufficient calcium intake.

REFERENCES

1. Margen S, Chu J-Y, Kaufmann NA, Calloway DH. Studies in calcium metabolism. 1. The calciuretic effect of dietary protein. Am J Clin Nutr 1974;27:584–589.
2. Parfitt AM. Dietary risk factors for age-related bone loss and fractures. Lancet 1983;2:1181–1185.
3. Heaney RP. Calcium in the prevention and treatment of osteoporosis. J Intern Med 1992;231:169–180.
4. Nordin BEC, Polley KJ, Need AG, Morris HA, Marshall D. The problem of calcium requirement. Am J Clin Nutr 1987;45:1295–1304.
5. Charles P, Jensen FT, Mosekilde L, Hansen HH. Calcium metabolism evaluated by 47Calcium kinetics :estimation of dermal calcium loss. Clin Sci 1983;65:415–422.
6. Heaney RP, Recker RR, Saville PD. Calcium balance and requirements in middle-aged women. Am J Clin Nutr 1977;30:1603–1611.
7. Goulding A. Effects of varying dietary salt intake on the fasting urinary excretion of sodium, calcium and hydroxyproline in young women. NZ Med J 1983;96:953–954.
8. Dawson-Hughes B. Calcium supplementation and bone loss: a review of controlled clinical trials. Am J Clin Nutr 1991;54:274S-80S.
9. Kochersberger G, Westlund R, Lyles KW. The metabolic effects of calcium supplementation in the elderly. J Am Geriatr Soc 1991;39:192–196.
10. Cosman F, Shen V, Xie F, Seibel M, Ratcliffe A, Lindsay R. Estrogen protection against bone resorbing effects of parathyroid hormone infusion. Assessment by use of biochemical markers. Ann Intern Med 1993;118:337–343.

11. Heaney RP, Skillman TG. Secretion and excretion of calcium by the human gastrointestinal tract. J Lab Clin Med 1964;64:29–41.

12. Mangaroo J, Glasser JH, Roht LH, Kapadia AS. Prevalence of bone demineralization in the United States. Bone 1985;6:135–139.

13. Johnson CC Jr. The relative importance of nutrition compared to the genetic factors in the development of bone mass. In: Buckhardt P, Heaney RP, eds. Nutritional Aspects of Osteoporosis, Proceedings of International Symposium. Lausanne, Switzerland, May 1991. Raven, New York, 1991.

14. Holbrook TL, Barret-Connor E, Wingard DL. Dietary calcium and risk of hip fracture: 14-year prospective population study. Lancet 1988;2:1046–1049.

15. Berga SL. Ways of optimizing calcium intake. Contemporary OB/GYN, June 1996;41:85–91.

16. Heaney RP. Estrogen calcium interactions in the post-menopause: a quantitive description. Bone Miner 1990;11:67–84.

17. Dawson-Hughes B, Dallal GE, Krall EA, Sadowski L, Sahyoun N, Tannenbaum S. A controlled trial of the effect of calcium supplementation on bone density in postmenopausal women. N Engl J Med 1990;323:878–883.

18. Nordin BEC, Need AG, Chatterton BE, Horowitz M, Morris HA. The relative contributions of age and years since menopause to postmenopausal bone loss. J Clin Endocrinol Metab 1990;70:83–88.

19. Reid IR, Ames RW, Evans EW, Gamble GD, Sharpe SJ. Effect of calcium supplementation on bone loss in postmenopausal women. N Engl J Med 1993;328:460–464.

20. Elders PJM, Netelenbos JC, Lips P, Van Ginkel FC, Khoe E, Leeuwencamp OR, Hackeng WHL, Vander Stelt PF. Calcium supplementation reduces vertebral bone loss in perimenopausal women: A controlled trial in 248 women between 46 and 55 years of age. J Clin Endocrinol Metab 1991;73:533–540.

21. Horowitz M, Need AG, Philcox JC, Nordin BEC. Effect of calcium supplementation on urinary hydroxyproline in osteoporotic postmenopausal women. Am J Clin Nutr 1984;39:857–859.

22. Need AG, Horowitz M, Morris HA, Nordin BEC. Effects of three different calcium preparations on urinary calcium and hydroxyproline excretion in postmenopausal women. Eur J Clin Nutr 1991;45:357–361.

23. Riis B, Thomsen K, Christiansen C. Does calcium supplementation prevent postmenopausal bone loss? N Engl J Med 1987;316:173–177.

24. Nordin BEC, Heaney RP. Calcium supplementation of the diet: justified by present evidence. Br Med J 1990;300:1056–1060.

25. Heaney RP, Recker RR, Saville PD. Menopausal changes in calcium balance performance. J Lab Clin Med 1978;92:953–963.

26. Kochersberger G, Bales C, Lobaugh B, Lyles KW. Calcium supplementation serum parathyroid hormone levels in elderly subjects. J Gerontol 1990;45:M159–M162.

27. Delmi M, Rapin CH, Bengoa JM, Delmas PD, Vasey H, Bonjour JP. Dietary supplementation in elderly patients with fractured neck of femur. Lancet 1990;335:1013–1016.

28. Calcium supplements. The Medical Letter 1996;38:108–109.

29. Bourgoin BP, Evan ER, Cornett JR, Lingard SM, Quattrone AJ. Am J Public Health 1993;83:1155–1160.

30. Deehr MS, Dallal GE, Smith KT, Taulbee JD, Dawson-Hughes B. Effects of different calcium sources on iron absorption in postmenopausal women. Am J Clin Nutr 1990;51:95–99.

31. Recker RR, Heaney RP. The effects of milk supplements on calcium metabolism, bone metabolism, and calcium balance. Am J Clin Nutr 1985;41:254–263.

32. Jensen FT, Charles P, Mosekilde L, Hansen HH. Calcium metabolism evaluated by 47Calcium-kinetics: a physiological model with correction for fecal lag time and estimation of dermal calcium loss. Clin Physiol 1983; 3:187–204.

33. Recker RR. Calcium absorption and achlorhydria. N Engl J Med 1985;313:70–73.

34. Pak CYC, Avioli LV. Factors affecting absorbability of calcium from calcium salts and food. Calcif Tissue Int 1988;43:55–60.

35. Brennan MJ, Duncan WE, Wartofsky L, Butler VM, Wray LH. In vitro dissolution of calcium carbonate preparations. Calcif Tissue Int 1991;49:308–312.

36. Mortensen L, Peder C. Bioavailibility of calcium supplements and the effect of vitamin D: comparisons between milk, calcium carbonate and calcium carbonate plus vitamin D. Am J Clin Nutr 1996;63:354–357.

37. Heaney RP, Weaver CM, Recker RR. Calcium absorbability from spinach. Am J Clin Nutr 1988;47:707–709.

38. Knox TA, Kassarjian Z, Dawson-Hughes B, Golner BB, Dallal GE, Arora S, Russel RM. Calcium Absorption in elderly subjects on high and low-fiber diets: effect of gastric acidity. Am J Clin Nutr 1991;53:1480–1486.

39. James WPT, Branch WJ, Southgate DAT. Calcium binding by dietary fibre. Lancet 1978;1: 638–639.
40. Thomsen K, Nilas L, Christiansen C. Dietary calcium intake and blood pressure in normotensive subjects. Acta Med Scand 1987;222:51–56.
41. Fraser DR. Fat-soluble vitamins — vitamin D. Lancet 1995:345:104–107.
42. Matsuoka LY, Wortsman J, Dannenberg MJ, Hollis BW, Zhiren LU, Holick MF. Clothing prevents ultraviolet-B radiation-dependent photosynthesis of vitamin D_3 . J Clin Endocrinol Metab 1992;75:1099–1103.
43. Kearney J, Giovannucci E, Rimm EB, Ascherio A, Stampfer MJ, Golditz GA, Wing A, Kampman E, Willett WC. Calcium, vitamin D, and dairy foods and the occurrence of colon cancer in men. Am J Epidemiol 1996;143:907–917.
44. Gennari C, Agnusdei D, Nardi P, Civitelli R. Estrogen preserves a normal intestinal responsiveness to 1,25–dihydroxyvitamin D_3 in oophorectomized women. J Clin Endocrinol Metab 1990;71:1288–1293.
45. Zerwekh JE, Sakhaee K, Glass K, Pak CY. Long-term 25–hydroxyvitamin D_3 therapy in postmeno-pausal osteoporosis: demonstration of responsive and nonresponsive subgroups. J Clin Endocrinol Metab 1983;56:410–413.
46. Chapuy MC, Arlot ME, Duboeuf F, Brun J, Crouzet B, Arnaud S, Delmas PD, Meunier PJ. Vitamin D_3 and calcium to prevent hip fractures in elderly women. N Engl J Med 1992;327:1637–1642.
47. Dawson-Hughes B, Dallal GE, Krall EA, Harris S, Sokoll LJ, Falconer G. Effect of vitamin D supple-mentation in wintertime and overall bone loss in healthy postmenopausal women. Ann Intern Med 1991;115:505–512.
48. Heaney RP. Thinking straight about calcium. N Engl J Med 1993;328:503–505.
49. Greaves JH, Redfern R, King RE. Some properties of calciferol as a rodenticide. J Hygiene 1974;73:341–351.
50. Hughes MR, Baylink DJ, Jones PG, Hanssier MR. Radiological Receptor assay for 25–hydroxyvitamin D_2/D_3 and 1α, 25–hydroxyvitamin D_2/D_3 . J Clin Invest 1976;58:61–70.

15   Phytoestrogens and Menopause

Geetha Matthews, MD
and Veronica A. Ravnikar, MD

CONTENTS

INTRODUCTION
CLASSIFICATION OF PHYTOESTROGENS
PHYTOESTROGENS STUDIED IN TISSUE CULTURE
CLINICAL AND IN VIVO STUDIES OF PHYTOESTROGENS —
    MENOPAUSAL SYMPTOMS
PHYTOESTROGENS AND OSTEOPOROSIS
PHYTOESTROGENS AND CARDIOVASCULAR DISEASE
PHYTOESTROGENS AND BREAST CANCER
CONCLUSION
REFERENCES

INTRODUCTION

Although women are aware of the reported benefits of hormone replacement therapy to their postmenopausal health and quality of life, many opt not to follow such a regimen, whether because of fears of negative effects or preferences for nonmedical or natural alternatives.

Dietary adjustments are one component of a nonmedical, lifestyle approach to the menopause. This approach has traditionally included increased calcium intake, lower dietary cholesterol, and regular exercise. More recently, however, a natural approach to the menopause has come to include dietary sources of estrogens, known as phytoestrogens.

Phytoestrogens are compounds produced by plants that have estrogenic properties when ingested by animals and humans. Medical interest in phytoestrogens originates in part from epidemiological studies that correlate national differences in the incidence of certain diseases with national variations in diet and lifestyle *(1)*. Specifically, these studies have attributed the lower incidence in East Asian societies of breast and prostate cancer, cardiovascular disease, and other hormonally associated problems like osteoporosis, to the phytoestrogen-rich soy-based diets traditionally consumed in these cultures *(2,3)*.

Phytoestrogens have gained an audience among those studying menopause because they offer a natural, dietary source of estrogen for the body. They have documented estrogen-like activities in vitro and in vivo and potential benefits similar to HRT in terms

From: *Contemporary Endocrinology: Menopause: Endocrinology and Management*
Edited by: D. B. Seifer and E. A. Kennard © Humana Press Inc., Totowa, NJ

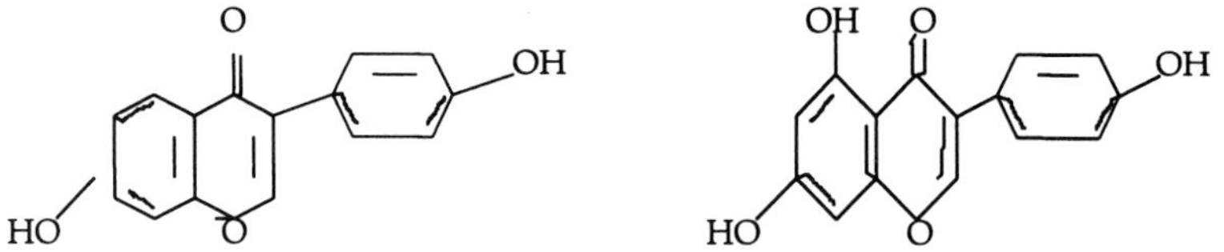

Daidzein   Genistein

Fig. 1. From *(19)* Messina MJ, Persky V, Setchell KDR, Barnes S. Soy intake and cancer risk: a review of the in vivo and in vitro data. Nutr Cancer 1994;21:113–131.

of symptomatic relief and protection from heart disease and bone fractures. Moreover, studies suggesting that dietary estrogens decrease the risk of breast cancer have increased their appeal as a topic of medical research in women's health.

The following brief review aims to consider the current state of knowledge on the physiological and medical relevance of phytoestrogens for women's health, particularly during and after menopause. Included with data from epidemiological studies and trials in humans are animal studies and in vitro experiments.

CLASSIFICATION OF PHYTOESTROGENS

More than 300 plant species have been found to contain phytoestrogens *(4,5)*. Chemically, phytoestrogens are classified as either lignans, isoflavones, or coumestans (*see* Fig. 1). They are produced in varying amounts in a plant in response to conditions of climate, soil fertility, and threats from pests and disease *(6,7)*. The production of these estrogen "impersonators" in the plant kingdom is theorized to exemplify the coevolutionary chemical "arms race" between plants' defensive strategies and their animal predators' adaptive abilities *(7)*.

Lignans are a class of phytoestrogens that form components of plant cell walls. They enter the gut as matairesinol and secoisolaricresinol and are metabolized by colonic bacteria into enterolactone and enterodiol, respectively. Enterodiol itself is a metabolic precursor of enterolactone. All four of these lignans can be absorbed from the gut *(8)*. Although lignans are found in a wide variety of fruits, vegetables, and cereals, they are found in highest concentrations in oilseeds like the linseed, which produces lignans in concentrations 100 times greater than those of other plants. Other diverse sources of lignans include lentils, dry seaweed, wheat, garlic, pears, and plums *(9)*.

The major isoflavones are genistein and daidzein (*see* Fig. 1). These enter the gut bound to a sugar moiety, which is removed by gut flora. Daidzein is formed from formonectin and is then metabolized into equol or O-desmethylangolensin, both of which are more potent estrogenically than their precursor. Genistein is formed from biochanin A and is metabolized into an inactive metabolite *(8)*. The major dietary source for isoflavones are soybeans and soy products, though some legumes such as peas and bean varieties, and the red clover herb, also contain appreciable amounts of isoflavones *(10,11)*.

Coumestans in the diet are found less commonly than the other two classes of phytoestrogens. Their main sources are byproducts of bean germination, like alfalfa and soybean sprouts. They are also found in clover *(11)*.

Metabolism of phytoestrogens varies between individuals, often depending on gastrointestinal flora, which is in turn influenced by gender, bowel pathology, and antibiotic

Table 1
Some Food Sources of Isoflavone
and Lignan Phytoestrogens

Isoflavones	Lignans
Roasted soybeans	Flaxseed flour
Soyflour	Lentil
Soy milk	Dried seaweed
Tempeh	Oat bran
Tofu	Wheat
Tofu yogurt	Wheat germ
Dry soy noodle	Barley
Lentils	Hops
Haricot beans	Rye
Kidney beans	Rice
Lima beans	Kidney beans
Chick peas	Cherries
	Apples
	Pears
	Carrots
	Sunflower seeds
	Fennel
	Vegetable oils

From refs. *9, 17*, and *14*.

use *(12)*. After absorption, differentially active metabolic pathways appear to be at work, leading to a variety of metabolites. Alternatively, once conjugated, these metabolites can enter the bile, undergo deconjugation in the gut, and reenter the enterohepatic circulation. In biological assays, isoflavones and lignans have been isolated in human plasma, urine, feces, semen, bile, saliva, and breast milk *(14)*.

As mentioned previously, variation in the phytoestrogen content of plants depends on the particular stresses encountered by the specific plant, as well as on the food-processing techniques employed. For example, second generation soy products such as soy noodles or soy yogurt, have been found to contain only 20% of the isoflavones found in soy beans as a whole *(15)* (*see* Table 1).

Whereas throughout Asia, consumption of phytoestrogen in a traditional diet is estimated to be about 25–45 mg/d of isoflavones, in Western countries it is estimated that less than 5 mg/d of isoflavones are consumed *(16)*.

It is worth mentioning that phytoestrogens are not the only dietary estrogens. Contaminants from pesticides like DDT, know as xenoestrogens, and resorcylic acid lactones produced by mold contaminants of cereal crops, known as mycoestrogens, are two other classes of estrogenically active compounds in the diet not discussed here. They gain entry into the food chain as contaminants of air, water, and food *(17)*.

PHYTOESTROGENS STUDIED IN TISSUE CULTURE

Studies of phytoestrogen activity in animal tissues have yielded an array of data enumerating the various ways in which these compounds exert their physiological effects. Phytoestrogens are much less potent than endogenous and synthetic estrogens. In human cell cultures, the potencies of bioassayed phytoestrogens were found to be at least 1000-

fold weaker relative to estradiol, with coumestrol = 0.00202, genistein = 0.00084, equol = 0.0061, diadzein = 0.00013, and formonetin = 0.000006 *(1,18)*.

Many studies conducted in human breast cancer cell lines have focused specifically on the behavior of genistein, an isoflavone whose dissociation constant has been measured at 100–10,000 times that of estradiol *(19)*. These cell culture studies have shown genistein's concentration-dependent activity to be biphasic, with growth stimulation at low concentrations (10 nM–μM), followed by growth inhibition at higher concentrations (20 μM). Moreover, in estrogen receptor-negative (ER–) cell lines, only the genistein's inhibitory activity at the higher concentration is observed, suggesting that the inhibitory mechanism is not mediated by the ER *(20,21)*. This may change in the future because more than one ER has been found and the older studies had antibiodies only to ER α receptors.

Independent of its actions at the human ER, genistein has also been shown to hinder tyrosine kinase activity *(22)*. Because of the role this enzyme plays in tumorogenesis via growth factors (GF) like epidermal GF, platelet-derived GF, insulin, and transforming GF alpha, it is hypothesised that the antityrosine kinase activity represents a key element in genistein's observed ability to inhibit breast cancer cell growth in culture. Other antiproliferative actions observed in vitro include genistein's inhibition of topoisomerase I and II, and of ribosomal s6 kinase, enzymes involved in the stabilization and translation of DNA, respectively *(14)*. Delay of endothelial cell proliferation in culture has also been documented, suggesting inhibition of angiogenesis by genistein *(23)*. Genistein, as well as daidzein, have demonstrated potent antioxidant properties *(24)*. Aromatase enzyme inhibition and increased sex hormone-binding globulin (SHBG) production are additional observed effects of genistein and other isoflavones in human cell lines *(25,26)*.

Other phytoestrogens have been studied in vitro, including the lignan enterolactone and the isoflavone Biochanin A, a precursor of genistein. Enterolactone was shown to inhibit ER+ breast cancer cells in the presence of estradiol, but to stimulate cell proliferation when acting alone, suggesting a mixed agonist/antagonist role at the ER *(27)*. This is in contrast to coumestrol and equol, which, unlike enterolactone, appear to act only as an ER agonist in mammalian cells, stimulating cell growth with increasing doses *(28)*.

Biochanin A, in a experimental system where the human estrogen receptor and two estrogen response elements were linked to the lacZ yeast gene, was shown to be antiestrogenic. Although biochanin was able to inhibit the activity of estradiol at the human estrogen receptor in a dose dependent fashion, it was completely ineffectual at blocking the stimulatory activities of either coumestrol or genistein at the same receptor, suggesting receptor conformational changes in the presence of these ligands *(29)*.

Extrapolation of the detailed in vitro data on phytoestrogen bioactivity to the in vivo context is not self-evident. Whereas tissue cultures demonstrating genistein's inhibition of tumor proliferation require a concentration of 10–100 mmol/L of genistein *(18,19)*, the highest serum genistein levels attained in humans after a high soy diet are only about 0.5–4 mmol/L *(30)*. Moreover, in vivo studies of phytoestrogens' effects have been shown to be species-specific. For example, although sheep exposure to equol precursors in the pasture flora led to the development of uterine inertia, uterine prolapse, abnormal mammary glands, and a cystic endometrium, this same diet, when fed in the same concentration to mares, did not result in any significant rise in reproductive pathology *(31)*.

CLINICAL AND IN VIVO STUDIES OF PHYTOESTROGENS — MENOPAUSAL SYMPTOMS

The health concerns surrounding menopause mainly relate to the decrease in circulating estrogens that results from follicular depletion of the ovaries. Short- and long-term morbidity secondary to this loss of estrogen includes vasomotor flushing and genitourinary atrophy as well as osteoporosis and ischemic heart disease.

The lower incidence of breast cancer, osteoporosis, and heart disease in Asian women consuming traditional phytoestrogen-rich diets (together with the less-frequent occurrence of menopausal hot flashes reported by them), when compared to the increasing incidence in these ailments among Asians who follow a Western diet, led to the evaluation of the potential benefits of dietary phytoestrogens during the after the menopause (1,2,32,33).

Results from short-term studies evaluating phytoestrogen-rich diets for evidence of estrogenic or therapeutic responses in menopausal women have varied. Overall, they demonstrate a small estrogenic response in vaginal cytology and a decrease in hot flashes, though not all studies conclusively agree. Arguably, much of the variation between trials derives from differences in sample size, phytoestrogen diet source, duration of evaluation, as well as the tendency of hot flashes to resolve over time (17).

Baird et al. (34) set out to test the hypothesis that a four-week diet rich in soy, providing 165 mg/d in phytoestrogens and equivalent in potency to 0.3 mg/d of steroidal estrogen, would provide estrogenic changes in 94 postmenopausal women. Compared to the control group, no significant increase in the amount of superficial vaginal cells were found. Similarly, the anticipated decreases in LH and FSH, and increase in SHBG were not found to be significant.

A 12-wk randomized, double-blind study by Murkies et al. (35), using unstated amounts of dietary phytoestrogens in 45 g of soy protein, found no significant change in vaginal cell maturation, but did find a significant 40% decrease in vasomotor flushing symptoms. This 40% decrease over a period of 12 wk is comparable with estrogen replacement therapy, where symptoms have been shown to decrease by 60% in 3 mo (36). This observed attenuating effect of phytoestrogens on the vasomotor symptoms of menopause has been attributed to phytoestogens' ability to decrease the responsiveness of the pituitary to GnRH, leading to decreased circulating LH (7).

Conclusive recommendations are lacking regarding the use of dietary phytoestrogens to treat common menopausal complaints. Because of its potential to help some symptomatic menopausal women, and because many patients express an interest in natural remedies for these symptoms, 30–50 mg/d of isoflavones in the diet has been suggested for those in search of minimally therapeutic estrogenic effects (37).

PHYTOESTROGENS AND OSTEOPOROSIS

To date, sufficient data from long-term studies on the possible benefit of phytoestrogens in preventing the osteoporetic changes associated with menopause are lacking. Again, indirect evidence derives from female Asian populations with diets high in phytoestrogens who have significantly lower rates of osteoporosis and hip fractures than women consuming a Western diet (38).

Animal studies have shown that ovarectomized rats fed dietary soybeans sustained significantly less bone loss than controls (39). Another study in ovarectomized rats demonstrated that genistein in low doses maintains trabecular bone mass in these animals at a rate equivalent to standard doses of conjugated equine estrogens. At higher doses, genistein had no retentive effects on the bone and instead appears to interfere with normal cell metabolism and kinetics in bony tissue *(40)*. Genistein's biphasic response in bony tissue is similar to that of Ipriflavone, a synthetic flavonoid that inhibits osteoclast recruitment and function and was shown to prevent bone loss at the distal radius in osteoporotic postmenopausal women at a dose of 600 mg/d *(41)*.

Another postmenopausal study revealed a significant increase in bone mineral content and density in postmenopausal women given a diet of 2.25 mg isoflavones/g protein for 6 mo *(42)*. Bone mineral content increased significantly as well in a trial of postmenopausal women fed 45 g/d of soy-enriched breads *(43)*. Although studies in both animals and humans seem to confirm the preventative role of phytoestrogens against osteoporosis, the clinical relevance of this evidence has yet to be delineated by longer-term studies.

PHYTOESTROGENS AND CARDIOVASCULAR DISEASE

Like osteoporosis, the incidence of heart disease rises in women postmenopausally, approaching the incidence seen in men of the same age. In postmenopausal women who use estrogen replacement therapy, the relative risk for ischemic heart disease is 0.56 *(44)*. The protection afforded by estrogen is thought to derive from its favorable impact on lipid profiles, as, simply put, it decreases low-density lipoprotein (LDL) and increases high-density lipoprotein (HDL); additionally, estrogen improves vasomotor tone and increases vessel wall compliance *(14)*.

As weak estrogen analogues, dietary phytoestrogens might be expected to provide cardioprotection though the same mechanisms as endogenous estrogens in premenopausal women and HRT in postmenopausal women. Additionally, given the other properties of phytoestrogens as antioxidants and inhibitors or platelet aggregation, their cardioprotective mechanisms could be slighter broader *(11,45)*. Epidemiological evidence to support the cardiovascular benefits of phytoestrogens again comes from the lower incidence of cardiovascular diseases in Asian populations where large amounts of phytoestrogens are consumed *(1)*.

Interestingly, whereas the antiatherogenic effects of soy protein have been recognized since 1941 *(46)*, the speculation that the phytoestrogen components of soy protein were largely responsible for lowering plasma cholesterol levels came much later *(47)*. Studies since then have demonstrated that the consumption of isoflavones in soy proteins favorably alters lipid levels. Anthony et al. *(48)*, using prepubertal rhesus monkeys fed a moderately atherogenic diet, also demonstrated that the isoflavones in soy protein were largely responsible for its hypocholesterolemic effects. Whereas one group was given soy protein isolate with phytoestrogen content intact, a second group received soy protein isolate from which the phytoestrogens had been removed through alcoholic extraction. In the first group, VLDL and LDL levels in both males and females decreased significantly by 30–40%, HDL increased significantly by 15% in females, and the total plasma cholesterol:HDL ratio decreased by 20% in males and by 50% in females. In a similar study by the same group of investigators, a postmortem exam of three randomized groups of male rhesus monkeys fed on either casein or soy protein with isoflavones, detected atheromatous plaques only in the former two groups *(49)*.

A meta-analysis of 38 published controlled clinical trials of soy protein consumption averaging 47 g/d (3 servings of soy products/d) calculated a 9.3% decrease in total cholesterol, 12.9% decrease in LDL and a 10.5% decrease in triglycerides, all statistically significant decreases *(50)*. This same review suggested that phytoestrogens alone in the soy protein accounted for 60–70% of these lipid profile changes. The hypocholesterolemic effects achieved with soy protein directly correlate to baseline, pretreatment cholesterol levels. For example, in patients with Type II hypercholesterolemia given soy protein diets, total cholesterol decreases an average of 20% *(51)*. A recent study on the cardioprotective effects in postmenopausal women of a 40-mg daily pill supplement of phytoestrogens, reported a 22% increase in HDL as the only significant lipid profile alteration *(52)*.

PHYTOESTROGENS AND BREAST CANCER

Women in Asia generally have a better prognosis when diagnosed with breast cancer than their Western counterparts. Japanese women have a higher number of cancers *in situ*, and have fewer nodal metastasis and less nodal spread than British or American women *(14)*. Japanese residents in the United States, however, have a higher incidence of breast cancer than those who live in Japan. The highest incidence rates, approaching those of Caucasian American women, occur among United States-born Japanese and those who immigrate early in life, indicating a strong environmental or lifestyle factor *(47)*.

Asian women's low risk of breast cancer has been associated with their high consumption of phytoestrogens, an intake that is estimated to be 30–50 times higher than that of Americans *(53)*. Numura *(54)* recorded the dietary habits of 6860 Japanese men in Hawaii as a representative substitute for their Japanese wives' diets from 1965–1968 and again from 1971–1975. During the second period, he found a significant inverse correlation between breast cancer incidence in premenopausal women and miso (soybean paste) soup intake. Another prospective investigation of 142,857 Japanese women over a 17-yr period demonstrated a significant graded inverse association between premenopausal breast cancer incidence and miso soup *(55)*. A diet high in soy protein was also inversely associated with breast cancer incidence in premenopausal women in a case-control study of Chinese women in Singapore. The relative risk of those eating a high soy diet was found to be 0.29 *(56)*. No similar protective effect of soy was found in postmenopausal women in any of these studies. A more recent case control study in Shanghai and Tainjin, China, moreover, has found no associations between soy intake and breast cancer incidence in any age group of women *(57)*.

Some have postulated that the decreased risk of breast cancer with high dietary phytoestrogen as seen in Asian countries is dependent on prepubertal exposure that leads to precocious breast tissue maturation and differentiation that lends protection from breast cancer in a manner similar to full-term pregnancy at a young age *(17)*. Conversely, when Western women expose themselves to high doses of these phytoestrogens postpubertally and without previous breast maturation, some argue that they could be increasing their breast cancer risks through estrogenic activity. A recent animal study in support of such a postulate showed that prepubertal rats given genistein develop significantly fewer mammary gland terminal-end buds, with more lobules than controls and fewer cells in the S-phase of the cell cycle at 50 d of age *(63)*.

Another study by Petrakis et al. *(58)*, which focused on differences in the characteristics of the nipple aspirate of women on high versus low phytoestrogen diets, yielded clinical findings suggestive of this latter point. Data were collected on the modifications of nipple aspirate fluid (NAF) in American women when exposed to 6 mo of daily soy protein isolate ingestion. The results, instead of confirming a hypothesis that the NAF's of American women would bear a closer resemblance to those of East Asian women, becoming smaller in volume and containing fewer hyperplastic or atypical epithelial cells (59), demonstrated a progressive increase in NAF volume in premenopausal women, with the appearance of hyperplastic epithelial cells in 30% of premenopausal women. Thus, the soy diet appeared to have a stimulatory effect on the premenopausal breast tissue of American women, with some hyperplasia, indicative of a modest increased risk for breast cancer (60).

Data from experimental mammary cancers in animal models on the effects of soy isoflavones have been mixed. X-ray-induced adenocarcinoma incidence was reduced in rats fed on a diet of raw soybeans compared with diets of casein or rat chow (61). Chemically induced breast tumors were similarly significantly reduced in number in rats fed soy and soy protein isolates, as were the tumors' estrogen receptors (19). Another animal model of chemically induced breast cancer demonstrated a 50% decrease in tumor incidence and a significant increase in tumor latency (61). Two other similarly organized studies, however, using soy protein isolate, showed no significant effect on carcinogenesis (19). Other laboratory studies have demonstrated the inhibition of mammary tumors in rats when fed dietary soy enriched with phytoestrogens, with no significant inhibition when phytoestrogen concentrations in the soy are minimal (62).

Breast cancer cell lines in tissue culture have demonstrated primarily that the inhibitory activity of genistein is present in both ER+ and ER– cell lines (64). Other studies have highlighted the biphasic character of ER+ cell growth in response to isoflavones, with stimulation of cell growth at lower concentrations and inhibition at higher concentrations (20). The relevance of in vitro data such as these to clinical medicine is unclear. This is especially true because more than one ER type has been identified.

CONCLUSION

The synthesis of data from cell culture, animal models, and human studies into clinically relevant conclusions about phytoestrogens represents a continuing challenge. Data accumulated thus far indicate that these dietary estrogens have an appreciable effect on the cardiovascular system through favorable changes in serum lipids. Data also exist showing an estrogenic benefit for symptomatic menopausal women and potentially for the prevention of osteoporosis. No studies to date have looked at the neurological effects of phytoestrogens to discern whether they afford protection comparable to the proposed beneficial effect of estrogen against Alzheimer's dementia.

As clinical data accrues, before serious recommendations may even be entertained regarding the array of potential benefits from phytoestrogens for postmenopausal woman, their actions on breast tissue need further clarification. Though epidemiological evidence in support of an antiproliferative effect from phytoestrogens exist, and though various in vivo and in vitro studies have not led researchers to speculate otherwise, one issue that deserves attention is the possible influence that female age exerts on this protection. As evidenced by in vivo studies, early premenarche exposure may be the key to phytoestrogens' anticancer activity.

REFERENCES

1. Adlercreutzt H. Western diet and western diseases: some hormonal and biochemical mechanisms and associations. Scand J Clin Lab Invest 1990;50:3S–23S.

2. Boulet MJ, Oddens BJ, Lehert P, Vemer HM, Visser A. Climacteric and menopause in seven south-east Asian countries. Maturitas 1994;19:157–176.

3. Rose DP, Boyar AP, Wynder EL. International comparisons of mortality rates for cancer of the breast, ovary, prostate and colon, and per capita food consumption. Cancer 1986;58;2363–2371.

4. Bradbury RB, White DC. Estrogens and related substances in plants. Vitamin Horm 1954;12:207–233.

5. Farnsworth NR, Bingel AS, Cordell GA, Crane FA, Fong HHS. Potential value of plants as sources of new antifertility agents II. J Pharm Sci 1975;64:717–754.

6. Eldridge AC, Kwolek WF. Soybean isoflavones: effect of environment and variety on composition. J Agri Food Chem 1983;31:394–396.

7. Chapin RE, Stevens JT, Hughes CL, Kelce WR, Hess RA, Daston GP. Endocrine modulation of reproduction. Fund App Toxicol 1996;29:1–17.

8. Setchell KDR, Adlercreutz H. Mammalian lignans and phytoestrogens. Recent studies on their formation, metabolism, and biological role in health and disease. In: Rowland IR, ed. Role of the Gut Flora in Toxicity and Cancer. Academic, London, 1993, pp. 315–345.

9. Thompson LU, Robb P, Serraino M, Cheung F. Mammalian lignan production from various foods. Nutr Cancer 1991;16:43–52.

10. Dwyer JT, Goldin B, Saul N. Tofu and soy drinks contain phytoestrogens. J Am Diet Assoc 1994;94:739–743.

11. Price Kr, Fenwick GR. Naturally occuring estrogens in foods — a review. Food Addit Contam 1985;2:73–106.

12. Kelly GE, Joannou GE, Reeder AY, Nelson C, Waring MA. The variable metabolic response to dietary isoflavones in humans. Proc Soc Exp Biol Med 1995;208:40–43.

13. Lu LJW, Anderson KE, Broemleing L, Doughty M, Hu DMC, Ramanujam VMS. Metabolism of soya isoflavones in healthy males after soymilk consumption (abs). J Nutr 1995;125:807–808.

14. Knight DC, Eden JA. A review of the clinical effects of phytoestrogens. Obstet Gynec 1996;87:897–904.

15. Wang H, Murphy P. Isoflavone content in commercial soybean foods. J Agri Food Chem 1994;42:1666–1673.

16. Coward L, Barnes NC, Setchell KDR, Barnes S. The isoflavones genistein and daidzein in soybean foods from American and Asian diets. J Agric Food Chem 1993;41:1961–1967.

17. Murkies AL, Wilcox G, Davis S. Phytoestrogens. J Clin End Metab 1998;83:297–302.

18. Markiewicz L, Garey J, Adlercreutz H, Gurpide E. In vitro bioassays of non-steroidal phytoestrogens. J Steriod Biochem Molec Biol 1993;45:399–405.

19. Messina MJ, Persky V, Setchell KDR, Barnes S. Soy intake and cancer risk: a review of the in vitro and in vivo data. Nutr Cancer 1994;21:113–131.

20. Zava DT, Blen M, Duwe G. Estrogenic activity of natural and synthetic estrogens in human breast cancer cells in culture. Env Health Persp 1997;105:637–644.

21. Wang TTY, Sathyamoorthy N, Phang JM. Molecular effects of genistein on estrogen receptor mediated pathways. Carcinogenesis 1996;17:271–275.

22. Akiyama T, Ishida J, Nakagawa S, et al. Genistein: a specific inhibitor of tyrosine-specific protein kinase. J Biol Chem 1987;262:5592–5595.

23. Fotsis T, Pepper M, Adlercruetz H et al. Genistein, a dietary derived inhibitor of in vitro angiogenesis. Proc Nat Acad Sci USA 1993;90:2690–2694.

24. Wei H, Bowen R, Cai Q, Barnes S, Wang Y. Antioxidant and antipromotional effects of the soybean isoflavone genistein. Proc Soc Expo Biol Med 1995;208:124–130.

25. Adlercreutz H, Banwart C, Wahala Kt. Inhibition of human aromatase by mammalian lignanas and isoflavanoid phytoestrogens. J Steriod Biochem Mol Biol 1993;44:147–153.

26. Mousavi Y, Adlercreutz H. Genistein is an effective stimulator of SHBG production in Hep-G2 human liver cancer cells and suppresses proliferation of these cells in culture. Ster 1993;58:301–304.

27. Mousavi Y, Adlercreutz H. Enterolactone and estradiol inhibit each other's proliferative effect on MCF-7 breast cancer cells in culture. J Steroid Biochem Molec Biol 1992;41:615–619.

28. Makela S, Davis VL, Tally WC, Korkman J, Salo L, Vihko R, Santti R, Korach KS. Dietary estrogens act through estrogen receptor-mediated processes and show no antiestrogenicity in cultured breast cells. Environ Health Perspec 1994;102:572–578.

29. Collins BM, McLachlan JA, Arnold SF. The estrogenic and antiestrogenic activities of phytochemicals with the human estrogen receptor expressed in yeast. Steroids 1997;62:365–372.

30. Morton MS, Wilcox G, Walqvist ML, Griffiths K. Determination of lignans and isoflavonoids in human female plasma following dietary supplementation. J Endocr 1994;142:251–259.

31. Molteni A, Brizio-Molteni L, Persky V. Vitro hormonal effects of soybean isoflavones. J Nutr 1995;125:751S–756S.

32. Ismael NN. A study of menopause in Malaysia. Maturitas 1994;19:205–209.

33. Tang GWK. The climacteric of Chinese factory workers. Maturitas 1994;19:177–182.
34. Baird DD, Umback DM, Lansdell L, Hughes CL, et al. Dietary intervention study to assess estrogenicity of dietary soy among postmenopausal women. J Clin Endo Met 1995;80:1685–1690.
35. Murkies AL, Lombard C, Strauss BJG, Wilcox G, et al. Dietary flour supplementation decreases post-menopausal hot flushes: effect of soy and wheat. Maturitas 1995;21:189–191.
36. Campbell S. Whitehead M. Oestrogen therapy and the menopausal syndrome. Clin Obstet Gynaecol 1977;4910:31–47.
37. Ahlgrimm M, Battistini M, Ravnikar V, Reed S, Schiff I. Nonhormonal treatments for menopausal symptoms. Patient Care 1998;32:28–54.
38. Cooper C, Campion G, Melton LJ, III. Hip fractures in the elderly: a world-wide projection. Osteoporos Int 1992;2:285–289.
39. Arjmandi BH, Alekel L, Hollis BW. Dietary soybean protein prevents bone loss in an ovarectomized rat model of osteoporosis. J Nutr 1996;126:161–167.
40. Anderson JJ. Ambrose WW. Garner SC. Biphasic effects of genistein on bone tissue in the ovariecto-mized, lactating rat model. Proc Soc Exper Biol Med 1998;217(3):345–350.
41. Agnusdei D, Adami S, Cervetti R, et al. Effects of ipriflavone on bone mass and calcium metabolism in postmenopausal osteoporoses. Bone Miner 1992;19:S43–S48.
42. Erdman JW, Stillman RJ, Lee KF. Short-term effects of soybean isoflavones on bone in postmenopausal women. Proc 2nd Int Symp Role of Soy in Preventing and Treating Chronic Disease. Sept 15–18, 1996. Brussels, Belgium.
43. Dalais FS, Rice GE, Wahlqvist ML, et al. Effects of dietary estrogens in postmenopausal women. Climacteric 1998; in press.
44. Stampfer MJ, Colditz GA. Estrogen replacement therapy and coronary heart. Prevenatative Med 1991;20(1):47–63.

16

General Care of the Postmenopausal Woman

Cynthia Evans, MD

Contents

INTRODUCTION

A multidisciplinary approach in a wellness clinic would be an ideal setting for the care of the perimenopausal and postmenopausal patient. In this setting, she could receive education about menopause, counseling regarding a heathy lifestyle, and integrated health care from physicians, psychologists, social workers, physiotherapists, and dieticians.

Prior to the first visit, the patient could be provided with a questionnaire detailing her past history and current concerns, to be completed in the privacy of her own home. Her first visit to the wellness clinic could include her partner, if possible. A nurse educator could be utilized to provide information in verbal, written, and video format regarding the hormonal changes of menopause, the benefits and risks of hormone replacement therapy (HRT), and counseling regarding an overall healthy lifestyle. Smoking cessation would be urged, as would modification of alcohol intake. Physiotherapists could be available to discuss relaxation methods, as well as stress the importance of aerobic exercise. Dieticians could offer individualized dietary counseling particularly regarding

From: *Contemporary Endocrinology: Menopause: Endocrinology and Management*
Edited by: D. B. Seifer and E. A. Kennard © Humana Press Inc., Totowa, NJ

an adequate calcium intake, a low-fat diet, and limiting caloric intake to avoid excess weight gain. Social work and psychology consults are helpful if issues of domestic violence are recognized.

Physician involvement at a first visit begins with a thorough history, incorporating the patient's self-questionnaire. Family history should be addressed particularly in regard to cancer, osteoporosis, Alzheimer's disease, and cardiovascular disease. It is important to inquire about tobacco and alcohol use as alcoholism may affect as many as 10% of older women. A sexual history must be taken to better understand her menopausal concerns and potentially identify domestic abuse. The patient should be asked about symptoms of urinary incontinence. Height, weight, and blood pressure are measured and a complete physical examination is performed. Laboratory evaluation, radiologic studies, endometrial biopsies, mammograms, and bone density studies should be performed as indicated. The physician should also discuss the benefits and risks of hormone therapy extensively with the patient and help her understand her individual risk profile for the diseases involved — cardiovascular disease, Alzheimer's disease, osteoporosis, colon cancer, breast cancer, and endometrial cancer.

If HRT is started at the first visit, it is important that a member of the medical team (the physician, or perhaps a nurse educator) spend time explaining the regimen to the patient and discuss possible side effects with her. Asking the patient to return to the clinic in three months to discuss her response to therapy significantly improves adherence. Adherence is also improved by providing pamphlets, books, and/or videos for the patient to study at home and by providing a phone line staffed by dedicated personnel to answer questions.

HYPERTENSION

As cardiovascular disease is by far the leading cause of mortality for women over age 50, wellness care should involve identifying various cardiovascular risk factors. As discussed earlier, lifestyle modification is essential. Patients should be encouraged to stop smoking and modify their alcohol intake. A low-fat diet of restricted caloric intake should be followed, and regular aerobic exercise is essential.

At each visit, the patients should be screened for hypertension. According to the recommendations of the Joint Commission on the Detection, Evaluation and Treatment of High Blood Pressure, a single diastolic blood pressure of 100 mm Hg should be rechecked in two months. If the repeat diastolic blood pressure is 100 mm Hg or greater, the patient should be further evaluated. A diastolic blood pressure greater than 120 mm Hg should be evaluated immediately, as should a systolic blood pressure over 160 mm Hg. An evaluation should include urinalysis, hemoglobin, serum creatinine, potassium, fasting blood sugar, fasting lipid profile, and an electrocardiogram (1). Initial therapy should consist of lifestyle modification. Dietary sodium restriction, weight loss, exercise, improved stress management, and smoking cessation should all be initiated. If hypertension persists, pharmacologic management is indicated.

CHOLESTEROL

Primary prevention trials for men have established that cholesterol reduction prevents coronary heart disease and suggest that it prevents death from the same. In men, for every 10 mg/dL increase in HDL, there is a 50% decreased risk of coronary heart disease (1). The association between cholesterol levels and death from coronary artery disease is not

Table 1
Risk Factors for Lung Cancer

Smoking
Age
Preexisting lung disease
Prior lung cancer
Occupational exposure to radon, asbestos, alkylating
    compounds, nickel, chromates, halo ethers, carcinogenic
    polyhydrocarbons.

as well established for women as it is for men, but cholesterol screening should be considered for postmenopausal women. The National Cholesterol Education Program (NCEP) of the National Heart, Lung and Blood Institute and the American Heart Association recommend that adults over age 20 have a total cholesterol and HDL measured every 5 yr. They recommend a full lipoprotein analysis for all patients with coronary heart disease. In patients without coronary heart disease, lipoprotein analysis should be performed if the total cholesterol is greater than 240 mg/dL, the total cholesterol is 200–239 mg/dL and the patient has two or more risk factors for coronary heart disease, or the patient has an HDL less than 35 mg/dL. The recommendation of the American College of Obstetricians and Gynecologists and the American College of Physicians are similar, but less detailed. They simply recommend a total cholesterol every five years after age 19. The Canadian Task Force on Periodic Health Examinations, however, states that there is insufficient evidence for the inclusion of universal screening for hypercholesterolemia in a periodic health examination (2). Importantly, total cholesterol and HDL can be measured in the nonfasting state, but LDL should only be measured after a 12-h fast. After eating, the LDL may be artificially lowered and the triglycerides may be artificially elevated.

LUNG CANCER

Lung cancer is the leading type of cancer-related deaths in the United States (*see* Table 1). Two screening tests have been proposed and evaluated: chest X-ray (CXR) and sputum cytology. Neither has been found to be sensitive enough to use as a screening test. Soda et al. retrospectively studied the value of an annual CXR. Of 305,934 participants, 206 lung cancers were found. Only 103 were Stage I. An overall sensitivity was noted to be 70%, but only 52% for squamous-cell carcinoma and only 50% for small-cell carcinoma. They concluded that the low detectability of Stage I adenocarcinoma on CXR and the late recognition of rapidly growing small-cell and squamous-cell carcinomas decrease the effectiveness of CXR for screening (37). The NCI Cooperative Lung Cancer Detection Program screened 30,000 asymptomatic smokers over age 45. They were followed for five years and offered annual CXR and sputum cytology every four months. CXR missed 33% of the cancers. Sputum missed 58% of the cancers. Neither test resulted in a reduced mortality from lung cancer (38–40).

The Mayo Clinic screened 10,933 male smokers from 1971 to 1976 with CXR and 3-d pooled sputum for cytology. Ninety-one cancers were found. The remaining 9211 patients were followed for 11 years with an annual CXR and sputum cytology every four months. The control group had no screening. Despite an improvement in five-year survival (35% vs 13%), no change in overall lung cancer mortality was detected. Many cancers were unresectable when detected (41–42).

Table 2
Risk Factors for Breast Cancer

Age (85% of breast cancer occurs after age 50)
Family history of breast cancer
Previous breast cancer
Alcohol consumption
First pregnancy after age 30
Menarche before age 12
Menopause after age 50
Obesity
High socioeconomic status
High fat consumption
History of endometrial or ovarian cancer

The NCI's Prostate, Lung, Colorectal, and Ovary trial will examine the benefit of annual CXR on lung cancer mortality. Until those results are available, the American Cancer Society, NCI, and the US Preventative Services Task Force do not recommend routine screening for lung cancer. All three agencies strongly support the primary prevention of encouraging patients to stop smoking.

BREAST CANCER

Among women in the United States, breast cancer is the most commonly diagnosed cancer and the second leading type of cancer-related death. Breast cancer is the leading cause of death for women age 40–49 in the United States. Screening for breast cancer in an attempt to diagnose and treat the disease at a more curable stage has, therefore, become a major public health concern (*see* Table 2).

To be effective, a screening test must offer high specificity, high sensitivity, be cost-effective, and lower mortality. Currently, there are three screening tests available for breast cancer: self-breast exam, clinical breast exam by a physician, and mammography. Self-breast examination (SBE) is simple, noninvasive, but not very sensitive. The Breast Cancer Detection Demonstration Project (BCDDP) found only a 26% sensitivity with SBE and no change in overall mortality. The BCDDP found only a 45% sensitivity with clinical breast examination by a physician, again with no overall change in mortality. In contrast, mammograms have been found to have a sensitivity ranging from 75 to 90% and a specificity of 90 to 95% (3).

There is good evidence from clinical trials that annual screening mammograms in women over age 50 reduce breast cancer mortality by 20 to 39%. However, considerable controversy has recently surrounded the issue of whether or not to screen women age 40–49. The data is mixed. In 1963, Shapiro started the first randomized-screening trial using mortality as a primary endpoint. Sixty-two thousand women, age 40–64 were offered usual care in the Health Insurance Plan (HIP) of Greater New York or a clinical breast exam plus a two-view mammogram annually. A published report from 1969 suggested a statistically significant 30% mortality reduction in women over age 50 in the study group. In 1986, after 18 yr of follow-up, a 23% decrease in mortality was noted in women age 50–59 at entry and a 24% decrease in mortality was noted in women age 40–49 of entry, but this did not appear until the eighth or ninth year of follow-up (4).

In 1992, the National Breast Screening Study (NBSS) was published. This "Canadian Trial" was specifically designed to study women age 40–49. The study group was screened with SBE, annual clinical breast examination by a physician, and mammography. They found no decrease in breast cancer mortality with regular mammograms *(5)*. This study has been criticized, however, as it recruited volunteers for subjects instead of randomly selected patients. The concern exists that this is a select group of patients. An increased number of women in the study group were found to have suspicious lymph nodes on prescreening physical exam when compared to the control group.

In 1973, the BCDDP was started by the American Cancer Society (and later joined by the NCI). Two hundred eighty thousand women were screened in 28 centers and this included 93,481 women age 40–49. The mammographic techniques used in the BCDDP trial were much better than that used in the HIP study. A 1982 report noted that minimal cancers (less than 1 cm of invasive cancer) made up 32.4% of cancers found and that more than 80% of the cancers detected had negative nodes *(3)*.

The Survillancy Epidemiology and End Results (SEER) program examined 104,351 breast cancer cases diagnosed between 1983 and 1989. They also found a trend toward earlier stage disease with mammographic screening. Of women age 40–49 when screened, there was a 216% increase in ductal carcinoma *in situ* (DCIS). The prevalence of invasive carcinoma with a tumor less than 1 cm with negative axillary nodes increased 80%. The prevalence of metastasized carcinoma (1–1.9 cm or greater than 2 cm) decreased by 38% and 23%, respectively *(6,7)*. Both the BCDDP data and the SEER data suggest that screening women age 40–49 resulted in a shift toward an earlier stage of disease at diagnosis and an increase in detection of smaller tumors.

The results of two randomized clinical trials in Sweden (Gothenberg and Mälmo) were recently released. The Gothenberg study concluded that screening women age 40–49 by mammography resulted in a 44% decrease in breast cancer mortality after 12 yr of follow-up *(8)*. The Mälmo study found a 36% decrease in mortality after 12 yr of follow-up *(9)*.

The metanalysis by Smart et al. of eight randomized clinical trials looked at all published or presented data, including the NBSS, and found a 16% reduction in breast cancer mortality among women screened by mammography beginning between age 40–49. This result was not statistically significant. When the same data were reanalyzed omitting the NBSS data (data that have been heavily criticized as mentioned earlier), the results are statistically significant. A 24% reduction in mortality was found *(10)*.

Based on the data from the Gothenberg and Mälmo studies, and the reduced mortality noted in Smart's metanalysis, the American Cancer Society recently revised its guidelines. They now recommend a monthly SBE beginning at age 20 and clinical breast examinations by a physician every 3 yr for women age 20–40 and yearly after age 40. Annual mammograms are now recommended beginning at age 40. The majority of the trials used a screening interval of 18–24 mo. Because premenopausal breast cancer tends to be more aggressive than postmenopausal breast cancer, the Society recommends annual mammograms hoping to lower the mortality rate even further than what was reflected in the trials.

The National Cancer Institute, however, recommends screening mammography every 1–2 yr for women age 40–49 followed by an annual mammography after age 50. Their more-conservative approach derives from the argument that although the randomized clinical trials did reveal a statistically significant reduction in mortality for women entering the study at age 40–49, that reduction was not seen until 7–10 yr after screening had started. They suggest that perhaps some of the observed decline in mortality was due

Table 3
Risk Factors for Colon Cancer

Personal or family history of colon cancer
Personal history of ovarian, endometrial, or breast cancer
Personal history of adenomatous polyps
History of familial adenomatous polyposis
Family history of nonpolyposis colorectal cancer syndrome or
    Lynch Syndrome II
History of inflammatory bowel disease
Age (90% of colorectal cancers occur after age 50)

to women screened after their 50th birthday. Unfortunately, these detailed data are not currently available in publication form.

This issue will be readdressed in Eurotrial-40. Eurotrial-40 is a randomized population-based trial begun in Europe in 1994. It will compare a control group receiving no mammograms with a study group receiving annual mammograms from age 40–49.

COLON CANCER

Colon cancer affects 1 out of 20 Americans by age 80 (*see* Table 3). It is an ideal candidate for screening for three reasons: most cancers slowly arise from precursor lesions (adenomas) over approximately 10 yr, methods of early detection are available, and local disease has a high 5-yr survival rate. The 5-yr survival rate for local disease is 91%, regional diseases 61%, but for distant disease, only 7%.

The World Health Organization (WHO) has promoted primary preventative measures in its 1985 recommendations. They recommend consumption of a balanced diet including 5 to 8 servings per d of fresh fruits and vegetables, whole grain cereals and breads, and a fat intake of less than 20% of the total caloric intake. They recommend avoiding excess calories and tobacco, and they also recommend a regular schedule of physical activity *(11)*. Currently, there are five possible screening methods available alone or in combination for detection of colorectal cancer: digital rectal exam, fecal occult blood testing (FOBT), flexible sigmoidoscopy, colonoscopy, and double-contrast barium enema.

The digital rectal exam is easily performed by a physician and fairly well tolerated by patients. It has never been tested in a controlled or randomized trial, however. Unfortunately, only 10% of colorectal cancers are within 7 to 10 cm of the anus, i.e., within the reach of an examining finger.

FOBT utilizes a guaiac-based card to test for the pseudoperoxidase activity of fecal heme. Unfortunately, peroxidase activity can also be found in fresh fruits and vegetables, bacteria, and animal hemoglobin. False positives can also be caused by an aspirin-induced gastritis. Vitamin C intake can cause a false-negative result, as can hemoglobin degradation by bacteria in the intestine, contamination by toilet water, and storage of slides more than five ds. It has been estimated that fewer than 30% of cancers and large polyps bleed enough to be detected by FOBT. In spite of these limitations, five controlled trials have examined the efficacy of FOBT for colorectal cancer screening.

In 1975, the Memorial-Sloan-Kettering Cancer Center in collaboration with the Strang Institute enrolled 21,756 patients over age 40. All received a digital rectal exam and 25 cm rigid sigmoidoscopic exam annually. The study group also received annual FOBT. If the

FOBT was positive, the patients received a double-contrast barium enema and a colonoscopy. The compliance rate for FOBT was 74% with a positivity rate of 1.7%. It was found to be 70% sensitive for detecting cancers and 98% specific. There were significantly more cancers, which were Duke's stage A&B in the study group. A 43% reduction in mortality from colorectal cancer was found in the screened group after 10 yr of follow-up, but this is not yet statistically significant (12).

Also, in 1975, the University of Minnesota enrolled 48,000 participants, age 50–80. They were randomly assigned to three groups: FOBT yearly, FOBT every other year, or control. Compliance was found to be 77% with 2.4% positivity rate. If the slide was positive, the patient had a sigmoidoscopy, barium enema, upper-gastrointestinal series, chest X-ray, electrocardiogram, and colonoscopy. The investigators found 48% fewer Duke's D tumors in the annually screened group compared to controls. In the annually screened group, the test was found to be 49.5% sensitive for detecting cancer, and 97% specific. A statistically significant 33% reduction in mortality was found among patients screened annually (13).

A study started in England in 1984 enrolled 156,000 participants, age 50–74. The patients were randomized to a control group or FOBT every other year. They found a compliance rate of 59% with 2.3% of tests positive. They found statistically significantly more Duke's Stage C or D tumors in the control group. A recently published update has reported a 15% mortality reduction in the screened group with an odds ratio of 0.85 (CI 0.74–0.98) (14).

The Swedish Study, started in 1982 and still in progress, enrolled 27,700 participants age 60–64. Two FOBT screenings were offered to the study group 16–22 mo apart. With a compliance rate of 66%, significantly more tumors were Duke's A or B in the study group. Sensitivity of the test was 52% (15).

In 1985, a study was begun in Denmark, enrolling 62,000 participants, age 45–74. The study group was offered FOBT every other year. They found that 1.1% of the slides were positive. In the study group, 81% of tumors found were Duke's A or B compared to only 42% of tumors found in the control group (16). Ten years after the study started, an 18% reduction in mortality was noted in the screened group.

In summary, these studies reveal a 50–70% compliance rate with FOBT and a 1–2% positivity rate for adults over age 50. Sensitivity was 50–70%. Most studies, however, show an approximate doubling of early detection of tumors from 30–40% Duke's A or B in the control groups to 70–80% in the study groups. Most importantly, however, three studies (University of Minnesota, England, and Denmark) found statistically significant reduction in mortality with FOBT. The greatest reduction in mortality was seen in the study from the University of Minnesota where annual FOBT was offered.

Only 10% of colorectal cancers are within reach of a digital rectal exam. A rigid sigmoidoscope, however, should be able to detect 25–35% of tumors and a 60 cm flexible sigmoidoscope should be able to detect 50–60% of tumors. Unfortunately, there are no prospective controlled trials to date that look at sigmoidoscopy as a screening method. However, in 1992, a retrospective case-control study of patients in the Kaiser Permanente Medical Care program was published that looked at the use of sigmoidoscopy in patients with colorectal cancer. No difference in mortality was found for patients with tumors located beyond the scope, but a significant 70% reduction in mortality was noted for patients with cancers within reach of the sigmoidoscope. Twenty-three patients in the control group died of rectosigmoid cancer, which was within reach of a scope. Certainly, this study supports the use of screening sigmoidoscopy *(17)*. Muller and Sonnenberg also published a retrospective study in 1995 and found a 60% reduction in colorectal cancer mortality in patients who had had one or more sigmoidoscopy *(18)*. The NCI is currently supporting a 16-yr multicenter randomized trial looking at performing a 60 cm flexible sigmoidoscopy every 3 yr on 148,000 participants age 60–74. Its effect on mortality will be determined.

Colonoscopy has been discussed as a screening method as well. It has a high specificity and sensitivity and can be both diagnostic and therapeutic. A screening interval of 10 yr has been suggested because of the slow growth of polyps. The National Polyp Study suggested that if patients with polyps are identified and if all polyps are removed at colonoscopy, the subsequent risk of colorectal cancer is reduced by 76–90% over the following 6 yr *(19)*. Unfortunately, colonoscopy is hampered by poor patient acceptance and compliance, an increased cost, and the increase in technical skill required for the procedure. It has been suggested that this method be reserved for high-risk patients.

Double-contrast barium enema has been found to be 90–95% sensitive for polyps over 1 cm in diameter, but unlike colonoscopy, biopsy, or polypectomy cannot be performed simultaneously. There are no studies looking at its effect on mortality.

The following recommendations were released in 1996 by the American Gastroenterological Association and endorsed by the American Cancer Society, American College of Gastroenterology, American Society of Colon and Rectal Surgeons, American Society for Gastrointestinal Endoscopy, and the Society of American Gastrointestinal Endoscopic Surgeons: screening for colorectal cancer and adenomatous polyps should be offered to all adults over age 50 regardless of risk factors. Options for screening average-risk patients include:

1. FOBT annually followed by colonoscopy if testing is positive;
2. Flexible sigmoidoscopy every 5 yr with biopsy of polyps smaller than 1 cm followed by colonoscopy if polyps larger than 1 cm, adenomatous polyps, or cancer is found;
3. Combine FOBT and sigmoidoscopy;
4. Double-contrast barium enema every 5–10 yr; or
5. Colonoscopy every 10 yr.

Patients with high-risk factors including: a first-degree relative with colorectal cancer; a family history of familial adenomatous polyposis; a family history of hereditary nonpolyposis colorectal cancer; a personal history of colorectal cancer or an adenomatous polyp; or patients with inflammatory bowel disease deserve much more careful screening with colonoscopy beginning at a young age. Genetic screening should be considered for some disorders *(20)*.

CERVICAL CANCER

Cervical cancer is the seventh most frequent cancer in the United States *(see* Table 4). Pap smears are a simple, inexpensive, well-established method to screen for this disease. An extensive analysis of large screening programs estimates that annual screenings could decrease the probability of developing invasive cervical cancer by 93.3% and that screening patients every three years would decrease the probability by 91.2% *(21)*.

The American Cancer Society, National Cancer Institute, American Medical Association, American Academy of Family Practioniers, and the American College of Obstetricians and Gynecologists (ACOG) recommend an annual pap smear for all women who

Table 4
Risk Factors for Cervical Cancer

Multiple sexual partners
First intercourse at an early age
Current or past HPV infection
Current or prior HSV infection
HIV infection
History of other sexually transmitted diseases
Smoking
History of cervical dysplasia
Lower socioeconomic status
History of partner whose previous partners had cervical cancer

are or ever have been sexually active and who have reached age 18. After three or more consecutive normal annual pap smears, the frequency may be reduced at the discretion of the patient's physician. ACOG recommends "more frequent" pap smears in patients with the following risk factors: multiple sexual partners; first intercourse at an early age; current or prior HPV infection; current or prior HSV infection; HIV infection; history of other sexually transmitted diseases; smoking; history of cervical dysplasia or cervical cancer; lower socioeconomic status; and history of a partner whose previous partners had cervical cancer (22).

An abnormal pap smear should be followed by a colposcopic examination with therapy based on biopsy findings.

ENDOMETRIAL CANCER

Unlike breast, colon, and cervical cancer, endometrial cancer typically presents with symptoms early in the disease process. As a result, 75% of patients are diagnosed in Stage I. Grade I, Stage I tumors have a 95% survival rate. Stage II tumors have a 5-yr survival rate less than 60%.

Because the diagnosis is almost always preceded by symptoms of postmenopausal bleeding, the incidence of asymptomatic cancer is estimated to be only 1.3–1.7 per 1,000 screened postmenopausal women (23). This limits the utility of routine screening for this disease. ACOG currently does not recommend routine screening of asymptomatic women (23). The American Cancer Society recommends an endometrial biopsy for all menopausal women and women with risk factors. They state that the frequency of biopsies is at the discretion of the physician (24). Certainly women with symptoms need to be evaluated (see Table 5).

Currently, methods of evaluation and/or screening include endometrial cytology, endometrial biopsy, dilatation and curettage (D&C) with or without hysteroscopy, and ultrasound. Endometrial cytology was studied in symptomatic patients in 1990. The Endopap Sampler is a 2 mm plastic instrument with distal notches. It was found to be 90% sensitive for cancer and only 58% sensitive for hyperplasia. The false-positive rate was 7.3% (25). It has never been studied in asymptomatic patients.

The endometrial biopsy is a well-accepted tool for evaluating postmenopausal bleeding in the office setting. It is fairly well-tolerated by patients with minimal morbidity. It has been reported to be almost as sensitive as a D&C. There are no randomized trials evaluating the effect on cancer mortality of routinely screening asymptomatic patients with endometrial biopsies.

Table 5
Risk Factors for Endometrial Cancer

Age (peak incidence is between ages 65 and 74)
Obesity
Diabetes
Hypertension
Early menarche
Chronic anovulatory bleeding
Estrogen-only replacement therapy
Previous breast cancer
Estrogen-secreting tumors
Delayed menopause
Chronic liver disease
Nulliparity

A D&C is associated with the risks of anesthesia, as it is usually done in a hospital setting, as well as the risk of uterine perforation. It is usually reserved for the evaluation (or possible treatment) of postmenopausal bleeding. A hysteroscopy will often be performed with a D&C in this setting. The availability of smaller scopes and the use of CO_2 distending medium allow the opportunity for hysteroscopy to be used in an office setting. Again, because of the low incidence of cancer in an asymptomatic population and the potential for complications with this procedure, hysteroscopy is usually reserved for symptomatic patients.

Transvaginal ultrasonography (TVUSN) has been evaluated as a possible tool for screening asymptomatic women. In contrast to the previous techniques, TVUSN involves minimal or no patient discomfort and minimal or no morbidity. In 1993, a Swedish study evaluated a random sample of 827 symptomatic women age 45–80. If the endometrium was less than or equal to 4 mm (a measurement that includes both endometrial layers at the thickest point), no further studies were performed. If the measurement was 5–7 mm or "nonmeasurable," the patient was reassessed in 1 yr. If the measurement was greater than or equal to 8 mm, a hysteroscopy and/or D&C was performed. Of the 827 women, 559 were postmenopausal and 183 (33%) were on some form of HRT. Eighty-two percent of the population had an endometrium less than or equal to 4 mm. One cancer was found (the thickness was 19 mm) and 23 cases of polyps were found (thickness 8–18 mm). No cases of hyperplasia were diagnosed *(23)*. This study does not support generalized screening of asymptomatic patients with TVUSN.

Similar conclusions were drawn from a study published in 1995 from Italy. They evaluated 2025 asymptomatic postmenopausal women. One hundred sixteen women (5.8% of their population) were found to have an endometrial thickness of at least 4 mm. Of the 116 women, 98 consented to an endometrial biopsy for evaluation. Sixty-six biopsies were completed and only three cases of cancer were found. They found a high rate of cervical stenosis (32 out of 98 attempted biopsies) and a very high cost of screening per cancer found. They noted no change in mortality rate based on routine screening with TVUSN *(26)*.

The "Nordic Trial" was slightly different from the previous trials in that they screened 1100 patients with symptomatic postmenopausal bleeding. Using a cutoff greater than 4 mm, they found a sensitivity of 96% and a specificity of 68%. This specificity, however, is simply for any pathologic abnormality and includes polyps, hyperplasia, or carcinoma *(27)*.

Table 6
Risk Factors for Ovarian Cancer

Age
Family history of ovarian cancer
Family history of breast/ovarian familial cancer
Syndrome or the Lynch II Syndrome (Hereditary Nonpolyposis
    Colorectal Cancer Syndrome)

Table 7
Decreased Risk for Ovarian Cancer

Pregnancy
Oral contraceptive use
? Breast feeding
? History of tubal ligation

Tamoxifen is a nonsteroidal antiestrogen that is commonly used today to delay recurrence and prolong survival in some breast cancer patients. The National Surgical Adjuvant Breast and Bowel Project (NASBP) trial suggested an increased risk of endometrial cancer in patients using this medication (28). Some studies have also suggested an increased risk of endometrial polyps, uterine sarcoma, and rapidly growing leiomyomata in these patients. A reliable screening protocol for these patients has not been established. Some authors recommend routine screening with TVUSN, but tamoxifen seems to cause some atypical ultrasound findings. Cystic-appearing areas are often seen, which seem to be endometrial, but when evaluated with hysterosonography, actually lie in the proximal myometrium. Likewise, endometrial biopsies appear to have a lower sensitivity in these patients. Currently, an accurate method for routinely screening these patients has not been developed.

In summary, routine screening of asymptomatic women for endometrial cancer is not currently recommended. Women with spontaneous postmenopausal bleeding, unexpected bleeding on HRT, or prolonged anovulatory bleeding deserve evaluation. Patients treated with estrogen-only replacement therapy need routine screening owing to its frequent association with the development of endometrial cancer, but the proper method and screening interval has not been established.

OVARIAN CANCER

Ovarian cancer is the leading cause of death from gynecologic malignancy (*see* Tables 6 and 7). Stage I ovarian cancer has a 70–90% 5-yr survival rate, whereas Stage IV cancer has a survival rate of less than 20%. Ovarian cancer would, therefore, seem to be a good candidate for screening. Screening has been hampered, though, by the poor specificity and/or sensitivity of the tests available and by the relatively low prevalence of the disease.

Currently available screening methods include pelvic examination, serum CA-125, TVUSN, and TVUSN plus color Doppler imaging. The annual pelvic exam as currently performed in the United States has a low detection rate for early ovarian cancer. When detected, the disease is typically quite advanced.

CA-125 is a serum tumor marker for ovarian cancer. Levels are greater than 35 U/mL in 80% of patients with ovarian cancer. Unfortunately, its usefulness as a screening tool is limited because more than 50% of patients with Stage I disease have normal CA-125 levels. Elevated CA-125 levels can be found in 6% of women with other diseases including cancers of the endometrium, pancreas, stomach, liver, lung, breast, colon, and, in pregnancy, pelvic inflammatory disease, endometriosis, and liver cirrhosis. One percent of patients with no apparent disease can have elevated CA-125 levels (29).

In 1988, Jacob et al. studied 1010 healthy postmenopausal women with a pelvic examination and a CA-125. If either were abnormal, the patients had an abdominal ultrasound. If that was abnormal, they were taken to surgery. Thirty-one patients had an abnormal CA-125. Only one case of ovarian cancer was detected. It was a Stage IA clear-cell carcinoma of the ovary. A follow-up report of 22,000 women found 41 elevated CA-125 levels. Eleven of 41 had ovarian cancer for a specificity of 99.9% and a sensitivity of only 78.6% at 1 yr and 57.9% at 2 yr. Additionally, eight of the remaining 21,959 patients with normal CA-125 levels developed ovarian cancer (30).

Einhorn et al. in Sweden studied 5550 women over age 40. He followed them with annual CA-125 levels. If an elevated level was found, a pelvic exam and a transabdominal ultrasound were performed. Six of the 175 women with elevated CA-125 levels had cancer, but only 2 were Stage I. Two patients had Stage II disease and two had Stage III disease at diagnosis. Six women with normal CA-125 levels subsequently developed ovarian cancer. He found a positive predictive value of only 3.4% for an elevated CA-125 (31). In summary, CA-125 levels are not sensitive enough nor specific enough for routine screening of asymptomatic women.

In 1991, Van Nagell et al. studied 1300 asymptomatic women with TVUSN. Thirty-three (2.5%) had abnormal ovaries on ultrasound. Twenty-seven consented to surgery. Three adenocarcinomas were found. One was metastatic from a previously known colon cancer, but two others were primary Stage I ovarian cancer (32). In 1991, Bourne et al. evaluated patients with a family history of ovarian cancer with TVUSN. Of 776 patients, 43 (5.5%) were referred to surgery because of an abnormal TVUSN. Thirty-nine had surgery and three Stage I ovarian cancers were found. None of these had an elevated CA-125 level. In 1993, they added a morphology index to their screening. Of the 3220 asymptomatic women screened, 44 (1.47%) had persistently abnormal ovaries. Three had primary ovarian carcinoma (33). Karlan et al. reviewed the results of several TVUSN screening programs. They found that 11,283 women had been screened, and 486 women had been taken to surgery. Nineteen cancers were found, 13 of which were Stage I. Of the patients who went to surgery, only 1 in 32 had Stage I cancer (34).

One possible future screening modality is TVUSN with color Doppler imaging. Tumor vessels have less smooth muscle in their walls and, therefore, less resistance to blood flow. A low resistance index (RI) or pulsatility index (PI) would be a sign of malignancy. In 1991, Kurjak et al. studied 14,317 asymptomatic or minimally symptomatic women. Each had an ultrasound with color Doppler. Abnormal ovaries were evaluated by surgery. Six hundred twenty-four masses were found to be benign. All except one (a chronic appendicitis with a hydrosalpinx) were found to have a normal RI. Fifty-six ovarian cancers were found. Fifty-four of the 56 were found to have a low RI. The RI was 96.4% sensitive and 99.8% specific (35). In 1993, Bourne et al. studied 1601 self-referred patients with a family history of ovarian cancer. All had TVUSN with color Doppler and a morphology index. Sixty-one patients had persistently abnormal ovaries. Six had primary ovarian cancer (3 had borderline tumors and 1 had Stage III disease), for an odds ratio of 1:9. If only patients with an elevated morphology index or low PI were taken to surgery, the odds ratio would have been 2:5 (36).

Because the evaluation of an abnormal screening test for ovarian cancer usually ultimately involves surgery, it is very important that the test used by highly specific. None of the screening methods to date meet this criteria. As a result, the US Preventative Task Force, American Cancer Society, ACOG, and the American College of Physicians do not recommend screening for ovarian cancer in the asymptomatic patient, other than a pelvic exam. The American College of Physicians suggests that the risks and benefits of screening be discussed with patients who have a family history of ovarian cancer (21).

As part of the Prostate, Lung, Colorectal, Ovary trial of the NCI, 148,000 women age 60–74 will be screened annually with a pelvic exam, CA-125, and TVUSN. The effect of the combination of these screening modalities on mortality will be assessed.

GENETIC SCREENING FOR CANCER RISK

It has been estimated that 3–7% of patients with ovarian cancer, 2–10% of patients with breast cancer (especially patients with early onset disease and/or bilateral disease), and 10–15% of patients with colon cancer appear to be from a family with a genetic predisposition. The goals of genetic counseling are to identify families at risk by the number and sites of cancer in a family. Each family is then studied to identify the mutation involved. This allows the testing of each family member to determine his/her individual risk for cancer. Finally, family members found to be carriers of the mutant gene are closely followed and screened to detect tumors as early as possible.

BRCA-1 has been mapped to chromosome 17q 12–21. Eighty-five percent of patients carrying this mutation will develop breast cancer. Forty-five percent will develop ovarian cancer (43). In 1997, Couch et al. found that 16% of women with breast cancer or a family history of breast or ovarian cancer (seen at a breast referral clinic) had BRCA-1 mutations. They found that only 7% of women with a family history of breast cancer but no ovarian cancer carried the mutation (44). Langton et al. found that 6% of women diagnosed with breast cancer before age 35 had a BRCA-1 mutation (45). Fitzgerald et al. found that 17% of women with the diagnosis of breast cancer prior to age 30 had BRCA-1 mutations (46). The mutations can be difficult to identify because this is a large gene. There are more than 80 different mutations.

BRCA-2 is on chromosome 13q 12 -13. In 1997, Krainer et al. found that only 2.7% of women with breast cancer diagnosed before age 32 had BRCA-2 mutations. There is a lesser risk of ovarian cancer with this gene (47).

Unfortunately, once patients at risk are identified, it is unclear how to screen or counsel these patients. Mammograms are much less sensitive in young women because of the dense breast tissue. Bilateral prophylactic mastectomy could be offered, but it is quite disfiguring and rare cases of breast cancer have been reported even after prophylactic mastectomy. Ovarian cancer screening is even more difficult. Prophylactic bilateral oophorectomy could be offered, but the patient is then committed to long-term HRT and cases of diffuse peritoneal carcinoma have been reported.

Patients with hereditary nonpolyposis colorectal cancer syndrome are at an increased risk of colorectal cancer, as well as cancer of the endometrium, ovary, ureter, kidney, stomach, liver, and small intestine. It has been linked to four genes, hMSH2 on chromosome 2, hMLH1 on chromosome 3, hPMS1 on chromosome 2, and hPMS2 on chromosome 7. Again, once susceptible patients are identified, the issues of screening and prophylactic treatment are unclear. Both sigmoidoscopy and colonoscopy

Table 8
Risk Factors for Osteoporosis

Early menopause
History of anorexia nervosa
Female hypogonadism
Hyperparathyroidism
Prolonged steroid use
History of anticonvulsants or antihypertensive early in life
Age
Smoking
Sedentary lifestyle
Low calcium intake
Family history
Alcohol abuse
Malabsorption

have been suggested as screening methods followed by prophylactic colectomy once polyps develop. As discussed earlier in this chapter, screening for ovarian and endometrial cancer is difficult. Some have suggested offering the patients a prophylactic hysterectomy and bilateral oophorectomy.

Screening for genetic predisposition for cancer is still early in its development. Even if all mutations were known, testing for susceptibility is a difficult decision for many patients. The emotional strain of knowing a patient is a carrier can be enormous for the patient and his family. There may be financial consequences from job pressures or medical insurance. Until adequate screening methods of cancer and prophylactic measures are instituted, widespread use of genetic screening is questionable.

OSTEOPOROSIS

Bone mineral density (BMD) as measured by dual energy X-ray absorptiometry (DEXA) is highest at the end of the third decade of life and gradually declines after age 45. Studies have shown that risk factors only identify 73% of women with low BMD and 66% of women with normal bone mass *(48)* (*see* Table 8).

Historically, there are four methods of determining bone mineral density: microdensitometry (MD), quantitative computed tomography (QCT), single-energy X-ray absorptiometry (SXA), or dual-energy X-ray absorptometry (DEXA). Because it has the highest degree of precision, DEXA is the currently recommended method for assessing BMD.

BMD testing is important to identify a patient's future risk of fracture. For each standard deviation decline in bone density (compared to a normal value for a 35-yr-old woman) the relative risk for fracture doubles *(49)*. Baseline testing can help in a patient's decision analysis for or against HRT. Repeat testing can be performed to assess a patient's response to therapy.

The "treatment" of osteoporosis actually begins with prevention. If a patient stops smoking, she can lower her risk of hip fracture by an estimated 25% and vertebral fractures by 300% *(50)*. Weight-bearing exercise is important to allow proper bone remodeling. Exercise allows better physical fitness and a lesser tendency to falls. Calcium supplementation is important. The National Institute of Health Consensus Development Panel recommends that a postmenopausal woman should consume 1000 to 1500 mg of calcium per d *(51)*. Pharmacologic prevention of osteoporosis was limited until recently, to estrogen replacement therapy (ERT). Estrogen therapy can increase or preserve bone density. Studies have shown a 50–60% reduction in osteoporotic fractures of the wrist and hip if therapy is started within 3 yr of menopause and continued for 6–9 yr. The risk of vertebral fractures is also significantly reduced *(52)*.

Other relatively new pharmacologic agents active against osteoporosis include calcitonin and the biophosphonates. Estrogen analogues (e.g., raloxofene) and sodium fluoride are still being tested.

Because many of these agents are relatively new, the active prevention of osteoporosis has been a new area of wellness care. The issue of whether postmenopausal women should be routinely screened with BMD testing is still being evaluated as is the proper interval for follow-up testing of both normal and abnormal results.

THYROID DISEASE

Estimates of the prevalence of hyperthyroidism in older adults vary from 0.5–10% of this population. In older patients, symptoms are often more subtle and therefore overlooked. The most frequent symptoms of hyperthyroidism in older adults are tachycardia, fatigue, and weight loss. Atrial fibrillation is common. In 1994, Faughnan screened 500 patients seen at a menopause clinic for thyroid disease. They were screened at their first visit. He found a 7.2% incidence of thyroid disease. He also found that a single thyroid-stimulating hormone (TSH) is sufficient as a screening tool *(53)*.

Screening for thyroid disease is simple yet essential. Hypothyroidism is associated with alterations in lipid profile, myocardial function abnormalities, and possibly an increased risk of coronary heart disease. Overtreatment of thyroid disease, however, can result in osteoporosis so therapy must be carefully monitored.

VACCINES

The Center for Disease Control (CDC) estimates that 41–84% of adults over age 60 may have insufficient immunity to diphtheria. Influenza is a major cause of morbidity and mortality in persons over age 65 with approximately 20,000 deaths/yr in the United States. There are also an estimated 40,000 deaths/yr due to pneumococcal infections in adults of this age group *(54)*.

Recommended vaccines are as follows:

1. Tetanus — diphtheria booster every 10 yr.
2. Influenza vaccine annually after age 55.
3. Pneumococcal vaccine — once at age 65 or earlier if the patient is a resident of a chronic-care facility or has a history of chronic cardiopulmonary disorders, metabolic, diseases (diabetes, hemoglobinopathies, immunosuppression, renal dysfunction) or sickle-cell disease, Hodgkin's Disease, asplenia, alcoholism, cirrhosis, or multiple myeloma *(1)*.

In summary, a multidisciplinary menopause clinic would be the ideal setting for the care of women over age 40. In this setting, health information can be given by nurse educators and the pros and cons of HRT can be discussed. Each patient needs to be evaluated on an individual basis. Cardiovascular risk factors need to be identified and corrected. Smoking cessation should be encouraged. Exercise and low-fat diets should be stressed. Each patient should be screened for hypertension and hypercholesteremia. Cancer screening should include yearly mammography after age 50 and at least every 1–2 yr for ages 40–49. Colon cancer screening should include annual FOBT plus sigmoidoscopy or colonoscopy periodically as discussed previously. Regular pap smears should be obtained and any atypical vaginal bleeding should be immediately evaluated. The issue of routine bone mineral density evaluation for all postmenopausal women is still being studied, but certainly protection against osteoporosis needs to be addressed. Routine TSH testing is probably indicated and finally, all vaccines should be updated. In an ideal setting, these needs are best met by a team approach, but hopefully will allow the "golden years" to truly be the best years of a woman's life!

REFERENCES

1. ACOG Tech Bull, Health Maintenance for Perimenopausal Women. Number 210, Aug. 1995.
2. Cholesterol Screening in Adults. U.S. Public Health Service, Washington, D.C., Am Family Phys. Jan. 1995, 129–136.
3. Baker, LH. Breast cancer detection demonstration project. Five-year summary report. Cancer 1982;32:194–225.
4. Shapiro S. Periodic Screening for Breast Cancer: The Health Insurance Plan Project and Its Sequelae, 1963–1986. Johns Hopkins University Press, Baltimore, MD, 1988.
5. Miller AB, Barnes CJ, To T, Wall C. Canadian National Breast Screening Study, 1: breast cancer detection death rates among women aged 40–49 years. Can Med Assoc J 1992;47:1459–1476.
6. Mettlin C. Encouraging trends in breast cancer incidence. Cancer 1993;72:637–638.
7. Swanson GM, Rayheb NE, Lin CS, et al. Breast cancer among black and white women in the 1980's: Changing patterns in the United States by race, age, and extent of disease. Cancer 1993;72:778–798.
8. Bjurstam N, Bjornel L, Duffy SW. The Gothenberg breast cancer screening trial: results from 11 years follow-up. In: Program and Abstracts. NIH Consensus Development Conference: Breast Cancer Screening for Women Ages 40 to 49. National Institutes of Health, Bethesda, MD, 1997.
9. Andersson I. Results from the Mälmo breast screening trial. In: Program and Abstracts. NIH Consensus Development Conference: Breast Cancer Screening for Women Ages 40 to 49. National Institutes of Health, Bethesda, MD, 1997.
10. Smart CR, Hendrick E, Rutledge JH, Smith RA. Benefit of mammography screening in women ages 40 to 49 years. Current evidence from randomized clinical trials. Cancer 1995;75(7):1619–1626.
11. Winawer SJ, StJohn DJ, Bond JH, Rosen P, Burt, RW, Waye, JD, Kronborg O, O'Brien MJ, Bishop DT, Kurtz, RZ, Shike M, Swaroop SV, Levin B, Fruhmorgan P, Lynch HT. Prevention of colorectal cancer: guidelines based on new data. Bull World Health Org 1995;73(1):7–10.
12. Winawer SJ, Flehinger BJ, Schottenfeld D, Miller G. Screening for colorectal cancer with fecal occult blood testing and sigmoidoscopy. J Natl Cancer Inst 1993;85(16):1311–1318.
13. Mandel JS, Bond JH, Church, TR, et al. Reducing mortality from colorectal cancer by screening for fecal occult blood. N Engl J Med 1993;328:1365.
14. Hardcastle JD, Chamberlain JO, Robinson MHE, Moss SM, Amar SS, Balfour TW, James PD, Mangham CM. Randomized controlled trial of fecal-occult-blood screening for colorectal cancer. Lancet 1996;348(30):1472–1477.
15. Kewenter J, Bjork S, Haglind E, Smith L, Svanvik J, Ähren C. Screening and rescreening for colorectal cancer. A controlled trial of fecal occult blood testing in 27,700 subjects. Cancer 1988;62(3): 645–651.
16. Krongberg O, Fenger C, Olsen J, Bech K, Sondrgaard O. Repeated screening for colorectal cancer with fecal occult blood test. A prospective randomized study at Funen Denmark. Scan J Gastro 1989;24(5):599–606.
17. Selby JV, Friedman GD, Quesenberry Jr. CP, Weiss NS. A case-control study of screening sigmoidoscopy and mortality from colorectal cancer. N Engl J Med 1992;326(10):653–657.
18. Muller AD, Sonnenberg A. Prevention of colorectal cancer by flexible endoscopy and polypectomy. A case-control study of 32,702 veterans. Ann Intern Med 1995;123:904–910.
19. Winawer SJ, Zauber AG, Ho MN, et al. Prevention of colorectal cancer by colonoscopic polypectomy. N Engl J Med 1993;329:1977–1981.

20. Winawer SJ, Fletcher FH, Miller L, Godlee F, Stolar MH, Mullow Cd, Woolf SH, Glick SN, Ganiats TG, Bond JH, Rosen L, Zapka JG, Olsen SJ, Giardiello FM, Sisk JE, VanAntwerp R, Brown-Davis C, Marciniak DA, Mayer RJ. Colorectal cancer screening: clinical guidelines and rationale. Gastroenterology 1997;112:594–642.

21. Warner EA, Parsons AK. Screening and early diagnosis of gynecologic cancers. Med Clinics North Am 1996;80(1):45–60.

22. ACOG Committee Opinion: recommendations on frequency of Pap test screening. Number 152. Int J Gynecol Obstet 1995;49:210–211.

23. Gull B, Karlsson B, Milsom I, Wikland M, Granberg S. Transvaginal sonography of the endometrium in a representative sample of postmenopausal women. Ultrasound Obstet Gynecol 1996;7(5):322–327.

24. Am Cancer Soc Doc #003251: Cancer Detection Guidelines. Feb. 1997.

25. Chambers JT, Chambers SK. Endometrial sampling: when? where? why? with what? Clin Obstet Gynecol 1992;35(1)28–39.

26. Ciatto S, Cecchini S, Bonardi R, Grazzini G, Mazzotta A, Zappa M. A feasibility study of screening for endometrial carcinoma in postmenopausal women by ultrasonography. Tumori 1995;81:334–337.

27. Karlsson B, Granberg S, Wiklan M, et al. Transvaginal ultrasonography of the endometrium in women with postmenopausal bleeding. A Nordic multicenter study. Am J Obstet Gynecol 1995;172(5):1488–1494.

28. Fisher B, Constantino JP, Redmond CK, Fisher ER, Wickersham DL, Cronin Wm. Endometrial cancer in Tamoxifen-treated breast cancer patients. Findings from the National Surgical Adjuvant Breast and Bowel Project (NSABP) B-14. J Natl Cancer Inst 1994;86(7):527–537.

29. Pearson VAH. Screening for ovarian cancer. A review. Pubic Health 1994;108:367–382.

30. Jacob I, Bridges J, Reynolds C et al. Multimodal approach to screening for ovarian cancer. Lancet 1988;i:268–271.

31. Einhorn N, Sjovall K, Schoenfeld DA et al. Early detection of ovarian cancer using the CA 125 radioimmunoassary. Proc Am Soc Clin Oncol 1990;9:157.

32. VanNagell JR, DePriest PD, Puls LE, et al. Ovarian cancer screening in asymptomatic postmenopausal women by transvaginal sonography. Cancer 1991;68:458–462.

33. Bourne TH, Whitehead MI, Campbell S, et al. Ultrasound screening for familial ovarian cancer. Gynecologic Oncology 1991;43:92–97.

34. Karlan BY, Platt LD. The current status of ultrasound and color Doppler imaging in screening for ovarian cancer. Gynecol Oncol 1994;55:528.

35. Kurjak A, Zalud I, Alfirevic Z. Evaluation of adnexal masses with transvaginal color ultrasound. J Ultrasound Med 1991;10:295–297.

36. Bourne TH, Campbell S, Reynolds KM, et al. Screening for early familiar ovarian cancer with transvaginal ultrasonography and colour blood flow imaging. Br Med J 1993;306:1025–1029.

37. Soda, H, Tomita H, Kohno S, et al. Limitations of annual screening chest radiography for the diagnosis of lung cancer. Cancer 72:2341–2346, 1993.

38. Fontana RS, Sanderson Dr, Woolner LB, et al. Lung cancer screening, The Mayo Program. J Occup Med 1986;28:746–750.

39. Tockman MS. Survival and mortality from lung cancer in a screened population. The Johns Hopkins Study. Chest 1986;89:324,325.

40. National Lung Program, Memorial Sloan-Kettering Cancer Center. Final report and data summary. Bethesda, MD, Natl Cancer Inst, 1984.

41. Fontana RS, Sanderson DR, Woolner, LB, et al. Screening for lung cancer. Cancer 1991;67(suppl):1155–1164.

42. Fontana RS, Sanderson DR, Taylor AWF, et al. Early lung cancer detection. Results of the initial (prevalence) radiologic and cytologic screening in the Mayo Clinic Study. Am Rev Respir Dis 1984;130:561–565.

43. Narod SA. Screening for cancer in high risk families. Clin Biochem 1995;28:367–372.

44. Couch FJ, DeShano ML, Blackwood MA, Calzone K, Stopfer J, Canpeau L, Ganguly A, Rebbeck T, Weber B. BRCA1 mutations in women attending clinics that evaluate the risk of breast cancer. N Engl J Med 1997;336(20):1409–1415.

45. Langton AA, Malone KE, Thompson JD, Daling JR, Ostrander EA. BRCA1 mutations in a population-based sample of young women with breast cancer. N Engl J Med 1996;334:137–142.

46. Fitzgerald MG, MacDonald DJ, Krainer M, et al. Germ-line BRCA1 mutations in Jewish and non-Jewish women with early-onset breast cancer. N Engl J Med 1996;334:143–149.

47. Krainer M, Silvo-Arrieta S, Fitzgerald MG, Shimada A, Ishioka C, Kanamanus R, MacDonald DJ, Unsal H, Finkelstein DM, Bowcock A, Isselbacher, KJ, Haber DA. Differential contributions of BRCA1 and BRCA2 to early-onset breast cancer. N Engl J Med 1997;336(20):1416–1421.
48. Ribot C, Pouilles JM, Bonnen M, Tremollieres F. Assessment of the risk of post-menopausal osteoporosis using clinical factors. Clin Endocrinol 1992;36:225–228.
49. Cummings SR, Black DM, Nevitt MC, et al. Bone density at various sites for prediction of hip fractures. Lancet 1993;341:72–75.
50. Law MR, Wald NJ, Meade TW. Strategies for prevention of osteoporosis and hip fracture. Br Med J 1991;303:453–459.
51. NIH Consensus Development Panel. Optimal calcium intake (Consensus Conference). JAMA 1994;272:1942–1948.
52. Josse RG. Effects of ovarian hormone therapy on skeletal and extra skeletal tissues in women. Can Med Assoc J 1996;155(7):929–934.
53. Faughnan M, LePage R, Fugére P, Bissonnette F, Brossard JH, D'Amour P. Screening for thyroid disease at the menopausal clinic. Clin Invest Med. 1995;18(1):11–18.
54. An Immunization Update for Primary Care Providers. Nurse Practioner 1995;20(6):52–65.

INDEX